# Immunosuppression in Transplantation

# Immunosuppression in Transplantation

### Edited by

**LEO C. GINNS, MD**
Associate Professor of Medicine
Harvard Medical School;
Medical Director
Lung Transplant Program
Massachusetts General Hospital
Boston, Massachusetts

**A. BENEDICT COSIMI, MD**
Claude E. Welch Professor of Surgery
Harvard Medical School;
Chief, Transplantation Unit
Massachusetts General Hospital
Boston, Massachusetts

**PETER J. MORRIS, MB, PhD, FRS**
Nuffield Department of Surgery
University of Oxford;
Oxford Radcliffe Hospital
Oxford, England

*b*
**Blackwell Science**

© 1999 by Leo C. Ginns, A. Benedict Cosimi, and Peter J. Morris

Editorial Offices:
Commerce Place, 350 Main Street, Malden, Massachusetts 02148, USA
Osney Mead, Oxford OX2 0EL, England
25 John Street, London WC1N 2BL, England
23 Ainslie Place, Edinburgh EH3 6AJ, Scotland
54 University Street, Carlton, Victoria 3053, Australia

Other Editorial Offices:
Blackwell Wissenschafts-Verlag GmbH, Kurfürstendamm 57, 10707 Berlin, Germany
Blackwell Science KK, MG Kodenmacho Building, 7–10 Kodenmacho Nihombashi, Chuo-ku, Tokyo 104, Japan

Distributors:

USA

Blackwell Science, Inc.
Commerce Place
350 Main Street
Malden, Massachusetts 02148
(Telephone orders: 800-215-1000 or 781-388-8250;
fax orders: 781-388-8270)

CANADA

Login Brothers Book Company
324 Saulteaux Crescent
Winnipeg, Manitoba, R3J 3T2
(Telephone orders: 204-224-4068)

AUSTRALIA

Blackwell Science Pty, Ltd.
54 University Street
Carlton, Victoria 3053
(Telephone orders: 03-9347-0300;
fax orders: 03-9349-3016)

OUTSIDE NORTH AMERICA AND AUSTRALIA

Blackwell Science, Ltd.
c/o Marston Book Services, Ltd.
P.O. Box 269
Abingdon
Oxon OX14 4YN
England
(Telephone orders: 44-01235-465500;
fax orders: 44-01235-465555)

The Blackwell Science logo is a trade mark of Blackwell Science Ltd., registered at the United Kingdom Trade Marks Registry

Acquisitions: Christopher Davis
Production: Kevin Sullivan
Manufacturing: Lisa Flanagan
Cover design by Leslie Haimes
Typeset by Best-set Typesetter Ltd., Hong Kong
Printed and bound by Braun-Brumfield, Inc.

Printed in the United States of America
99 00 01 02 5 4 3 2 1

Library of Congress Cataloging-in-Publication Data
Immunosuppression in transplantation / edited by
  Leo C. Ginns, A. Benedict Cosimi, Peter J. Morris.
    p.  cm.
  Includes index.
  ISBN 0-632-04445-4
  1. Immunosuppressive agents.
2. Immunosuppression.  3. Transplantation
immunology.  4. Transplantation of organs, tissues, etc.
I. Ginns, Leo C.  II. Cosimi, A. Benedict.
III. Morris, Peter J., 1943–    .
  [DNLM: 1. Transplantation Immunology.
2. Immunosuppression—methods.
3. Immunosuppressive Agents—therapeutic use.
WO 680 I332   1999]
RM373.I46  1999
617.9′5—DC21
DNLM/DLC
for Library of Congress                    99-24601
                                              CIP

To Nancy, Sara, Laura, Rebecca, Mildred, Jean, Al

**LCG**

To my wife and children, Pat, Lisa, Gregg, and Beth, to my parents, and to Cathy for all their support

**ABC**

To the pioneers who made it happen

**PJM**

This book is also dedicated to all those transplant patients who have allowed us to gain the knowledge over the years on which this book is based.

# C O N T E N T S

**Sir Roy Y. Calne, FRS**
Emeritus Professor of Surgery
Department of Surgery
Cambridge University
Cambridge, United Kingdom

**Lucienne Chatenoud, MD**
Department of Clinical Immunology
Hôpital Necker
Paris, France

**A. Benedict Cosimi, MD**
Claude E. Welch Professor of Surgery
Harvard Medical School;
Chief, Transplantation Unit
Massachusetts General Hospital
Boston, Massachusetts

**Barry D. Kahan, MD, PhD**
Division of Immunology and Organ Transplantation
The University of Texas Medical School at Houston
Houston, Texas

**Paul A. Keown, MB, CHB**
Professor and Director of Immunology
Vancouver Hospital and Health Sciences Center
Vancouver, British Columbia
Canada

**Goran B. Klintmalm, MD, PhD, FACS**
Department of Transplantation
Baylor University Medical Center
Dallas, Texas

**Stephen C. Rayhill, MD**
Assistant Professor of Surgery
University of Iowa Hospitals and Clinics
Iowa City, Iowa

**Ferda Senel, MD**
Division of Immunology and Organ Transplantation
The University of Texas Medical School at Houston
Houston, Texas

**Hans W. Sollinger, MD, PhD**
Folkert O. Belzer Professor of Surgery
Chair, Division of Organ Transplantation
University of Wisconsin School of Medicine
Madison, Wisconsin

**Mark Waer, MD, PhD**
Professor of Nephrology
Director, Laboratory for Experimental Transplantation
University of Leuven
Leuven, Belgium

**Rowan G. Walker, MD, BS, FRACP**
Department of Nephrology
Royal Melbourne Hospital
Melbourne, Australia

## COMMENTATORS

**Christina Brattström, MD, PhD**
Attending Surgeon
Department of Transplantation Surgery
Karolinska Institute
Huddinge Hospital
Stockholm, Sweden

**John J. Fung, MD**
Department of Surgery
Presbyterian University Hospital
Pittsburgh, Pennsylvania

**Carl G. Groth, MD, PhD**
Professor of Transplantation Surgery
Department of Transplantation Surgery
Karolinska Institute
Huddinge Hospital
Stockholm, Sweden

**Henri Kreis, MD**
Service de Transplantation
Hôpital Necker
Paris, France

**J. A. Myburgh, MD**
Department of Surgery
University of Witwatersand Medical School
Johannesburg, South Africa

**Jean-Paul Soulillou, MD**
Institut National de la Sante et de la Recherche Medicale
(INSERM)
C.H.U. Hotel-Dieu
Nantes, France

**Thomas E. Starzl, MD, PhD**
University of Pittsburgh;
Department of Surgery
Presbyterian University Hospital
Pittsburgh, Pennsylvania

**Karl Wagner, MD**
Leitender Arzt der IV. Medizinischen Abteilung
Nieren-und Hochdruckkrankheiten
Allgemeines Krankenhaus Barmbek
Rübenkamp, Hamburg,
Germany

For patients ravaged by a variety of diseases resulting in organ failure, the replacement of the exhausted body part by healthy tissue offers the opportunity to improve the quality of life and to extend life expectancy. The successful transplantation of each tissue or organ, however, demands that several barriers be overcome, including graft rejection. Strategies to achieve this goal depend upon a thorough knowledge of basic immunologic principles, as well as an understanding of the mechanisms of action of immunosuppressive agents and their clinical effects. We are pleased to have assembled an internationally recognized group of contributors to address salient aspects of immunosuppressive therapy.

*Immunosuppression in Transplantation* should prove useful not only for transplant physicians and surgeons, but also for immunologists, pharmacologists, nurses, and others interested in the transplant recipient's response to immune modification. Practical strategies for immunomodulation derived from our current understanding of immunosuppressive agent activity and side effects are reviewed. Conventional immunosuppressive protocols, as well as agents about to become available, for the prevention and treatment of organ rejection are discussed. These include cyclosporine,

azathioprine, steroids, tacrolimus, mycophenolate mofetil, new small molecule agents, biologic modifiers, and irradiation. Our hope is that this book will provide the basis for understanding molecular and cellular principles of immunosuppressive therapy for those who are new to the field, and will offer deeper insight and perspective for those who are more experienced. Also included in this work are selected commentaries from a variety of experts whose views both enrich the text and lend to its balance.

The editors are most grateful to the contributors and commentators who have helped to prepare *Immunosuppression in Transplantation*. We appreciate the assistance of our Executive Editor, Chris Davis, and his Senior Editorial Assistant, Karin Commeret, from Blackwell Science. Finally, we acknowledge our own patients, from whom we always learn while we strive to help them, and we recognize all of the donor families and individuals upon whom so much of transplantation depends.

**LCG**
**ABC**
**PJM**

# Molecular and Clinical Therapeutics of Cyclosporine in Transplantation

PAUL A. KEOWN

## MECHANISMS OF ACTION

The cyclosporine family comprises some 25 natural lipophilic cyclic undecapeptides and more than 2000 derivatives originally obtained from the fermentation products of the fungal species *Tolypocladium inflatum Gams* (1). Several analogues exhibit diverse in vitro biologic activities, but only cyclosporin A (CsA) and the natural analogues (Thr²)-cyclosporin C (CsC), (Val²)-cyclosporin D (CsD), (Nval²)-cyclosporin G (CsG), and (Nva²)-cyclosporin M (CsM), produced by substitution of the $\alpha$-aminobutyric acid at the 2 position, cause selective inhibition of the immune response in vivo.

The unique molecular structure and physiochemical properties of these analogues are integral to their biologic actions and pharmacologic behavior. They consist of 10 known aliphatic amino acids and one novel C9 amino acid [4-butenyl-4-methyl-threonine (MeBmt)] arranged in a cyclic structure, producing a molecular weight of approximately 1200 kd (Fig. 1.1). Solid state x-ray diffraction and nuclear magnetic resonance studies in nonaqueous solution show that the molecule is characterized by two structural motifs (1). Residues MeBmt (AA1) to MeLeu (AA6) comprise an antiparallel $\beta$-sheet that is stabilized by three transannular hydrogen bonds (dotted lines in Fig. 1.1), while the residues Ala (AA7) to MeVal (AA11) form a loop in which the 9–10 peptide bond is in the *cis* position. An additional extra-annular hydrogen bond links the NH of DAla (AA8) to the carbonyl oxygen of MeLeu (AA6) (see Fig. 1.1).

The immunosuppressive cyclosporines possess two regulatory domains. Residues 1, 2, 9, 10, and 11 represent the receptor-binding domain, while the antipodean residues 4 to 8 function as the effector domain. Molecular substitution within either of these regions substantially alters the biologic effects of the compound.

CsA binds to several proteins in the eukaryotic cell, the most important of which are the cyclophilins (2). The principal cytoplasmic isoform, cyclophilin A (CyPA), is abundantly expressed in mammalian tissues and binds CsA with high affinity [dissociation constant ($K_D$) of 6 nmol/L]. This 18-kd enzyme facilitates tertiary protein folding through its peptidyl-prolyl *cis*-trans isomerase function, a function that is abrogated by CsA, although this now appears to be incidental to the immunosuppressive action of the drug and occurs only at much higher concentrations (3).

Several other mammalian cyclophilin isoforms have now been isolated. They contain rotamase domains and exhibit substantial homology with cyclophilin A, but differ in subcellular localization and CsA-binding affinity. The 21-kd protein CyPB ($K_D$ = 9 nmol/L) appears to reside within the endoplasmic reticulum and may mediate translocation into this structure. The 23-kd CyPC ($K_D$ = 6 nmol/L), while also expressed predominantly within the same organelle, shows restricted tissue distribution and is found principally in the kidney (4). Whether this is related to the unique renal toxicity of the cyclosporins is not yet known. A fourth mammalian isoform, CyCD, possesses a signal sequence thought to target it to mitochondria. Finally, a 40-kd cytoplasmic protein termed CyP-40 has recently been identified that is a component of the inactive steroid receptor. This structure contains subunits that can bind with three distinct classes of immunosuppressive agents: glucocorticoids, cyclosporins, and macrolides (tacrolimus and sirolimus). The relevance of this and other binding proteins—such as the 150-kd NK-TR, a component of the putative tumor recognition complex, or the immunophilins expressed in greater concentration in the brain (5)—remains to be determined.

The cyclosporins exert diverse biologic effects that influence many aspects of cell growth and differentiation. For example, selective inhibition of the multiple disease

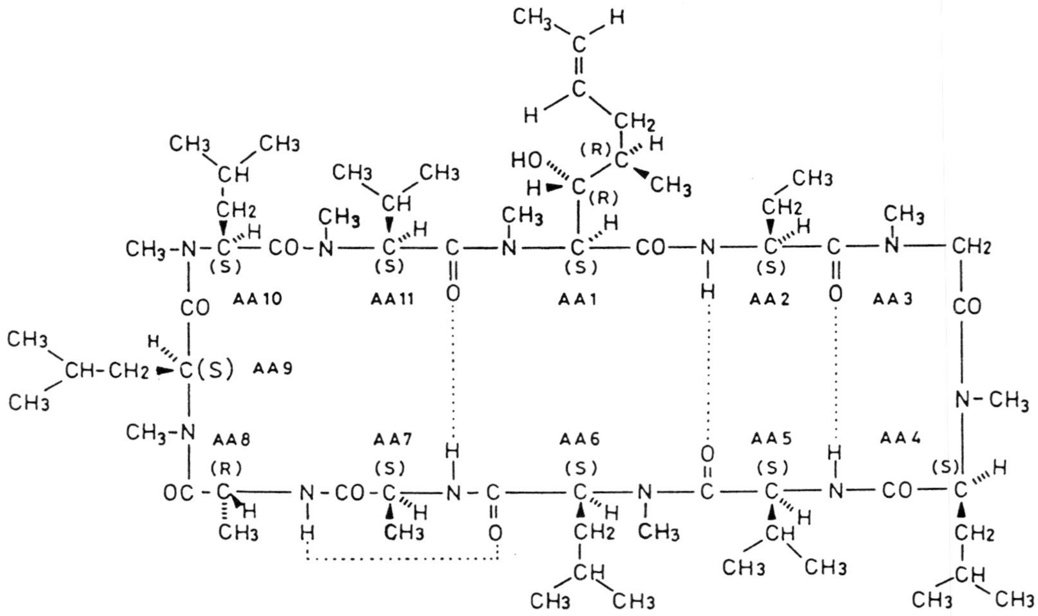

**FIGURE 1.1.**    *Structure of cyclosporine, an 11-amino-acid cyclic peptide. Amino acid residues 1–6 are held together by transannular hydrogen bonds (dotted lines). These, together with the hydrogen bond linking the open loop residues 7–10 to residue 6, contribute to the rigidity of the CsA skeleton.*

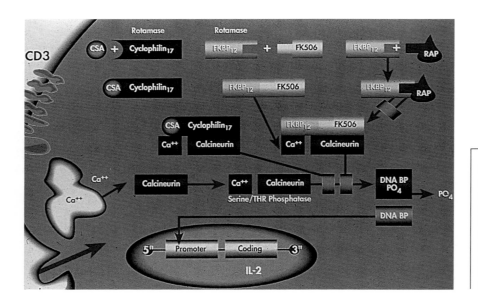

**FIGURE 1.2.**    *Schematic representation of the mechanism of action of CsA, compared with tacrolimus (FK506). CsA bound to cyclophilin (or FK506 to its binding protein, FKBP) complexes with and blocks the enzymatic function of the calcium-activated calcineurin. This prevents dephosphorylation and, therefore, activation of DNA-binding proteins. Thus, IL-2 synthesis is prevented. Sirolimus (RAP) also binds to FKBP (see Chapter 6).*

resistance gene product p-glycoprotein, a leading cause of drug resistance in malignant cells (6), is an action most effectively mediated by [3′-keto-Bmt1]-Val2 cyclosporine, a non-immunosuppressive cyclosporin D derivative (7). Another recent recognition is that CsA and certain nonimmunosuppressive cyclosporine analogues compete with the Gag polyproteins of the human immunodeficiency virus for binding to cyclophilin A, thereby preventing incorporations of this isomerase into the virions and resulting in a linear reduction of reverse transcription after T-cell infection (8,9).

The most important and extensively studied function, however, is the selective inhibition of lymphocyte signal transduction, a function that appears to be uniquely restricted to those analogues with immunosuppressive potency identified above. The bimolecular complex interacts via the CsA effector domain with the calcium- and calmodulin-dependent serine/threonine phosphatase calcineurin (Fig. 1.2), now recognized as a rate-limiting step in lymphocyte activation (10,11). Blockade of the enzymatic functions of calcineurin prevents dephosphorylation of the

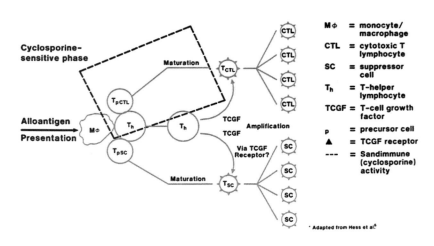

**FIGURE 1.3.** *Cyclosporine's effect on the immune response. Inhibition of IL-2 and other growth factor synthesis attenuates the maturation from precursor cells to cytotoxic T cells, and possibly favors the development of suppressor cells.*

antigen-inducible transcription factors NFAT1, elk-1, and the cAMP-response element binding protein (CREB) (12,13), also termed DNA-binding proteins (see Fig. 1.2). Translocation to the nucleus is thereby prevented, abrogating transcription of the cytokine gene complex and of the proto-oncogenes c-*myc*, c-*fos*, and n-*ras*. CsA may also directly inhibit the expression of G0/G1 switch genes through an as yet unknown mechanism (14).

As a consequence of these events, entry into the cell cycle is arrested at the G0 or G1 phase, DNA, RNA, and protein synthesis are inhibited, and growth factor production is abrogated. Activation structures are not expressed on the lymphocyte surface, and the generation of specific antibody and cytotoxic T lymphocytes directed against donor antigens is attenuated (Fig. 1.3). CsA also impedes the downstream organization of inflammatory events within the graft by blocking the dynamic upregulation of adhesion molecules and MHC determinants on the high endothelial venule, as occurs under the influence of interferon gamma (IFN-γ), tumor necrosis factor (TNF), and other inflammatory cytokines. Lymphocyte trafficking and accumulation within the graft is attenuated, preventing the T-cell clustering necessary for interaction between graft antigen and the T-cell receptor and the resulting cascade of inflammatory events (15).

## CLINICAL PHARMACOLOGY

The intravenous formulation of CsA is stabilized with Cremophor at a concentration of 100 mg/mL, and is administered by either intermittent or continuous infusion over 4 to 24 hours. The oral liquid and gel caplets previously were formulated in corn oil (Sandimmune; Novartis). Advances in pharmaceutical chemistry have now resulted in a new stable microemulsion that combines a lipophilic solvent, a hydrophilic solvent, and a surfactant. This new form is available in both liquid and gel caplet form (Neoral; Novartis) (16). Several generic products are also in the process of clinical evaluation (17).

## Absorption

Cyclosporine is absorbed preferentially from the upper intestine via a zero-order process in which the rate of absorption is constant and independent of drug concentration at the absorption site. Presystemic metabolism occurs in the intestinal epithelium under the influence of cytochrome P450-IIIa, reducing the amount of parent drug available for uptake (18). A variable proportion is also recycled into the gut lumen by the multiple drug resistance gene product p-glycoprotein in the epithelial cell membrane (19). The residual unchanged parent compound is absorbed into the portal system (Fig. 1.4); only a small amount is transported via the lymphatics (20).

Absorption following oral administration of Sandimmune is slow, incomplete, and unpredictable, with a lag time of 30 to 60 minutes and an absorption half-life ($t_{1/2}$) of approximately 60 minutes. Peak concentration ($C_{max}$) in blood or plasma is reached within 3 to 4 hours (mean 2.5 hours), although delayed and secondary peaks are common (21). Uptake is incomplete, with a mean of 30% reaching the systemic circulation (22). Absorption is bidirectionally influenced by food, particularly grapefruit juice (23), and is markedly impaired by reduced bile flow, delayed gastric emptying, intestinal dysmotility, accelerated gastrointestinal transit, or reduced absorptive area, resulting in a high between- and within-subject variability (24–26).

Absorption from Neoral is more rapid, complete, consistent, and dose-linear due to the homogeneous dispersion of uniform particles ($<0.15\mu$) at the absorptive surface (27–30). The absorption lag is virtually eliminated, and the time to peak concentration ($t_{max}$) is significantly reduced. $C_{max}$ occurs at 1.5 hours, and delayed or secondary absorption peaks are uncommon (31). While the trough concentration does not differ from that with the oil formulations, $C_{max}$ is increased by more than 60%, and overall bioavailability is increased by 30% to 50% with Neoral (32). Between- and within-patient variability in $t_{max}$, $C_{max}$, and exposure throughout the dosing interval ($AUC_{0-12}$) are also reduced by up to 75% (33,34).

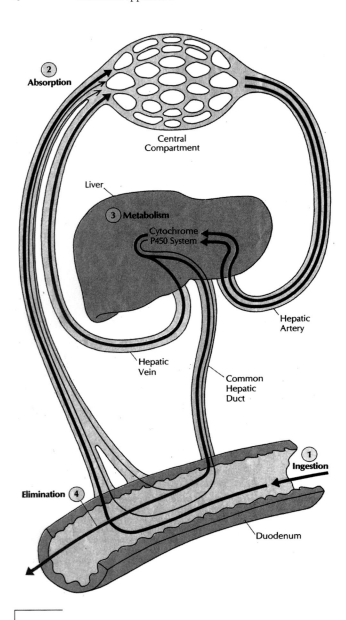

**FIGURE 1.4.**    *Unlike other lipophilic agents, cyclosporine initially bypasses the hepatic portal system. After absorption through intestinal lacteal lymphatics, it goes into the thoracic duct and then to the central blood compartment. From there, cyclosporine enters the liver, where it is metabolized into numerous metabolites (more than 25 have been identified). These metabolites recirculate in the blood, return to the liver, and then move out through the biliary tree into the bowel, where they may be reabsorbed or eliminated. A small amount of the parent compound is probably excreted as well.*

## Metabolism

Disposition of CsA is independent of the formulation employed. Partitioning within the blood compartment obeys a temperature-dependent equilibrium in which approximately 50% is bound to erythrocytes, 10% to leukocytes, and 30% to 40% to plasma proteins; only 1% to 6% normally exists in the free state (35). In plasma, 33% to 46%

is associated with high-density lipoprotein (HDL), 28% to 35% with low-density lipoprotein (LDL), and 6% to 19% with very-low-density lipoprotein in a ratio inversely reflecting their clearance rates (36). The remaining 11% to 23% of CsA is associated with the nonlipoprotein fraction.

CsA accumulates readily in the body fat, liver, pancreas, heart, lung, kidney, spleen, lymph nodes, and blood. However, it does not readily cross the blood-brain barrier or placenta. Drug concentrations are low in the cerebrospinal fluid, brain, and spinal cord, and the concentration in the fetus represents less than 5% of the maternal drug load (37). Significant concentrations of CsA will accumulate in breast milk, so breast feeding is contraindicated to protect the neonatal immune system (38).

Metabolism of CsA occurs in the liver and bowel under the influence of cytochrome P450-IIIA (39) by demethylation of derivatives on the molecular face opposite the cyclophilin binding site. More than 25 metabolites have been documented in human blood, bile, and urine, all of which retain the cyclic oligopeptide structure (40). The first oxidation products are the primary metabolites M1, M9, and M4N. Further oxidation then produces a second group of metabolites including M19, M49, or M4N9. Other secondary derivatives, such as M4N69 and M69 found in human urine, may represent further oxidation products of M4N9 and M9, respectively. CsA is the major component in plasma, while M1 and M9 are present in high concentration in erythrocytes and other tissues. M1 is the major component in urine, where unchanged CsA represents only 0.1% of the administered dose. An acid derivative of M1 predominates in bile, where CsA is present in only trace amounts. All natural and synthetic metabolites are less immunosuppressive than the parent molecule. CsA is eliminated primarily by biliary excretion, with a median half-life of 6 to 8 hours.

Clearance is higher in children and slower in females (41), reflecting partly the accumulation of the drug in body fat. Alterations in lipid profile modify the distribution and metabolism of CsA; CsA increases lipoprotein concentration, thereby reciprocally modulating its own distribution (36). Clearance of CsA is significantly impaired in patients with liver disease, and the elimination half-life may be prolonged fourfold. Thus, longer dosing intervals or a substantial reduction in dose are necessary in the presence of hepatic dysfunction.

## Drug Interactions

Pharmacokinetic interactions (Table 1.1) are commonly due to modulation of cytochrome P450 enzyme activity, which alters the metabolism and clearance of CsA (42). Phenytoin, rifampin, and nafcillin are prototypic of drugs that induce mixed function oxidases—they cause a fall in CsA levels within 72 hours of administration, and may lead to graft rejection unless the interaction is recognized and corrected. Less commonly, drugs such as cholestyramine or the

**Table 1.1.**    Drug Interactions with Cyclosporine

| Agent | Pharmacokinetic Action | Consequences |
|---|---|---|
| Carbamazepine<br>Nafcillin<br>Phenobarbital<br>Phenytoin<br>Rifampin | Induce cytochrome P450 enzymes | Decrease half-life, blood levels, and immunosuppressive effect |
| Colchicine<br>Diltiazem<br>Fluconazole<br>Fluoroquinolones<br>Ketoconazole<br>Macrolide antibodies<br>Oral contraceptives<br>Verapamil | Inhibit cytochrome P450 enzymes | Increase half-life, blood levels, and toxicity or immunosuppression |
| Aminoglycosides<br>Amphotericin B<br>Cimetidine<br>Nonsteroidals<br>Sulfur | Interact at a glomerular or tubular level | Increase nephrotoxicity |

somatostatin analogue octreotide influence CsA absorption through direct or indirect means. In contrast, erythromycin, ketoconazole, diltiazem, colchicine, and certain fluoroquinolones inhibit the cytochrome P450 enzyme system. These agents increase CsA exposure within days and may cause acute nephrotoxicity requiring a reduction in CsA dose by 50% or more (43).

Less potent interactions have been reported with the macrolide derivatives josamycin, ponsinomycin, and roxithromycin, and with fluconazole and verapamil. Nifedipine and nitrendipine have no demonstrable influence on CsA pharmacokinetics. Oral contraceptives are weak inhibitors of cytochrome P450 enzymes (44) and may increase CsA concentration in recipients of renal and liver transplants. CsA and prednisolone are metabolized by the same hepatic microsomal enzymes, and human liver microsomal studies show a bidirectional inhibition of CsA and corticosteroid metabolism (45). High-dose intravenous methylprednisolone may transiently increase CsA trough levels (46), but this interaction is of uncertain clinical importance.

Pharmacodynamic drug interactions may also influence the immunosuppression or toxicity of CsA. Median effect analysis in experimental animals shows that immune suppression is additive with azathioprine and mycophenolate, and synergistic with sirolimus (47). In contrast, ciprofloxacin antagonizes CsA in vitro by increasing interleukin (IL)-2 gene transcription, and may increase the risk of acute rejection in vivo (48).

Nonsteroidal anti-inflammatory drugs (NSAIDs) reduce intra-renal blood flow by inhibiting the production of vasodilatory prostaglandins, and may lead to acute renal dysfunction in patients receiving CsA. NSAIDs are generally to be avoided, although short courses may be required for treatment of acute gout or other rheumatologic conditions. Septra, cimetidine, and ranitidine may also elevate serum creatinine, although this occurs by inhibition of tubular secretion rather than by impairment of glomerular filtration (49).

## CLINICAL USE OF CYCLOSPORINE

Cyclosporine may be administered intravenously until gastrointestinal function is reestablished. There is little data to determine whether continuous or intermittent infusion is preferable, but in either case the dose should be adjusted to achieve an average concentration ($C_{av} = AUC_{0-t}/t$) above 500 $\mu$g/L throughout the dosing interval to minimize the risk of rejection (50). Oral therapy is normally commenced at a dose of 4–5 mg/kg twice daily, although a higher dose or a shorter dosing interval may be required in children and in patients with external bile drainage, gastrointestinal disease, or a decreased elimination half-life (51). Pretransplant pharmacokinetic monitoring may be useful to identify patients with inadequate drug exposure who are at risk of rejection and graft loss, and to predict the dose and dosing interval required (52). Aerosolized CsA has been used in the attempt to reverse acute lung rejection (53); however, demonstration of consistent efficacy awaits larger trials.

Prospective, concentration-controlled studies in kidney and liver transplant recipients suggest that Neoral reduces the need for intravenous CsA (54), decreases the risk or severity of acute rejection (55,56), and enables more predictable and cost-effective therapy (57,58). In the international renal study comparing Neoral and Sandimmune, the mean administered CsA dose was 8% lower at 3 months in patients receiving the microemulsion (4.5 versus 4.9 mg/kg/day), although trough levels were comparable at all times. CsA absorption was 49% greater by 2 weeks after transplant ($AUC_{0-12h}$: 7155 vs. 5221 ng·hr/mL) in these patients, and remained significantly superior throughout the period of follow-up (55). Patient and graft survival were essentially identical for both formulations (98% and 91%, respectively), but acute rejection was significantly less frequent in patients receiving Neoral (42% versus 60%, $P = 0.04$), without any evidence of increased nephrotoxicity, hepatotoxicity, hypertension, or other adverse effects. The UK multicenter study confirmed these results (56). Target CsA levels were achieved more quickly (2 versus 4 days), while the incidence of both first (35.9% versus 52%) and recurrent rejection (9.7% versus 18.4%) were significantly reduced in patients receiving the microemulsion. Interestingly, the risk of acute rejection was lowest among those who did not receive intravenous cyclosporine (27%, $P = 0.026$).

Neoral is particularly important in liver transplantation, where external biliary drainage reduces CsA bioavailability from the oil vehicles to less than 5% (59). Absorption is enhanced by two- to sixfold with the new formulation and is closely correlated with age ($r = 0.87$, $P = 0.02$), while total body clearance (12 mL/min/kg) and volume of distribution ($Vd_{ss}$: 2.2 L/kg) are unchanged (60). Blood levels are comparable to those achieved with intravenous administration within the first 48 hours, and within- (31%) and between-patient variability (17%) are low (61). Intravenous therapy may thus be avoided in 90% of patients (62), while achieving graft survival above 90% and a reduced frequency ($P = 0.02$) and severity ($P = 0.027$) of acute rejection without evidence of incremental toxicity (63,64).

Preliminary studies in pancreas, heart, lung, and heart–lung transplantation confirm these observations, and exposure is increased by approximately twofold and $C_{max}$ by threefold in patients with cystic fibrosis on treatment with Neoral (65–68).

Several large-scale studies have demonstrated that stable patients may be converted safely from Sandimmune to Neoral, offering consistent and predictable immunosuppression at lower cost (69–71). Conversion is normally performed at a 1:1 dose ratio, although the mean dose of CsA must then be reduced by approximately 5% to 12% to maintain constant trough levels. The most extensive pharmacoepidemiologic study encompassed 1097 stable patients randomized 2:1 to receive Neoral or continue on Sandimmune (72). CsA absorption was significantly greater within the first 4 hours after dosing in the Neoral group (3032 ± 1039 versus 1978 ± 934 ng·hr/mL, $P < 0.001$), without any significant change in the trough concentration (203 ± 85 versus 202 ± 95 ng·hr/mL). The magnitude of increase observed was not simply proportional in all patients, but was maximal in the group of patients who experienced the lowest bioavailability from Sandimmune (more than 1 SD below the mean) and were hence at greatest risk of immunologic injury. All of these patients became good or excellent absorbers when converted to Neoral. In contrast, patients who had good bioavailability on Sandimmune saw little incremental improvement in CsA exposure after conversion to Neoral, and thus were not placed at greater risk of toxicity. Apart from a mild and transient increase in serum creatinine in the first month after conversion in the Neoral group, there was no evidence of incremental toxicity throughout the 18 months of follow-up (73). The incidence of acute rejection was similar during the period of observation (5%); the incidence of chronic rejection was slightly lower among patients receiving Neoral (8% versus 11%), but this did not reach statistical significance due to the relatively small cohort size.

Therapeutic monitoring of CsA is widely employed to assist dose adjustment, to detect drug interactions, and to recognize noncompliance with therapy. Adequate bioavailability and consistency of exposure, measured using full pharmacokinetic profiles, have been shown respectively to correlate closely with freedom from acute rejection and chronic rejection (74,75). Because sequential pharmacokinetic profiling is impractical in many settings, the trough ($C_0$) blood level has been generally accepted for long-term therapeutic monitoring. However, the assumption that this accurately reflects drug exposure has now been shown to be false with Sandimmune ($R^2 = 0.43$) and only marginally superior with Neoral ($R^2 = 0.5$–$0.8$) (76).

The use of limited sampling strategies to predict exposure throughout the dosing interval, first developed by Johnston et al (77), has now been expanded by other researchers using time points selected from both the absorption and the elimination phases of the dosing interval (78–80). Kahan and colleagues, using a two-point sampling protocol (2 hr and 6 hr post dose) showed a 92% to 99% correlation with full AUC in patients receiving Neoral (82). The Canadian Study Group, for practical purposes of clinical management, has confined the sampling period to the first 4 hours of the dosing interval. In these studies, a four-point protocol with sampling at 0, 1, 2, and 4 hours provided a greater than 97% correlation with the full 12-hour AUC, while selection of just two points at 0 and 2 hours showed a correlation of 94.5% and a mean predictive error of <10% (34). Because of the greater heterogeneity of absorption in the first 2 weeks after transplant, three-point sampling may prove superior during this time, following which two-point sampling using one of several time combinations appears to provide an excellent prediction of drug exposure (83). It is expected that this approach will, for the first time, allow the accurate separation of the transplant population into two groups: those who have excellent and consistent absorption with Neoral and in whom the frequency of monitoring can be markedly reduced or eliminated, and the small but critical population with inadequate or inconsistent exposure who require special attention.

## Mycophenolate Mofetil

The use of mycophenolate mofetil (MMF) in combination with CsA has dramatically reduced both the incidence and the severity of acute rejection (84). Initial studies in Canada, Australia, Europe, and the United States were conducted using Sandimmune (85–87), but extensive experience has since been gained with MMF in combination with Neoral. The risk of biopsy-proven acute rejection has declined below 20%, and the frequency of resistant rejection has decreased to almost 5% (84). As a result, this drug is replacing azathioprine as standard therapy for many transplant units.

Apart from an increase in risk of viral infection, largely controlled by routine prophylaxis, there appears to be little cumulative toxicity of these agents. Unfortunately, the rate of chronic graft injury is unaltered, despite the lower incidence of acute rejection episodes following use of this combination. Chronic renal allograft damage remains at 15% to 20% by 3 years, which is in contrast to the early promise of experimental studies (88). Chapter 5 presents a more detailed review of MMF.

## Sirolimus (Rapamycin)

Sirolimus (Rapamune, Wyeth-Ayerst) and CsA act at discrete molecular sites (see Fig. 1.2). Sirolimus selectively inhibits a later stage in the immune activation cascade, blocking the downstream effects of the IL-2 receptor signal (89). The two drugs are potently synergistic in experimental animal studies of heart and kidney transplantation, where sirolimus may retard chronic vascular injury (90,91). Phase II studies in human kidney transplantation show that the incidence of acute rejection is reduced to approximately 10% when using optimal combinations of both drugs (92). In addition, sirolimus potentiates the pharmacokinetic exposure to CsA when the two drugs are administered simultaneously (93).

Sirolimus is not nephrotoxic, but may cause thrombocytopenia and hypercholesterolemia, complications also attributed to CsA. Phase III studies now underway will determine the risks and benefits of this combination. A detailed discussion of sirolimus is presented in Chapter 6.

## Basiliximab and Daclizumab

Two monoclonal antibodies directed against the IL-2 receptor, basiliximab (Simulect, Novartis) and daclizumab (Zenapax, Hoffman-LaRoche) (94,95), have recently been tested in phase III studies with CsA (see Chapter 8). Both bind to the α-chain of the IL-2 receptor and cause a rapid depletion of cells bearing this structure from the peripheral circulation.

Basiliximab, a chimeric murine monoclonal, is administered on days 0 and 4 post-transplant. The humanized monoclonal daclizumab is given 5 times at 2-week intervals throughout the first 2 months. When combined with CsA microemulsion, both agents produce excellent graft and patient survival (>95% at 6 months). They also provide a significant reduction in the incidence of biopsy-proven acute rejection (basiliximab: 33% versus 51% placebo control, *P* = 0.001; daclizumab: 28% versus 47% placebo control, *P* = 0.0001), without any measurable increase in infections, malignancy, or specific toxicity.

## MAJOR ADVERSE EFFECTS OF CYCLOSPORINE

The side effects of cyclosporine are summarized in Table 1.2.

## Renal

Nephrotoxicity is unquestionably the most worrying side effect of CsA and is of particular concern in renal transplant recipients, in whom it has to be distinguished from rejection as a cause of deteriorating renal function. This disadvantage became evident very soon after its initial clinical use. For this reason, investigators have advocated the use of

**Table 1.2.** Major Adverse Effects of Cyclosporine Therapy

| Effect | Clinical Presentation | Frequency and Severity |
|---|---|---|
| Nephrotoxicity* | | |
| Acute | Increased BUN, Cr | Very common (35% to 50%); mild, usually reversible |
| | Hemolytic uremia | Uncommon; severe, occasionally reversible |
| Chronic | Increased BUN, Cr Proteinuria, B.P. | Uncommon (7% to 10%); severe, progressive |
| Cardiovascular | Hypertension* | Very common (70% to 90%) |
| | Intravascular coagulation | Rare |
| Neurotoxicity* | Tremor, hyperesthesia | Common (25% to 30%) |
| | Headache | Usually transient |
| | Seizures | Uncommon (<5%) |
| | Severe neurotoxicity (cortical blindness, quadriplegia, seizures, coma, white matter changes on CT or MRI) | Uncommon |
| Metabolic | Hyperkalemia* | Very common |
| | Hyperuricemia* | Common |
| | Hyperglycemia* | Common |
| | Hyperlipidemia* | Common |
| | Hypomagnesemia | Uncommon |
| Gastroenterologic | | |
| GI upset | Nausea, anorexia, cramps, diarrhea | Common; mild, transient |
| Hepatotoxicity* | Increased SGOT, SGPT, alkaline phosphatase, bilirubin | Uncommon; mild, transient, dose-related |
| Mucocutaneous | Hirsutism* | Common, often severe |
| | Gingival hyperplasia* | Common, mild |
| | Facial dysmorphism | Common (infants) |
| | Acne, brittle fingernails | Very uncommon |
| | Decreased scalp hair | Very uncommon |
| Neoplastic* | PTLD | Uncommon (1% to 8%) |
| | Epithelial malignancies | Common |

\* The most commonly cited side effects (often referred to as the "three Ns" and "eight Hs"). Cr, creatinine, B.P., blood pressure.

CsA only in patients whose kidneys were diuresing after transplantation (96).

Three clinical types of nephrotoxicity are observed with CsA. The first type occurs immediately after transplantation, usually in a kidney already damaged by ischemia, and is more commonly associated with use of intravenous CsA. The incidence of delayed function after renal transplantation has generally tended to be higher in patients treated with CsA than in those given azathioprine and steroids (97), although there is no general agreement about this (98). The implications of the possible additive effects of CsA nephrotoxicity on an ischemic kidney are important because they suggest that protocols that delay the administration of

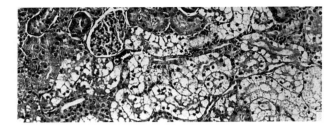

**FIGURE 1.5.**    *Acute CsA nephrotoxicity in a patient with allograft dysfunction 3 weeks after initiation of CsA therapy. Note the extensive proximal tubular vacuolization and sparse cellular infiltrate that are characteristic of CsA nephrotoxicity rather than acute rejection.*

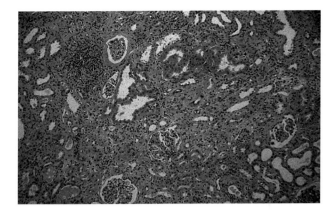

**FIGURE 1.6.**    *Chronic CsA nephrotoxicity. Note the severe ("striped") interstitial fibrosis and diffuse cellular infiltrate. Although intimal proliferation in this biopsy is not dramatic, the histopathologic changes of chronic rejection are often quite similar.*

CsA until adequate renal function is established may be desirable.

The second type of nephrotoxicity is seen any time after the first 2 or 3 weeks and is accompanied by deteriorating renal function, usually but not always associated with high CsA blood levels. This is the type of nephrotoxicity that must be differentiated from an acute rejection episode. Although high serum or blood CsA trough levels are often associated with nephrotoxicity and low levels with rejection, there are numerous exceptions to this. Percutaneous biopsy or fine-needle aspiration of the kidney is essential for making the correct diagnosis. Mild focal infiltrates, tubular vacuolization, and arteriopathy (Fig. 1.5) are characteristically seen, although differentiation from rejection is frequently difficult. This type of nephrotoxicity recovers rapidly with a CsA dose reduction. Another possible uncommon manifestation of acute CsA nephrotoxicity is a hemolytic-uremia–like syndrome that occurs in the first several weeks after transplantation. Biopsies show striking arteriolopathy and even thrombosis. Despite the striking nature of the histologic findings, a return of renal function has been reported with cessation of CsA or the use of streptokinase and heparin (99).

The third type of nephrotoxicity is a chronic condition in which there is a slow but steady deterioration in renal function. The histology of the kidney typically reveals severe interstitial fibrosis (Fig. 1.6). This type may show some improvement in renal function with a decrease in the CsA dosage, but it tends to be relatively short lived. It seems likely that many of the changes observed result from chronic rejection, on which is superimposed some element of CsA nephrotoxicity. After cardiac transplantation, this steady deterioration in renal function of patients on CsA has resulted in some patients requiring hemodialysis or renal transplantation (100).

### Mechanism

The mechanism of CsA nephrotoxicity has not yet been clarified, but it would seem that a direct toxic action on proximal tubular cells is not a significant factor. Instead, a decrease in renal blood flow with an increased renal vascular resistance at the level of the glomerular afferent arteriole is the primary cause of the nephrotoxicity (101). That acute nephrotoxicity is reversed so rapidly after cessation of CsA is compatible with the concept of renal vasoconstriction as the primary cause of the nephrotoxicity.

Other reports have postulated that the effect of CsA on the production of renal prostaglandin might be responsible for the vasoconstriction as well as the changes in intravascular coagulation (102). The prostaglandins are potent renal vasodilators and are thought to play an important role in modulating the influence of various renal vasoconstrictor factors. There is some evidence that CsA inhibits the production of the prostaglandin metabolites, but CsA may also increase the production of thromboxane, which is a potent vasoconstrictor. Thus, this effect of CsA on the arachidonic acid metabolic pathway within the kidney could explain most of the observed functional and morphologic changes of nephrotoxicity.

Prostaglandins of the E series have immunosuppressive properties and, theoretically, are attractive agents to combine with CsA in order to reduce its nephrotoxicity. Some investigators have shown that misoprostol (a prostaglandin $E_1$ analogue) improves renal function and safely reduces the incidence of acute rejection in renal transplant recipients treated concurrently with CsA and prednisone (103). However, others have not been able to demonstrate any advantage to the concurrent use of this agent with CsA (104). This strategy has not, therefore, gained universal acceptance.

It has been reported that calcium channel blockers reduce the incidence of primary nonfunction in patients on CsA. Diltiazem has been associated with a marked reduction in CsA dosage with fewer episodes of primary nonfunction and less severe rejection episodes (105). Verapamil resulted in the need for lower CsA doses but equivalent blood levels, but there was no reduction in nephrotoxicity or incidence of rejection (106).

## Cardiovascular

Hypertension is commonly associated with the use of CsA. Cyclosporine appears to have complex effects on intravascular coagulation, and there have been reports of an increased incidence of renal artery and vein thrombosis (107,108) and an increase in the incidence of deep venous thrombosis (109). Although it is tempting to attribute these complications, as well as the microangiopathy and hemolytic-uremic syndrome, to CsA's effect on the arachidonic acid metabolic pathway (as discussed earlier), the evidence is too uncertain as yet to draw any firm conclusions.

## Neurologic

A variety of neurologic complications have been reported with CsA use, including tremor, headache, convulsions, various paresthesias of the limbs, mania, and depression. Although the relationship with CsA is not always clear, there is sufficient evidence that such neurologic syndromes can be attributed to CsA toxicity in many instances, because they are typically associated with high blood levels and reverse on lowering the CsA dosage. Evidence suggests that CsA-induced hypomagnesemia may contribute to these neurologic complications, especially the convulsions.

## Metabolic

Hyperkalemia is common in patients on CsA and is readily reversible by lowering the dosage or discontinuing the drug. The mechanism is unclear, but the decreased potassium excretion may be a result of decreased serum aldosterone levels or a primary tubular defect (110).

Hyperglycemia may occur in patients on CsA, and is often associated with a raised urine glucose level. The glycosuria is undoubtedly a manifestation of nephrotoxicity, but the hyperglycemia may reflect a toxic effect of CsA on $\beta$ cells of the pancreas. The condition does appear to be reversible.

Renal handling of uric acid is also affected by the use of CsA, leading to higher serum urate levels even after correction for elevated serum creatinine. These high urate levels slowly return to normal over several weeks after the drug is discontinued. Again, this probably reflects a tubular defect associated with CsA nephrotoxicity. Gout occasionally occurs as a byproduct of the hyperuricemia. Urate levels may need to be lowered with allopurinol, and the leukocyte count needs to be monitored carefully if the patient is also on azathioprine.

Hyperlipidemia is a significant management issue in immunosuppressed allograft recipients. Post-transplant hyperlipidemia has been linked to cardiovascular disease, with its high morbidity and mortality rate. Along with steroid therapy, CsA has been implicated in contributing to hyperlipidemia (111), and conversion from CsA to tacrolimus has been shown to lower cholesterol, LDL, and apolipoprotein B in hyperlipidemic recipients (112).

Hypomagnesemia is due to an increased magnesium clearance in patients on CsA and is usually associated with high blood levels of CsA. This reflects another manifestation of CsA nephrotoxicity. Convulsions, mentioned previously as another possible manifestation of CsA toxicity, have been attributed to hypomagnesemia.

## Gastroenterologic

Cyclosporine is unpleasant to take and cannot be adequately disguised, even when taken with flavored drinks such as chocolate milk. Consequently, some patients may experience nausea and anorexia, particularly with large doses. In general, this has been less of a problem with current preparations such as Neoral. The development of the gelatin capsule for CsA has been welcomed by most patients. However, as the capsules are large and difficult to swallow, some patients may prefer to remain with the liquid form.

Hepatotoxicity has been observed in patients on CsA after renal, cardiac, and bone marrow transplantation. Generally this manifests as a temporary elevation of liver function tests that regresses on dosage reduction. No histologic changes have been described in association with these biochemical changes, but high doses of CsA in the rat produce ultrastructural changes and a deterioration in liver function (113). Cyclosporine may be contraindicated in patients with abnormal liver function tests before renal transplantation, because they may be at risk for the development of frank cirrhosis. Furthermore, because CsA is metabolized in the liver, depressed liver function may alter blood levels of the drug.

## Mucocutaneous

Mucocutaneous side effects of CsA have been recognized since the drug's introduction. The most common of these side effects are gingival hyperplasia and hypertrichosis. Although plaque control has been shown to be of benefit for gum hypertrophy, gingival surgery has occasionally been necessary. Recently, treatment with azithromycin has been recommended (114), but conversion to tacrolimus is almost always effective in reversing this condition. This approach typically controls hypertrichosis as well.

In children, facial dysmorphism (which was not seen in patients on azathioprine and steroids) can be striking. Again, conversion to tacrolimus, with the admitted increased risk of post-transplant lymphoproliferative disorder (PTLD), is the usual treatment.

## Neoplastic

An apparent increased incidence of lymphomas in the early patients treated with CsA caused considerable alarm (115). With time, however, the incidence of lymphoma in renal and cardiac allograft recipients was found to be no greater than expected in recipients treated with conventional immunosuppressive therapy. Indeed, most of the patients who have developed lymphomas have received other drugs as well, such as prednisolone and antilymphocyte globulin, suggesting that the occurrence of lymphoma is due to excessive immunosuppression rather than specifically to CsA.

Skin cancer is a major complication after transplantation, particularly in the sun-blessed countries such as Australia. It appears to be just as common among users of CsA as with other types of immunosuppression.

## CONCLUSION

Cyclosporine has transformed whole organ transplantation from an experimental procedure with serious morbidity and mortality to a highly successful and economically viable treatment that is universally recognized as the optimal clinical therapy for most patients with end-stage organ failure. Its incorporation into therapeutic protocols has not only improved survival rates for recipients of extra-renal allografts but has also allowed for the reduction of steroid therapy and the accompanying side effects.

European and Canadian clinical trials were among the first to herald this transition (97,116,118), although the highly lipophilic nature of CsA proved a difficult challenge in pharmaceutical chemistry. The formulations initially employed for delivery of CsA resulted in incomplete and erratic absorption, and thus wide variations in exposure occurred within and between individuals. These pharmacokinetic limitations had serious clinical consequences, increasing the risks of both acute and chronic rejection and reducing the value of therapeutic drug monitoring. The introduction of a new microemulsion vehicle has overcome most of these difficulties, cementing the role of CsA as the cornerstone of clinical immunosuppression for renal transplantation.

In the next decade, optimal immunosuppression for organ transplantation must achieve five clinical goals:

1. Patient survival greater than 95%
2. Graft survival exceeding 90%
3. Rejection rate less than 10%
4. Incidence of infection less than 10%
5. Incidence of lymphoma less than 1%

There is now compelling cumulative evidence that the combination of CsA with agents to inhibit nucleotide synthesis, growth factor receptor expression, or growth signal transduction can move renal transplantation over this new threshold of safety and success.

## REFERENCES

1. Wenger RM. Structures of cyclosporine and its metabolites. Transplant Proc 1990;22:1104–1109.
2. Fruhman DA, Burakoff SJ, Bierer BE. Immunophilins in protein folding and immunosuppression. FASEB 1994;8:391–400.
3. Bierer BE, Somers PK, Wandless TJ, et al. Probing immunosuppressant action with a non-natural immunophilin ligand. Science 1990;250:556–558.
4. Friedman J, Weissman I. Two cytoplasmic candidates for immunophilin action are revealed by affinity for a new cyclosporine: one in the presence and one in the absence of CsA. Cell 1991;66:799–806.
5. Snyder SH, Sabatini DM, Lai MM, et al. Neural actions of immunophilin ligands. Trends Pharmacol Sci 1998;19:21–26.
6. Demeule M, Beliveau R, Wenger RM. Molecular interactions of cyclosporin A with P-glycoprotein. Photolabeling with cyclosporin derivatives. J Biol Chem 1997;272:6647–6652.
7. Archinal-Mattheis A, Cohen D, Bair KW, et al. Analysis of the interactions of SDZ PSC 83([3′-keto-Bmt1]-Val2]-Cyclosporine), a multidrug resistance modulator, with P-glycoprotein. Oncol Res 1997;7:603–610.
8. Braaten D, Luban J, Phares W, et al. Cyclosporine A-resistant human immunodeficiency virus type 1 mutants demonstrate that Gag encodes the functional target of cyclophilin A. J Virol 1996;70:5170–5176.
9. Bartz SR, Malkovsky M, Rich DH, et al. Inhibition of human immunodeficiency virus replication by nonimmunosuppressive analogs of cyclosporin A. Proc Natl Acad Sci USA 1995;92:5381–5385.
10. Cardenas ME, Muir RS, Breuder T, Heitman J. Targets of immunophilin-immunosuppressant complexes are distinct highly conserved regions of calcineurin A. EMBO J 1995;14:2772–2783.
11. Batiuk TD, Kung L, Halloran PF. Evidence that calcineurin is rate-limiting for primary human lymphocyte activation. J Clin Invest 1997;100:1894–1901.
12. Sugimoto T, Stewart S, Guan KL. The calcium/calmodulin-dependent protein phosphatase calcineurin is the major Elk-1 phosphatase. J Biol Chem 1997;47:29415–29418.
13. Kruger M, Schwaninger M, Blume R, et al. Inhibition of CREB- and cAMP response element-mediated gene transcription by the immunosuppressive drugs cyclosporin A and FK506 in T cells. Naunyn Schmiedebergs Arch Pharmacol 1997;356:433–440.
14. Cristillo AD, Heximer SP, Russell L, Forsdyke DR. Cyclosporin A inhibits early mRNA expression of G0/G1 Switch Gene 2 (G0S2) in cultured human blood mononuclear cells. DNA Cell Biol 1997;16:1449–1458.
15. Borel JF, Baumann G, Chapman I, et al. In vivo pharmacological effects of ciclosporin and some analogues. Adv Pharmacol 1996;35:115–245.
16. Otto MG, Mayer AD, Clarien PA, et al. Randomized trial of cyclosporine microemulsion (Neoral) versus conventional cyclosporine in liver transplantation: MILTON study. Multicentre International Study in Liver Transplantation of Neoral. Transplantation 1998;66:1632–1640.
17. First MR, Alloway R, Schroeder TJ. Development of Sang-35: a cyclosporine formulation bioequivalent to Neoral. Clin Transplant 1988;12:518–524.
18. Kolars JC, Merion RM, Awni WM, Watkins PB. First-pass metabolism of cyclosporin by the gut. Lancet 1991;338:1488–1490.
19. Lown KS, Watkins PB, Benet LZ, et al. Role of intestinal P-glycoprotein (mdr1) in interpatient variation in the oral bioavailability of cyclosporine. Clin Pharmacol Ther 1997;62:48–60.
20. Freeman DJ. Pharmacology and pharmacokinetics of cyclosporine. Clin Biochem 1991;24:9–14.
21. Primmett D, Levine M, Wrishko R, Keown P. A pharmacokinetic study of cyclosporine A: factors affecting the usefulness of trough levels in predicting drug exposure in renal transplant patients. Clin Drug Invest 1997;13:23–36.
22. Kahan BD, Kramer WG, Wideman C, et al. Demographic factors affecting the pharmacokinetics of cyclosporine estimated by radioimmunoassay. Transplantation 1986;41:459–464.
23. Brunner LJ, Munar MY, Vallian J, et al. Interaction between cyclosporine and grapefruit juice requires long-term ingestion in stable renal transplant recipients. Pharmacotherapy 1998;18:23–29.
24. Gupta SK, Manfro RC, Tomlanovich SJ, et al. Effect of food on the pharmacokinetics of cyclosporine in healthy subjects following oral and intravenous administration. J Clin Pharmacol 1990;30:643–653.
25. Lindholm A, Henricsson S, Dahlqvist R. The effect of food and bile acid administration on the relative bioavailability of cyclosporine. Br J Pharmacol 1990;29:541–548.
26. Naoumov NV, Tredger JM, Steward CM, et al. Cyclosporin A pharmacokinetics in liver transplant recipients in relation to biliary T-tube clamping and liver dysfunction. Gut 1989;30:391–396.
27. Mueller EA, Kovarik JM, van Bree JB, et al. Pharmacokinetics and tolerability of a microemulsion formulation of cyclosporine in renal allograft recipients: a concentration-controlled comparison with the commercial formulation. Transplantation 1994;57:1178.
28. Kovarik JM, Mueller EA, van Bree JB, et al. Within day consistency in cyclosporine pharmacokinetics from a microemulsion formulation in renal transplant patients. Ther Drug Monit 1994;16:232–237.

29. Kovarik JM, Mueller EA, van Bree JB, et al. Cyclosporine pharmacokinetics and variability from a microemulsion formulation: multicenter investigation in kidney transplant patients. Transplantation 1994;58:1–5.

30. Mueller EA, Kovarik JM, van Bree JB, et al. Improved dose-linearity of cyclosporine pharmacokinetics from a microemulsion formulation. Pharmacol Res 1994;11:301–304.

31. Keown PA for the National and International Neoral Study Groups. Use of cyclosporine microemulsion (Neoral) in de novo and stable renal transplantation: clinical impact, pharmacokinetic consequences and economic benefits. Transplant Proc 1996;28:2147–2150.

32. Kovarik JM, Mueller EA, Richard F, et al. Evidence for earlier stabilization of cyclosporine pharmacokinetics in de novo renal transplant patients receiving a microemulsion formulation. Transplantation 1996;62:759–763.

33. Kovarik JM, Mueller EA, van Bree JB, et al. Reduced inter- and intraindividual variability in cyclosporine pharmacokinetics from a microemulsion formulation. J Pharmaceut Sci 1994;83:444–446.

34. Keown P, Landsberg D, Halloran P, et al. A randomized, prospective multicenter pharmacoepidemiologic study of cyclosporine microemulsion in stable renal graft recipients. Report of the Canadian Neoral Renal Transplantation Study Group. Transplantation 1996;62:1744–1752.

35. Lindholm A, Henricsson S. Intra- and inter-individual variability in the free fraction of cyclosporine in plasma in recipients of renal transplants. Ther Drug Monitor 1989;11:623–630.

36. Wasan KM, Pritchard PH, Ramaswamy M, et al. Differences in lipoprotein lipid concentration and composition modify the plasma distribution of cyclosporine. Pharmaceutical Res 1997;14:1613–1620.

37. Nandakumaran M, Eldeen AS. Transfer of cyclosporine in the perfused human placenta. Dev Pharmacol Ther 1990;15:101–105.

38. Behrens O, Kohlhaw K, Gunter H, et al. Detection of cyclosporin A in breast milk—is breast feeding contraindicated? Geburtshilfe Fraunenheilkunde 1989;49:207–209.

39. Kronbach T, Fisher V, Meyer UA. Cyclosporine metabolism in human liver: identification of a cytochrome P-450III gene family as the major cyclosporine-metabolizing enzyme explains interactions of cyclosporine with other drugs. Clin Pharmacol Ther 1988;43:630–635.

40. Keown PA. Pharmacokinetics, drug interactions and analytical measurements of cyclosporin. In: Bach J-F. T-cell directed immunointervention. Oxford: Blackwell Scientific, 1993:51–76.

41. Ptachcinski RJ, Venkataramanan R, Burckart GJ. Clinical pharmacokinetics of cyclosporin. Clin Pharmacokinet 1986;11:107–132.

42. Freeman DJ, Laupacis A, Keown PA, et al. Evaluation of cyclosporine-phenytoin interaction with observations on cyclosporin metabolites. Br J Clin Pharmacol 1984;18:887–893.

43. Martell R, Heinrichs D, Stille CR, et al. The effect of erythromycin in patients treated with cyclosporine. Ann Intern Med 1986;104:660–661.

44. Orme ML, Back DJ, Breckenridge AM. Clinical pharmacokinetics of oral contraceptive steroids. Clin Pharmacokinet 1983;8:95–136.

45. Yee GC. Pharmacokinetic interactions between cyclosporine and other drugs. Transplant Proc 1990;22:1203–1207.

46. Klintmalm G, Sawe J. High dose methylprednisolone increases plasma cylosporin levels in renal transplant recipients. Lancet 1984;1:731.

47. Tu Y, Kahan BD, Chou TC, Stepkowski SM. The synergistic effects of cyclosporine, sirolimus, and brequinar on heart allograft survival in mice. Transplantation 1995;59:177–183.

48. Wrishko RE, Levine M, Primmett DRN, et al. Investigation of a possible interaction between ciprofloxacin and cyclosporine in renal transplant patients. Transplantation 1997;64:996–999.

49. Campana C, Molinaro M, Buggia I, Regazzi MB. Clinically significant drug interactions with cyclosporin. An update. Clin Pharmacokinet 1996;30:141–179.

50. Kahan BD, Grevel J. Optimization of cyclosporine therapy in renal transplantation by pharmacokinetic strategy. Transplantation 1988;46:631–644.

51. Cooney GF, Hoppu K, Habucky K. Cyclosporin pharmacokinetics in paediatric transplant recipients. Clin Pharmacokinet 1997;32:481–495.

52. Lindholm A, Kahan BD. Influence of cyclosporine pharmacokinetics, trough concentrations, and AUC monitoring on outcome after kidney transplantation. Clin Pharmacol Ther 1993;54:205–218.

53. Iacono AT, Smaldone GC, Keenan RJ, et al. Dose-related reversal of acute lung rejection by aerosolized cyclosporine. Am J Respir Crit Care Med 1997;155:1690–1698.

54. Levy GA, Neuhaus P, Jamieson NV, et al. Neoral in de novo liver transplantation: adequate immunosuppression without intravenous cyclosporine. Liver Transpl Surg 1997;3:571–577.

55. Keown P, Niese D. Cyclosporine microemulsion increases drug exposure and reduces acute rejection without incremental toxicity in de novo renal transplantation. Kidney Int 1998;54:938–944.

56. Lodge JPA, Pollard SG. Neoral vs. Sandimmune: interim results of a randomized trial of efficacy and safety in preventing acute rejection in new renal transplant recipients. Transplant Proc 1997;29:272–273.

57. Kingma I, Ludwin D, Dandavino R, et al. Economic analysis of Sandimmune Neoral in de novo renal transplant patients in Canada. Clin Transplant 1997;11:42–48.

58. Keown PA, Landsberg D, Lawen J, et al. Economic Analysis of Sandimmune Neoral in Canadian stable renal transplant patients. Transplant Proc 1995;27:1845–1848.

59. Trull AK, Jamieson NV, Alexander GJ, et al. Absorption of cyclosporin from conventional and new microemulsion oral formulations in liver transplant recipients with external biliary diversion. Br J Clin Pharmacol 1995;39:627–631.

60. Dunn SP, Meligeni J, Elder CA, et al. Absorption characteristics of a microemulsion formulation of cyclosporine in de novo pediatric liver transplant recipients. Transplantation 1995;60:1438–1442.

61. Rasmussen A, Kirkegaard P, Heslet L, et al. Induction of immunosuppression by microemulsion cyclosporine in liver transplantation. Transplantation 1996;62:1031–1033.

62. Hemming AW, Levy GA, Aljumah AA, et al. A microemulsion of cyclosporine without intravenous cyclosporine in liver transplantation. Transplantation 1996;62:798–1802.

63. Winkler M, Pichlmayr R, Neuhaus P, et al. A new oral formulation of cyclosporine for early oral immunosuppressive therapy in liver transplant recipients. Transplantation 1996;62:1063–1068.

64. Graziadei IW, Krom RA, Steers JL, et al. Neoral compared to Sandimmune is associated with a decrease in histologic severity of rejection in patients undergoing primary liver transplantation. Transplantation 1997;64:726–731.

65. van der Pijl JW, Cohen AF, van der Woude FJ, et al. Pharmacokinetics of the conventional and microemulsion formulations of cyclosporine in pancreas-kidney transplant recipients with gastroparesis. Transplantation 1996;62:456–462.

66. White M, Carrier M, Jesina C, et al. Pharmacokinetic, hemodynamic, and metabolic effects of cyclosporine Sandimmune versus the microemulsion Neoral in heart transplant recipients. J Heart Lung Transplant 1997;16:787–794.

67. Kesten S, Scavuzzo M, Chaparro C, Szalai JP. Pharmacokinetic profile and variability of cyclosporine versus Neoral in patients with cystic fibrosis after lung transplantation. Pharmacotherapy 1998;18:847–850.

68. Tan KK, Wallwork J, Uttridge JA, Trull AK. Relative bioavailability of cyclosporin from conventional and microemulsion formulations in heart-lung transplant candidates with cystic fibrosis. Eur J Clin Pharmacol 1995;48:285–289.

69. Neumayer HH, Luft FC, Waiser J, et al. Substitution of conventional cyclosporin with a new microemulsion formulation in renal transplant patients: results after 1 year. Nephrol Dial Transplant 1996;11:165–172.

70. Pescovitz MD, Wong RL, Wombolt DG, et al. Safety and tolerability of cyclosporine microemulsion versus cyclosporine: two-year data in primary renal allograft recipients: a report of the Neoral Study Group. Transplantation 1997;63:78–80.

71. Pasha TM, Wiesner RH, Dahlke LM, et al. An open-label study of the safety and tolerability of converting stable liver transplant recipients to Neoral. Liver Transpl Surg 1998;4:410–415.

72. Keown P, Parfrey P, Belitsky P, et al. A randomized, prospective multicenter pharmacoepidemiologic study of cyclosporine microemulsion in stable renal graft recipients. Report of the Canadian Neoral Renal Transplantation Study Group. Transplantation 1996;62:1744–1752.

73. Cole E, Keown P, Landsberg D, et al. Safety and tolerability of cyclosporine microemulsion during 18 months of follow-up in stable renal transplant recipients: a report of the Canadian Neoral Renal Study Group. Transplantation 1998;65:505–510.

74. Kasiske BL, Heim-Duthoy K, Venkateswara R, Awni WM. The relationship between cyclosporine pharmacokinetic parameters and subsequent acute rejection in renal transplant patients. Transplantation 1988;46:716–722.

75. Kahan BD, Welsh M, Schoenberg L, et al. Variable oral absorption: a biopharmaceutical risk factor for chronic renal allograft rejection. Transplantation 1996;62:599–606.

76. Keown PA, Halloran P, Kahan BD, et al. Optimization of cyclosporine therapy with new therapeutic drug monitoring strategies. Transplant Proc 1998 (in press).

77. Johnston A, Sketris I, Marsden JT, et al. A limited sampling strategy for the measurement of cyclosporine AUC. Transplant Proc 1990;22:1345–1346.

78. Grevel J, Kahan BD. Abbreviated kinetic profiles in area-under-the-curve monitoring of cyclosporine therapy. Clin Chem 1991;37:1905–1908.

79. Cantarovich M, Besner JG, Barkun JS, et al. Two-hour cyclosporine level determination is the appropriate tool to monitor Neoral therapy. Clin Transplant 1998;12:243–249.

80. Melter M, Rodeck B, Kardorff R, Hoyer PF, Brodehl J. Pharmacokinetics of cyclosporine in pediatric long-term liver transplant recipients converted from Sandimmune to Neoral. Transpl Int 1997;10:419–425.

81. Rial M de C, Frias S, Argento J, et al. Convenience of level of cyclosporine-Neoral at time 3 to determine the area under curve in renal transplant. Transplant Proc 1997;29:292–293.

82. Amante AJ, Kahan BD. Abbreviated AUC strategy for monitoring cyclosporine microemulsion therapy in the immediate post-transplant period. Transplant Proc 1996;28:2162–2163.

83. Primmett DRN, Levine M, Kovarik JM, et al. Cyclosporine monitoring in renal transplant patients: two- or three-point methods that estimate area under the curve are superior to trough levels in predicting drug exposure. Ther Drug Monit 1989;20:276–283.

84. Halloran P, Mathew T, Tomlanovich S, et al. Mycophenolate mofetil in renal allograft recipients: a pooled analysis of three randomized double-blind clinical studies in prevention of rejection. Transplantation 1997;63:39–47.

85. The Tricontinental Mycophenolate Mofetil Renal Transplant Study Group. A blinded, randomized clinical trial of mycophenolate mofetil for the prevention of acute rejection in cadaveric renal transplantation. Transplantation 1996;61:1029–1037.

86. Sollinger HW for the US Renal Transplant Mycophenolate Mofetil Study Group. Mycophenolate mofetil for the prevention of acute rejection in primary cadaveric renal allograft recipients. Transplantation 1995;60:225–232.

87. European Mycophenolate Mofetil Cooperative Study Group. Placebo-controlled study of mycophenolate mofetil combined with cyclosporine and corticosteroids for prevention of acute rejection. Lancet 1995;345:1321–1325.

88. The Tricontinental Mycophenolate Mofetil Study Group. A blinded, randomized multicentre study of mycophenolate mofetil (mmf) in cadaveric renal transplantation: results at three years. Transplantation 1989 (in press).

89. Kelly PA, Kahan BD, Behbod F, Gruber SA. Sirolimus, a new, potent immunosuppressive agent. Pharmacotherapy 1997;17:1148–1156.

90. Stepkowski SM, Kahan BD, Chou TC, et al. Synergistic mechanisms by which sirolimus and cyclosporine inhibit rat heart and kidney allograft rejection. Clin Exp Immunol 1997;108:3–68.

91. Morris RE, Berry GJ, Shorthouse R, et al. Studies in experimental models of chronic rejection: use of rapamycin (sirolimus) and isoxazole derivatives (leflunomide and its analogue) for the suppression of graft vascular disease and obliterative bronchiolitis. Transplant Proc 1995;27:2068–2069.

92. Kahan BD. Concentration-controlled immunosuppressive regimens using cyclosporine with sirolimus or brequinar in human renal transplantation. Transplant Proc 1995;27:33–36.

93. Kaplan B, Kahan BD, Napoli KL, Meier-Kriesche HU. The effects of relative timing of sirolimus and cyclosporine microemulsion formulation coadministration on the pharmacokinetics of each agent. Clin Pharmacol Ther 1998;63:48–53.

94. Nashan B, Moore R, Amlot P, et al. Randomized trial of basiliximab versus placebo for control of acute cellular rejection in renal allograft recipients. Lancet 1997;350:1193–1198.

95. Vincenti F, Kirkman R, Light S, et al for the Daclizumab Triple Therapy Study Group. Interleukin-2 receptor blockade with Daclizumab to prevent acute rejection in renal transplantation. N Engl J Med 1998;338:161–165.

96. Calne RY, White DJ. The use of cyclosporin A in clinical organ grafting. Ann Surg 1982;196:330–337.

97. The Canadian Multicentre Transplant Study Group. A randomized trial of cyclosporine in cadaveric renal transplantation. N Engl J Med 1983;309:809–815.

98. Fletchner SM, Payne WD, Van Buren L, et al. The effect of cyclosporine on early graft function in human renal transplantation. Transplantation 1983;36:268–272.

99. Remuzzi G, Bertani T. Renal vascular and thrombotic effects of cyclosporine. Am J Kidney Dis 1989;13:261–272.

100. Goldstein DJ, Zuech N, Sehgal V, et al. Cyclosporine-associated end-stage nephropathy after cardiac transplantation. Transplantation 1997;63:664–668.

101. Remuzzi G, Perico N. Cyclosporine-induced renal dysfunction in experimental animals and humans. Kidney Int Suppl 1995;52:S70–74.

102. Neild GH, Rocchi G, Imberti L, et al. Effect of cyclosporin A on prostacyclin synthesis by vascular tissue. Thromb Res 1983;32:373–379.

103. Moran M, Mozes MF, Maddux MS, et al. Prevention of acute graft rejection by the prostaglandin E1 analogue misoprostol in renal transplant recipients treated with cyclosporine and prednisone. N Engl J Med 1990;322:1183–1188.

104. Pouteil-Noble C, Chapuis F, Berra N, et al. Misoprostol in renal transplant recipients: a prospective, randomized, controlled study on the prevention of acute rejection episodes and cyclosporin A nephrotoxicity. Nephrol Dial Transplant 1994;9:552–555.

105. Chrysostomon A, Walker RG, Russ GR, et al. Diltiazem in renal allograft recipients receiving cyclosporine. Transplantation 1993;55:300–304.

106. Pirsch JD, D'Alessandro AM, Roecker EB, et al. A controlled, double-blind, randomized trial of verapamil and cyclosporine in cadaver renal transplant patients. Am J Kidney Dis 1993;21:189–195.

107. Canadian Multicentre Transplant Study Group. A randomized clinical trial of cyclosporine in cadaveric renal transplantation. N Engl J Med 1986;314:1219–1225.

108. Rigotti P, Flechner SM, VanBuren CT, et al. Increased incidence of renal allograft thrombosis under cyclosporine immunosuppression. Intern Surg 1986;71:38–41.

109. Vanrenterghem Y, Roels L, Lerut J, et al. Thromboembolic complications and haemostatic changes in cyclosporin-treated cadaveric kidney allograft recipients. Lancet 1985;1:999–1002.

110. Bantle JP, Nath KA, Sutherland DER, et al. Effects of cyclosporine on the renin-angiotensin-aldosterone system and potassium excretion in renal transplant recipients. Arch Intern Med 1985;145:505–508.

111. Satterthwaite R, Aswad S, Sunga V, et al. Incidence of new-onset hypercholesterolemia in renal transplant patients treated with FK506 or cyclosporine. Transplantation 1998;65:446–449.

112. McCune TR, Thacker LR, Peters TG, et al. Effects of tacrolimus on hyperlipidemia after successful renal transplantation. Transplantation 1998;65:87–92.

113. Thomson AW, Whiting PH, Simpson JG. Pathobiology of cyclosporin A in experimental animals. In: Cyclosporin A, White DJ, ed. Amsterdam: Elsevier Biomedical, 1982:177.

114. Nash MM, Zaltzman JS. Efficacy of azithromycin in the treatment of cyclosporine-induced gingival hyperplasia in renal transplant recipients. Transplantation 1998;65:1611–1615.

115. Bird AG, McLachlan SM, Britton S. Cyclosporin A promotes spontaneous outgrowth in vitro of Epstein-Barr virus-induced B cell lines. Nature 1981;289:300–301.

116. Gomez R, Moreno E, Colina F, et al. Steroid withdrawal is safe and beneficial in stable cyclosporine-treated liver transplant patients. J Hepatol 1998;28:150–156.

117. Cyclosporine as sole immunosuppressive agent in recipients of kidney allografts from cadaver donors: preliminary results of a European multicentre trial. Lancet 1982;2:57–69.

118. Beveridge T, Calne RY. Cyclosporine (Sandimmune) in cadaveric renal transplantation. Transplantation 1995;59:1568–1570.

# Azathioprine

Roy Y. Calne

The use of azathioprine as an immunosuppressant for solid organ grafts was a watershed in the development of clinical transplantation. In the Tuckahoe Laboratories of Burroughs-Wellcome, Hitchings and Elion started a program to develop synthetic chemical agents that would be valuable in the treatment of cancer. They deliberately substituted purines and pyrimidines to produce molecules that would act in a fraudulent manner, becoming incorporated in vital biologic processes but then poisoning the cells and preventing their division (1). One of the agents they produced was the thiopurine 6-mercaptopurine (6-MP), which was recognized as valuable in the treatment of certain leukemias.

Schwartz and Damashek (2), working at Tufts Medical School in Boston, used 6-MP in experiments to inhibit the clonal proliferation of lymphocytes that occurs in response to an antigenic stimulus. Rabbits challenged with a foreign protein were treated for 2 weeks with daily doses of 6-MP. This prevented the expected primary and later secondary response to that specific protein, but after the 14-day period of treatment the animals could react against other proteins. The 2-week course of 6-MP appeared to have conferred a specific inhibition of antibody production, determined by the challenging protein at the commencement of the treatment. Of special interest was the observation that this effect lasted for a long time after the 6-MP treatment had stopped. Thus, for a simple foreign protein the drug 6-MP was able to produce tolerance.

At the time, the only clinical success with kidney transplants was between identical twins and very closely matched sibling donors who had been treated with total body irradiation. Many patients within the same irradiation protocol but with less well-matched kidneys developed uncontrollable rejection of the organs or died from the side effects of the irradiation. Infection was a major cause of death. Some clinicians persisted with this treatment, despite the almost universal failure. Developing a safer and more effective form of immunosuppression was essential if organ transplantation was to become established.

Following Schwartz and Damashek's rabbit study, I investigated the effect of this drug in dogs receiving renal allografts, in hope of obtaining similar tolerance to organ grafts. Although tolerance could not be produced, several animals had markedly prolonged survival without rejection of their grafts (3). Similar observations were made independently by Zukoski and Hume, which led to investigations using a variety of antiproliferative drugs, including corticosteroids, for control of the immune process (4).

My quest for a more specific agent than 6-MP led me to a visit to Tuckahoe and discussions with Hitchings and Elion. They gave me a variety of compounds including thiopurines and pyrimidines that they felt were worthy of investigation. I studied these in Joseph Murray's laboratory in Francis Moore's department of surgery at the Peter Bent Brigham Hospital in Boston and found that an imidazole-linked 6-MP, later called azathioprine, was slightly superior to the parent compound (5).

The first use of thiopurines in clinical transplants was in England and France using the parent drug 6-MP (6). Following the observations on azathioprine, however, this agent became part of a new protocol that Murray and his colleagues began to use at the Peter Bent Brigham Hospital in 1962. The early results showed that azathioprine was a superior immunosuppressant to total body irradiation, but alone it did not appear to be sufficiently effective for major clinical development.

In 1960 Goodwin (7) showed that an acute rejection crisis in a clinical renal transplant could be reversed by a large dose of corticosteroids, and that corticosteroids combined with azathioprine was a drug protocol that could give better results in renal allografts than azathioprine alone.

Working in Denver, Starzl and his colleagues performed a series of renal allografts using azathioprine and corticosteroids for immunosuppression. These results were the best that had so far been produced in the clinical setting (8). Rejection crises that continued to occur were treated by higher doses of steroids.

There was a danger that overimmunosuppression would cause infection. Side effects of steroids could be very severe, particularly in children. They caused stunted growth and cushingoid facies, turning the children into monsters who could not socialize in a normal manner. Adults often developed aseptic necrosis of bone from a high steroid dose. The chief side effect of azathioprine was bone marrow suppression, and also some patients had an idiosyncratic hepatotoxic reaction. Long-term treatment with azathioprine may be associated with hypertrophic nodular hepatic adenomata, while macrocytic anemia was another rare complication.

Despite these risks, azathioprine and steroids were used with success throughout the Western world and Australasia. Some of the early patients are still alive, 30 years after renal allografting. This mode of immunosuppression was also used in transplants of the heart, liver, and pancreas. There were some notable good long-term results with grafts of these organs, but the high failure rate did not give confidence to clinicians. We had to await the introduction of cyclosporine to clinical transplantation before transplants of the heart, liver, and pancreas could be considered appropriate therapeutic undertakings (9). Continuing good results have now led to a shortage of organs, which grows more serious every year.

## MODE OF ACTION

Azathioprine inhibits both DNA and RNA synthesis, and so interferes with the precursors of purine synthesis and suppresses de novo purine synthesis. It has an effect on both B and T lymphocytes when they are in the process of proliferating. It suppresses both primary T-cell and secondary antibody synthesis, but it does not affect the production of lymphokines. It also has anti-inflammatory action, probably mainly due to its effect on proliferating cells. In addition to marrow suppression and hepatic dysfunction, azathioprine can also cause gastrointestinal disturbance.

The dosage depends on whether azathioprine is being used with other potent agents. Initially, when it is used only with corticosteroids, 3–5 mg/kg/day is given from the time of transplantation. It is usually well tolerated orally, and maintenance doses can often be lowered to 1–3 mg/kg/day. Patients already suffering from liver impairment may require much lower doses or, in some cases, azathioprine may have to be stopped and substituted by another agent such as cyclophosphamide. Azathioprine can also be given intravenously at a similar or slightly lower dose than orally.

When cyclosporine was introduced into clinical organ transplantation, this new agent was used alone or in combination with corticosteroids. Later, it was combined with azathioprine (and corticosteroids) in a triple-drug regimen. In some centers, antilymphocyte antibodies, polyclonal or monoclonal, were given together with the three drugs. To treat a patient with four different immunosuppressive agents requires very careful clinical monitoring, as overimmunosuppression, with accompanying infections and risks of malignancy (particularly B-cell lymphomas), is a hazard. Although the exact immunosuppressive protocol followed by different centers varies in detail, for the past decade triple therapy with cyclosporine, azathioprine, and steroid has been the most common form of treatment.

Currently, the situation is changing. The new powerful purine analogue mycophenolate mofetil (MMF) is thought to have a more specific action on T cells, interfering with their division more than that of other cells. Mycophenolic acid has been used in patients with autoimmune disease, and the MMF derivative has been compared in large multicenter trials with azathioprine. MMF appears to have a better effect in reducing the incidence of acute rejection, although to date there has been no statistically significant improvement in survival of patients or their grafts. Longer follow-up of these studies is now being undertaken.

In summary, for 20 years azathioprine was the lynch-pin of immunosuppression for recipients of solid organ allografts. It was preferred to other antimitotic agents as having a better therapeutic index. Today, however, it may well be replaced by other, more specific agents such as mycophenolate mofetil.

## REFERENCES

1. Elion GB, Bieber S, Hitchings GH. The fate of 6-mercaptopurine in mice. Ann NY Acad Sci 1955;60:297–303.
2. Schwartz R, Damashek W. Drug-induced immunologic tolerance. Nature 1959;183:1682–1683.
3. Calne RY. The rejection of renal homografts. Inhibition in dogs by using 6-mercaptopurine. Lancet 1960;1:417.
4. Zukoski CF, Lee HM, Hume DM. The prolongation of functional survival of canine renal homograft by 6-mercaptopurine. Surg Forum 1960;11:470.
5. Calne RY. Inhibition of the rejection of renal homografts in dogs with purine analogues. Transplant Bull 1961;28:445.
6. Hopewell J, Calne RY, Beswick I. Three clinical cases of renal transplantation. Brit Med J 1964;1:411.
7. Goodwin WE, et al. Human renal transplantation: clinical experiences with 6 cases of renal homo-transplantation. J Urol 1963;89:13.
8. Starzl TE, Marchioro TL, Von Kaulla KN, et al. Homotransplantation of the liver in humans. Surg Gynecol Obstet 1963;117:659.
9. Calne RY, White DJG, Thiru S, et al. Cyclosporin A in patients receiving renal allografts from cadaver donors. Lancet 1978;2:323.

# Steroids and Transplantation

Rowan G. Walker

From the days of early clinical renal transplantation in the 1960s, steroids (glucocorticoids) provided at least part of the basis of immunosuppressive therapy. For the next 20 to 25 years, steroids would provide the backbone of maintenance immunosuppression, particularly in combination with azathioprine, and virtually stood alone as the treatment for acute rejection. Their major role in maintenance immunosuppression therapy has clearly been lessened by the advent of cyclosporine (early 1980s) and the other calcineurin blockers. Also, to some extent the role of steroids in the treatment of acute rejection episodes has been supplemented, at least in part, by the availability of antilymphocyte serum preparations, particularly the monoclonal anti-T cell antibodies.

Thus, prednisolone, or prednisone in conjunction with azathioprine, has come to be known as "conventional immunosuppression" (1). Although cyclosporine—alone, in combination with steroids, or in triple combination with prednisolone and azathioprine—has probably become the major and most effective form of maintenance immunosuppression, there remains a very significant number of patients for whom steroids are an integral part of the long-term treatment. For these patients, the major problem remains finding the optimal dose and planning for withdrawal of the steroids, with the aim of minimizing the steroids' long-term toxic effects.

## HISTORY

As far back as the 1920s, steroids were known to affect the immune system. Their first successful use in renal transplantation was in Boston in 1960, when cortisone was used to reverse a rejection episode in a living-related donor transplant recipient who had been immunosuppressed by whole body irradiation.

In 1961, Elion et al (2) synthesized azathioprine, an imidazole derivative of 6-mercaptopurine (6-MP), which had been found to be less toxic than 6-MP in dogs (3). The development of azathioprine led quite quickly to the undertaking of regular clinical renal transplantation in 1961 (4,5), and steroids were added to azathioprine as maintenance therapy in most centers after 1962 (6). However, following the early observation of successful reversal of acute rejection with large doses of prednisone (7), for many years several centers employed only steroids for the treatment of such episodes (8). Although initially prednisone was the steroid most commonly used, most units replaced it relatively soon with prednisolone.

## PHARMACOLOGY

The pharmacology of steroids and their effects on the immune system are known to be extremely complex (9). Steroids affect the immune response in innumerable ways, especially in high doses, and their effects are especially seen on T lymphocytes. Corticosteroids have been shown to block $Ca^{2+}$ ionophore-induced lymphocyte proliferation, which is an in vitro model of postreceptor events occurring after interaction of the T-cell receptor with antigen (10). Although cyclosporine also inhibits $Ca^{2+}$ ionophore-induced proliferation, the mechanism is different (11). The cooperation between monocytes and lymphocytes in the proliferative response is also inhibited by steroids (12).

The block to the activation of T-cell proliferation by steroids has subsequently been shown to be associated with blocking the activation of certain cytokine genes. In particular, steroids block activation of the interleukin 2 (IL-2) gene in T cells (13), and also block activity of IL-1 (14) and IL-6 genes in other cells such as macrophages (15). It has been argued that the ability of steroids to prevent or suppress the fever associated with allograft rejection probably derives from the blocking of the release of these pyrogenic cytokines. As IL-2 is largely dependent on the presence of IL-1 and IL-6, corticosteroids have indirect as well as direct effects on IL-2 production from T cells.

Apart from the inhibition of lymphokines described above, steroids clearly reduce the migration of monocytes toward sites of inflammation. These broad and powerful anti-inflammatory actions of steroids also play an important role in the rejection process. This is particularly evident in the treatment of rejection episodes with high doses of prednisolone (or methylprednisolone) where the clinical effect is most often evident within 1 or 2 hours, which is quite clearly far too rapid to be adequately explained as a true immunosuppressive effect.

## MAINTENANCE STEROID REGIMENS

There are virtually no situations where steroids would be used alone as maintenance immunosuppression, except in patients who are intolerant to all other agents or in whom the overall immunosuppression burden needs to be reduced (e.g., a patient developing severe neoplasia where continued use of other agents might hasten the neoplastic disease process). From the early days of clinical renal transplantation, it became increasingly apparent that there was a need to use steroid together with azathioprine; as the pharmacology of these two agents became established, they demonstrated quite different but additive effects (10).

### Azathioprine and Steroids

Dual "conventional" immunosuppression maintenance therapy regimens consisting of azathioprine and steroids were used at most centers for the 25 years leading up to the mid-1980s. For the most part, such regimens consisted of:

1. an azathioprine dosage of 2–3 mg/kg/day, given as a single daily dose and reduced only if specifically indicated by complications (mainly leucopenia).
2. a prednisolone dosage, initially quite high (50–100 mg/day) then reduced slowly to a maintenance dose of approximately 10 mg/day over 6 to 7 months, and possibly as low as 5 mg/day over the longer term.

This general type of regimen (with minor variations) was the most common, but a number of exceptions gradually evolved, the most important of which has been the use of low-dose maintenance steroids.

#### Perioperative Therapy

Virtually all immunosuppressive regimens were established empirically. Whether steroids are given as part of dual (or even triple or quadruple) therapy, a typical perioperative regimen would be preoperative methylprednisolone, 1 gram IV, followed by postoperative hydrocortisone, 100 mg IV

every 6 hours until oral therapy could be commenced. There is some evidence to support the approach of administering steroids before antigen exposure, particularly in suppression of humoral immunity. However, in a small controlled clinical trial, Kauffman et al (16) were not able to demonstrate any benefit of perioperative intravenous methylprednisolone. Regardless of the nature of the other immunosuppressive agents in the chosen regimen, many clinicians would continue to use the above approach or something similar.

#### High-Dose or Low-Dose Steroids

In the late 1970s and early 1980s, McGeown (17,18) consistently achieved excellent graft survival and a low incidence of steroid-related complications with a single daily prednisolone dose of 20 mg/day. The steroid was given from the day of transplantation, with gradual reduction after 6 months. The Necker group deliberately avoided the use of steroids in living donor recipients until the first rejection episode had occurred and discovered that 53% of HLA-identical grafts never developed rejection (19). Although this approach was attempted with cadaveric grafts, nearly all patients developed rejection episodes and subsequently required steroids. These observations strongly suggest that the degree of total immunosuppression, particularly the steroid dosage provided by a typical high-steroid azathioprine regimen, was unnecessary and was associated with an unacceptable rate of complications, especially steroid-related complications.

Eventually, the group at Oxford undertook a prospective trial (20–22). A typical high-dose regimen was compared with a relatively low-dose regimen. The low-dose group received prednisolone, 30 mg/day (as a single morning dose) for the first 60 days with subsequent slow reduction. This was supplemented by methylprednisolone, 1 gram IV on days 6, 7, and 8 after transplantation. Importantly, the study results showed a halving of the rate of steroid-related complications in the low-dose group with preservation of similar patient and graft survival rates to those achieved in patients receiving high-dose steroid. Unfortunately, the number of patients studied (39 on high-dose, 32 on low-dose) was too small to confidently exclude a real difference in graft survival being present in a larger sample. Although other groups (23–25) subsequently reported similar trials and results, there were problems with the relatively small numbers of patients in most of these studies. Nonetheless, the trend of the findings further support the hypothesis that low-dose steroids cause less complications and achieve similar graft survival rates to high-dose steroids (26).

#### The Influence of Azathioprine Dose

An important Australian multicenter trial (189 patients), showed a significantly worse graft survival in low-dose steroid–treated patients (27). This trial directly compared the original McGeown low-dose steroid regimen with each participating center's standard high-dose steroid therapy—azathioprine dosage was not mandated and each center was at liberty to use its own standard azathioprine dosage protocol.

The results ultimately indicated that the effects of the two steroid regimens could not be considered independently from the azathioprine dosage even after 4 years (28), at

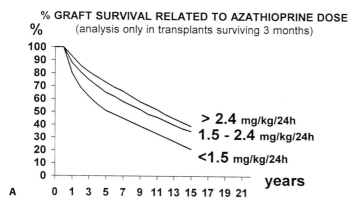

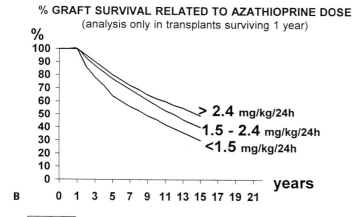

**FIGURE 3.1.** *Effects of azathioprine (AZA) dose on primary cadaveric graft survival, evaluated at 3 months (**A**) and 12 months (**B**) after transplant. The effect of AZA dose is examined only on grafts that had survived the early post-transplant period. No attempt was made to determine the reason(s) for an AZA dose <1.5 mg/kg/24 h. [Data from the Australian and New Zealand Dialysis and Transplantation Registry (ANZDATA), 1978.]*

which time the apparent differences between the high- and low-steroid regimens demonstrated at 12 months were no longer apparent. It was clear that the combination of low doses of both agents provided inadequate immunosuppression and a poor graft survival, whereas higher doses of azathioprine allowed the use of low-dose steroid without significantly more graft losses than occurred with high-dose steroid. High doses of steroid could compensate to only a variable extent for lower azathioprine doses.

This study (27,28) almost certainly helps to explain the poor results achieved in some units with low-dose steroid regimens. It also indicates that, provided the azathioprine dose is adequate (greater than approximately 2 mg/kg/24 h), it would be possible to exclude any detrimental effect of low-dose steroid on graft survival of 10% or greater with a confidence of 95%.

In patients receiving only the combination of azathioprine and steroids, the important influence of an adequate azathioprine dose can also be demonstrated by analysis of the Australian and New Zealand Dialysis and Transplantation Registry data (Fig. 3.1 and Table 3.1), where the relationship between azathioprine dose and graft survival can be clearly observed irrespective of the steroid dose, even 10 to 15 years after transplantation. Interestingly, the relative importance of azathioprine dose has not been seen subsequently in immunosuppressive regimens that contain cyclosporine (29).

It seems that among "conventional" azathioprine/steroid dual-immunosuppression therapy regimens, the high-azathioprine/low-steroid regimen of the McGeown group is the best option available because it reduces steroid-related complications (28) without risking extra graft losses.

## Cyclosporine and Steroids Versus Cyclosporine, Azathioprine, and Steroids

Steroids may form part of an immunosuppressive regimen that contains the key immunosuppressive agent cyclosporine (see Chapter 1). Since the introduction of cyclosporine in the late 1970s and early 1980s, it is interesting to reflect that graft outcome (3-year survival) is virtually identical for all

**Table 3.1.** Effects of Azathioprine (AZA) Dose on Primary Graft Survival (Data Shown in Figure 3.1)

| | Evaluated 3 Months After Surgery | | | Evaluated 12 Months After Surgery | | |
|---|---|---|---|---|---|---|
| | | Number of Patients at Risk | | | | Number of Patients at Risk | |
| AZA Dose (mg/kg/24 h) | 3 Months | 10 Years | AZA Dose (mg/kg/24 h) | 1 Year | 10 Years |
| <1.5 | 342 | 110 | <1.5 | 308 | 112 |
| 1.5–2.4 | 941 | 400 | 1.5–2.4 | 843 | 386 |
| >2.4 | 288 | 140 | >2.4 | 166 | 83 |

Source: Australian and New Zealand Dialysis and Transplantation Registry (ANZDATA), 1978.

regimens, provided that cyclosporine forms one of the components (30). Comparing cyclosporine alone; cyclosporine and steroids; cyclosporine and azathioprine; and cyclosporine, azathioprine, and steroids, the most notable difference is that the relative mean dose of cyclosporine (at 1 year) was lower in the regimen employing all three immunosuppressive agents (so-called "triple" therapy). Of all these regimens, triple therapy is far and away the most popular (31–33), as it allows flexibility in the regimen and a low dose of the potentially nephrotoxic cyclosporine (34,35). Importantly, it also offers the opportunity for tapering the steroid dose to very low maintenance dose levels or even complete withdrawal of steroids (34,35).

It is not yet clear which of the cyclosporine-containing regimens is the optimal maintenance immunosuppressive regimen. One thing that is perhaps clear is the relationship between poor long-term graft outcome (function and survival) and the number and severity of acute rejection events. To what extent a steroid component of the regimen influences these episodes is difficult to determine precisely, particularly in triple-therapy regimens where the dose of cyclosporine is typically reduced compared to monotherapy (cyclosporine alone) or dual therapy (cyclosporine and steroids). The situation has become even more complicated with the introduction of new antiproliferative agents, particularly mycophenolate mofetil (MMF), which in three large multicenter controlled trials (36–38) was shown to reduce the incidence of acute rejection episodes during the early post-transplant months in patients who were simultaneously receiving cyclosporine and steroids (see Chapter 5).

A high proportion of patients receiving monotherapy (cyclosporine alone) require prednisolone (or azathioprine) to be added to the regimen because of immunologic instability. Unfortunately, this approach is not always successful in reversing the rejection process. The alternative approach is to commence with a broader immunosuppression regimen (triple therapy) and consider withdrawing steroids and/or azathioprine sequentially in patients in whom rejection has not proven to be a problem.

## Variables Affecting Maintenance Steroid Dose

### Patient Size

Children excluded, it is not common for steroid doses to be tailored to body size. Normally, the aim of dose adjustment according to weight would be to give doses in proportion to a patient's metabolic rate. Although surface area most closely reflects metabolic rate, weight is a reasonable guide in adults and is generally easier to measure. However, the correlation between weight and surface area is poor, and it particularly underestimates dosages in children and in small adults (<40 kg) in whom body surface area should be used.

### Bioavailability

Prednisone and prednisolone are generally absorbed rapidly from the gastrointestinal tract, with peak plasma concentra-

tions occurring within 1 to 3 hours (39). Prednisone is metabolized by the liver to prednisolone and the efficiency of this conversion is very variable. An average bioavailability of approximately 80% of that achieved by prednisolone (40) is the result of the conversion. Prednisolone is bound partly by the cortisone-binding globulin and also weakly by albumin. Although the binding affinity of albumin is relatively low, it is quantitatively the most important at pharmacologic concentrations of steroids.

Because only free steroid is available to interact with cytosol receptors, conditions that alter the level of plasma binding have marked effects on bioavailability. For example, pregnancy is associated with an increased plasma-binding capacity; consequently, there is reduced bioavailability of steroids in pregnant women. In hypoalbuminemia, the reverse is true—bioavailability is increased, thus explaining the increased incidence of steroid side effects reported in hypoalbuminemic patients (41).

Steroids are almost exclusively inactivated by the liver, so alterations in hepatic functional capacity will influence the half-life. The normal half-life of prednisone is about 60 minutes and that of prednisolone is 200 minutes (42). However, it should be remembered that prednisone is converted to prednisolone, thus the therapeutic effect lasts considerably longer than the half-life would suggest. Chronic liver disease (cirrhosis) can result in a doubling of steroid half-life (41), and certain commonly used drugs such as phenytoin barbiturates and rifampicin shorten the half-life by induction of hepatic enzymes (39).

### Renal Function

As steroid metabolism is hepatic, serum activity, and consequently toxicity, is not changed in renal failure.

### Timing of Drug Administration

In the era of "conventional" immunosuppression (azathioprine and steroids), it was originally common practice to administer steroids as divided doses (usually twice daily) in adult transplant patients. However, many centers have used a single daily dose, and those particularly concerned with pediatric transplantation have occasionally been inclined to use alternate-day steroids. The aim of single and alternate daily doses of steroid is obviously to reduce the incidence of steroid-related complications, without reducing their effectiveness as antirejection agents.

The logic of using single daily doses is that they be given in the morning to coincide with the cortisol peak, which is subject to diurnal rhythm. Certainly, the suppression of the hypothalamic-pituitary-adrenal axis is less using single morning steroid doses than single evening doses or divided daily doses (43,44). Similarly, there is also less suppression of the axis if steroids are given as a double dose on alternate days (1,45–47). Apart from relative sparing of the adrenal-pituitary axis, it is not clear that other steroid side effects are reduced by single daily doses. The benefits of alternate-day doses are more evident, with less growth retardation, cushingoid characteristics (46), serious infectious complications, and osteonecrosis (48), and these benefits are achievable without detectable loss of anti-inflammatory activity (45,46,49).

There is no appreciable difference in the immunosuppressive efficacy of twice- and once-daily steroids, but alternate-day steroids are definitely less suppressive as judged by their capacity to suppress delayed hypersensitivity skin testing to recall and/or to de novo antigens (49). At a clinical level, although it has not been subjected to trial, single and divided doses seem equally effective; however, many clinicians would argue that compliance is likely to be enhanced with the use of single daily dosing.

In patients receiving azathioprine and steroids, alternate-day prednisolone would predictably be associated with an intensified immune response. Indeed, in more than one study a changeover from daily to alternate-day steroids has been associated with increased rejection events (50–52). However, two prospective trials have not demonstrated a higher incidence of rejection or loss of function (48,53). In trying to interpret this apparent dichotomy, it should perhaps be emphasized that a failure to demonstrate a difference cannot necessarily be extrapolated to the assumption that the two therapies are equally effective, unless the numbers of patients studied are very large.

It has also been suggested that the changeover from daily to alternate-day steroids should be made within a few months of transplantation in children (54). Again, these recommendations were based on experience obtained using a high-dose steroid regimen and cannot be automatically considered to hold true with a low-dose steroid regimen, particularly as the recommended time of changeover is well before the steroid dose is actually down to a "maintenance" level. Growth in pubertal children is particularly sensitive to steroids compared to prepubertal children (55).

One might conclude that, in conventional dual therapy using azathioprine and steroids, in adults low-dose steroid given as a single morning dose would be the optimal regimen, although some would still argue for alternate-day therapy (56). The higher level and the nature of the side effects of daily steroids in children potentially outweigh the possible disadvantages of alternate-day therapy. In regimens containing cyclosporine (and prednisolone) it has been common practice to give the steroid as a single daily dose taken in the morning.

## Steroid Withdrawal

Although immunosuppressive therapy including steroids has been discontinued successfully in the long-term in some patients (sometimes inadvertently), it was generally the case that such a practice was often followed by rejection (57). In contrast to complete cessation of immunosuppression in patients on azathioprine and steroids, reduction of the daily dose of azathioprine of stable patients from about 2.0–2.5 mg/kg to 1.5–2.0 mg/kg after 2 years may be relatively safe—the evidence is that azathioprine, rather than the small

dose of steroid, contributes to the high risk of malignancy in long-term transplant recipients.

When cyclosporine was first used in clinical transplantation (58) it was suggested that it could be used as sole therapy—thus effectively eliminating the need for maintenance steroid therapy. This view was gradually modified with the recognition that cyclosporine was not only nephrotoxic (59,60), but that the nephrotoxicity was in part dose dependent (61,62). In addition, several studies showed that adding prednisolone and lowering cyclosporine doses reduced toxicity and rejection episodes (63,64). Yet cessation of steroids at 6 or 12 months was likely to be associated with rejection (65,66).

The constant desire to reduce the individual toxicity of the various immunosuppressants eventually led to the development of low-dose "triple therapy" regimens (cyclosporine, azathioprine, and steroids). The synergism between cyclosporine and azathioprine (67) encouraged some clinicians to again consider complete steroid withdrawal. Although this may be achievable in more than 60% of patients (34,68), without rejection and without any adverse effect on graft function or outcome, in the remaining patients rejection episodes still may be observed. As suggested above, incorporation of the newer pharmacologic agents, including MMF (see Chapter 5) and tacrolimus (see Chapter 4), may allow more successful withdrawal of steroids (69). Nevertheless, a steroid-withdrawal approach to immunosuppression is certainly not universally practiced.

Interestingly, the proportion of patients who ultimately require steroids to be introduced into regimens not employing steroids from the outset (70) is strikingly similar to the proportion of patients from whom steroids cannot be successfully withdrawn when steroids are used from the outset.

## TREATMENT OF REJECTION EPISODES

Despite the increasing use of antilymphocyte globulin and monoclonal anti-T cell antibodies as antirejection therapy, steroids continue to be the most important first-line treatment of acute rejection. In the treatment of rejection the important issue is not so much the choice of agent but the certainty of the diagnosis. The treatment of rejection is certainly important, but there is no evidence that delaying therapy for 24 hours to make certain of the diagnosis has a detrimental effect on the final outcome. At least 60% of acute rejection episodes can be reversed with oral or intravenous prednisolone (71), although success rates are lower if rejection occurs very early (within the first week) or if the clinical course is complicated by delayed function.

Once the diagnosis of rejection is established, treatment with oral or intravenous "bolus" methylprednisolone (equivalent to 3–15 mg/kg/day) is usually instituted (72). Interestingly, the use of high-dose oral prednisolone (e.g., 200 mg/day for 3 days) as a short course has not been shown to be inferior to intravenous methylprednisolone (0.5–1.0 gram daily for 3 days) in terms of the rate of rejection reversal. The oral regime is simpler, cheaper, and probably better tolerated by patients (73), but intravenous methylprednisolone appears to remain the treatment of choice.

For steroid-resistant rejection, treatment with OKT-3 (71) or antithymocyte globulin (ATG) should be instituted with a high expectation of reversal in the short term (see Chapter 8). For the prednisolone treatments, the incidence of major complications appears to be similar between intravenous and high-dose oral prednisolone therapies. Kauffman et al (74) compared high-dose (30 mg/kg/day) and low-dose (3 mg/kg/day) intravenous methylprednisolone regimens, and established that there was no advantage in high-dose therapy. When high-dose oral prednisolone courses are prolonged, a higher incidence of side effects may be anticipated (75,76).

It is virtually universal practice to repeat a course of high-dose steroid (oral or intravenous) after 3 to 5 days if there is a failure to respond, an incomplete response, or a relapse. The risk of serious complications undoubtedly escalates quite markedly with repeated courses of antirejection therapy. As indicated above, virtually all steroid-resistant rejection episodes respond to polyclonal ATG or a monoclonal T-cell antibody (OKT-3). Common practice is to use OKT-3 or ATG in rejection episodes unresponsive to steroids, and then to repeat the steroid course should the episode either respond and subsequently relapse, or only partially respond. In refractory rejection, an increasing role for other agents such as mycophenolate mofetil or tacrolimus (see Chapter 4) is being progressively established (77,78).

Various forms of in vitro testing of steroid sensitivity have been shown to predict a subsequent response to steroids during acute rejection in the clinical setting. However, the use of such techniques as a guide to immunosuppressive therapy has not gained much acceptance among clinicians (79,80).

## COMPLICATIONS AND SIDE EFFECTS

Although it is often possible to ascribe responsibility for particular complications to particular immunosuppressants, many complications are due to the combined immunosuppressive effect of the drug regimen. Because of the nature of those complications, clinicians have always wanted to reduce the steroid burden whenever possible. This desire resulted in enthusiasm for the use of low-dose steroid regimens and steroid-withdrawal protocols when it became clear that the former was probably as effective in preventing graft rejection as conventional high-dose regimens (28), and the latter could be successfully achieved in 60% to 70% of patients taking cyclosporine (34) or in most patients on triple therapy (81).

### Complications of Steroids Alone

#### Growth Retardation
Growth retardation with subsequent failure to reach adult height is one of the most unfortunate features of pediatric renal transplantation. Growth rates prior to the availability

of recombinant human growth hormone were no better after transplantation than those seen in children on dialysis (82). Many factors potentially influence the final outcome: renal failure itself is a cause of growth retardation owing to impaired somatomedin activity, as are hyperparathyroidism and renal rickets. Similarly, some causes of renal failure, such as cystinosis, are themselves potent causes of growth retardation.

It has been suggested that any improvement in growth velocity occurring after transplantation may be enhanced by the use of alternate-day rather than daily steroids (54). Other important factors include complete normalization of renal function and transplantation prior to the onset of puberty. Puberty is frequently delayed in chronic renal failure, and it may occur soon after transplantation with rapid epiphyseal closure and minimizing of further growth. As stated previously, during puberty, sensitivity of skeletal growth to steroids is marked.

Although the growth velocity after transplantation may reach normal, there is rarely any significant catch-up growth (82). Thus, the degree of growth retardation present before transplantation is some guide to the ultimate best outcome. Immunosuppression regimens containing cyclosporine may offer the best prospects of improved growth (see Chapter 1) after transplantation. The use of recombinant growth hormone before and after transplantation in growth-retarded children (especially prepubertal children) has been so successful that growth retardation is clearly diminishing as a problem in pediatric transplantation. Concerns still remain, however, as to the possible role of recombinant human growth hormone in rejection events (83,84).

#### Wound Healing
Steroids reduce the rate of wound healing, and this situation is exacerbated by chronic renal failure.

#### Bone Disease
Steroids are an important predisposing factor in the development of osteoporosis and avascular necrosis (AVN).
**Avascular Necrosis**   The incidence of AVN is as high as 10% to 15% in patients treated with "conventional" high-dose steroid regimens and probably as low as 1% to 2% in patients receiving low-dose steroid. The incidence seems to be more closely related to the level of maintenance steroid than to the short courses ("pulses") of high doses given for rejection. Patients with secondary hyperparathyroidism at the time of transplantation may be at higher risk of developing AVN (85). The AVN lesion most commonly affects the hips and is frequently bilateral (Fig. 3.2). AVN may also affect other joints including the wrists, elbows, knees, ankles, and shoulders.

Pain, often very severe, is the usual presenting symptom. Radiologic changes are typically absent in the early stages. Pain is also the symptom that ultimately is most likely to lead to surgery. Initial treatment is the avoidance of weight-bearing on the affected joint, but compliance with this is difficult to achieve, especially when pain subsides. Contin-

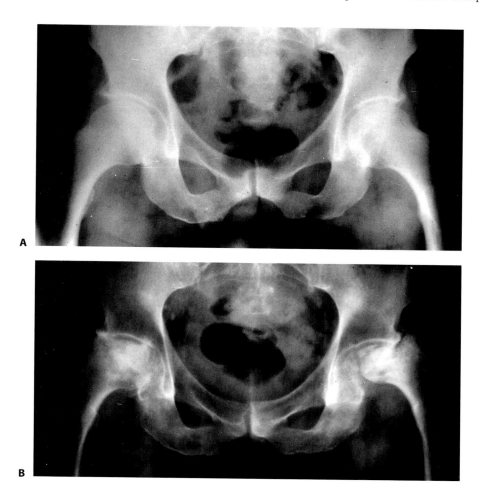

**FIGURE 3.2.**    *Radiographic appearance of a 24-year-old renal transplant recipient developing the early symptoms of aseptic necrosis, with minimal radiologic changes. The patient's condition 6 months after transplant (**A**) progressed to almost total destruction of both hips (femoral heads) 30 months later (**B**). The patient had received large doses of intravenous corticosteroids for early acute rejection episodes, along with prolonged oral high-dose maintenance prednisolone.*

ued weight-bearing on the joint results in crushing of the femoral head, with a resulting limp. Ultimately, most patients will require surgery (total hip replacement), which is often undertaken relatively early to maximize rehabilitation.

**Osteoporosis**    Osteoporosis associated with steroid use may lead to pathologic fractures. Loss of bone density after transplantation (especially early after transplant) is now well described (86,87) and may be very rapid (88). While glucocorticoids are important (89), the structure of the skeleton is likely to depend on a number of other effects (especially in renal transplant recipients) including exacerbation or remission of hyperparathyroidism, resolution of amenorrhea, increased physical activity, and changes in the renal tubular handling of phosphate (67,90,91).

### Cataracts

The incidence of posterior lenticular cataracts is probably as high as 10% in patients receiving high-dose steroid, especially in the peritransplant period (92). The majority of cataracts are small and usually central, and they normally do

not cause a very severe handicap. Less frequently (in about 1% to 2% of cases), the cataract is large and necessitates lens removal.

### Diabetes

In patients on high-dose steroid regimens, glycosuria in the first 6 months after transplant occurs in about 60% of cases. Most often this is of renal origin, and in only about 20% of patients will hyperglycemia clinically be present. After the first 6 months, when the steroid dose is at maintenance level, glycosuria is much less common (5% of patients). Overall, only 5% to 10% of patients actually require therapy, usually oral hypoglycemic agents, and in many cases this need is transient. One report has suggested that post-transplant glucose intolerance is more likely to be associated with the same HLA-B locus antigens (B8, B18, BW 15, and BW 16) that are associated with juvenile-onset diabetes mellitus (93). There is a clear difference in the incidence of diabetes in patients receiving cyclosporine, where the incidence is low, and those receiving tacrolimus (FK506), where the incidence is high (see Chapter 4). The contribution of prednisolone to the latter is uncertain.

### Weight Gain and Obesity

Steroids are frequently associated with a marked increase in appetite, which, coupled with a cessation of dialysis diet restrictions, may result in excessive weight gain (obesity). The problem usually begins to become apparent 2 to 3 months after transplant, and it is most effectively managed using preventative measures rather than by attempts to lose the extra weight. The appetite settles to normal as the steroid dose is reduced. The problem ought to be less marked with a low-dose steroid regimen, but our own experience (28) did not confirm this.

### Hyperlipidemia

Hyperlipidemia has been increasingly recognized as a common problem following organ transplantation. Interest particularly centers on hyperlipidemia as a cause of accelerated atherosclerosis and post-transplant coronary and cerebrovascular events (94). In addition, hyperlipidemia may play a role in chronic rejection and late renal graft loss.

The precise cause of post-transplant hyperlipidemia is uncertain. In patients treated with prednisolone (and azathioprine), hypertriglyceridemia is the most common finding but is frequently accompanied by hypercholesterolemia. The abnormal lipid profiles are evident early and tend to persist (95). The hypertriglyceridemia probably results from an increased consumption of calories (carbohydrate and fat) following reversal of kidney failure accompanied by glucose intolerance secondary to the steroid administration. In contrast, patients treated with cyclosporine tend to have hypercholesterolemia, which, unlike hyperglycemia, is more severe in cyclosporine- than tacrolimus-treated recipients (see Chapter 4).

The initial therapeutic approach to hyperlipidemia in the transplant recipient is to impose dietary calorie-fat restrictions. The role of pharmacologic lipid-lowering agents in the cyclosporine era is being established (96).

### Cushingoid Features

The characteristic features of Cushing's syndrome, including moon face, acne, altered hair distribution, and truncal obesity with thin extremities, are common with high-dose steroid regimens. The severity of the problem is highly variable. Myopathy can be severe, especially in the elderly and in the early post-transplant months.

### Peptic Ulceration

Although there has always been debate about whether steroids cause peptic ulcers, there is clearly an increased incidence and risk in transplant patients, particularly in the early post-graft period when steroid doses are relatively high. Many units use prophylactic $H_2$ antagonists (e.g., cimetidine) in symptomatic patients or during the period when steroid doses are above 20–30 mg/day. Anecdotal reports suggest

that this has been associated with a reduced incidence of peptic ulcers.

Most important for avoiding the potentially fatal complications of peptic ulcers is thorough investigation of all dialysis patients with indigestion prior to transplantation, using elective gastroscopy and/or radiologic studies (barium meal), followed by treatment if any lesions are detected. Silent ulcers are not uncommon in dialysis patients; many patients show minor lesions on gastroscopy, particularly those with hyperparathyroidism. Ulcers detected prior to transplantation should be treated medically first, and then surgically if medical treatment fails.

### Colonic Perforation

Colonic perforation is a rare but potentially lethal complication of transplantation. The role of steroids is unclear. In many cases, it is a complication of preexisting diverticulosis, and it may also be seen in overt cytomegalovirus (CMV) infection. Although it is uncommon, its importance lies in the fact that it causes very high mortality in transplant patients. Historically, some units have investigated all potential transplant recipients by barium enema or colonoscopy to exclude diverticular disease. Some units have considered prophylactic surgery, but this is probably not justified in the era of cyclosporine, except perhaps in the occasional patient with a history of recurrent active diverticulitis.

### Pancreatitis

Pancreatitis represents another complication in whose etiology the role of steroids is arguable. It is extremely uncommon, and is usually the result of an acute viral infection (e.g., mumps, CMV), preexisting gallstones, or pancreatic disease. Azathioprine should be considered as a possible causative agent in patients receiving the drug as part of the immunosuppression regimen.

### Hypertension

Steroids may contribute to the high incidence of post-graft hypertension (at least 50%), but they are rarely the sole cause. The major contributors are the native kidneys, as demonstrated by the low incidence in patients who have been bilaterally nephrectomized; other agents, such as cyclosporine; and transplant arterial disease—either renal artery stenosis or chronic vascular obliteration due to rejection.

### Psychiatric Disturbance

Mood changes, most commonly euphoria, are a common side effect of high-dose steroids. Frank psychosis is not rare, but it is almost invariably based on an underlying psychiatric disorder that may not have been readily evident prior to transplantation. Sleep disorders, particularly insomnia, are also a common complaint in the early period; however, such disturbances (particularly involving nightmares) are more often a result of β-blockers for hypertension, rather than steroids.

## Combined Effects of Steroids and Other Immunosuppression

### Infections

Infection in transplant patients remains a relatively common and potentially serious problem. The incidence of infections in "conventional" low-dose steroid regimens appears to be less than that found with high-dose regimens (28). Anti-lymphocyte agents, used either at induction or for the treatment of acute rejection, increase the susceptibility of the patient to infection, especially viral infections such as CMV, herpes simplex, and herpes zoster. Most episodes of acute rejection will have been treated by large bolus doses of prednisolone before the introduction of the antilymphocyte agents.

### Malignancy

The incidence of virtually all malignancies, especially skin cancer, increases dramatically in immunosuppressed renal transplant recipients (97).

### Skin Disorders

The skin is the site of a variety of complications following transplantation. Skin cancers may manifest, but many of the skin problems seen after a transplant are the result of infections (e.g., acne, warts, herpes simplex, and herpes zoster). The etiology is less certain in other skin disorders (98). Steroids induce thinning of the dermis by loss of collagen, a problem most often found in female patients. This common, readily detectable condition creates a risk of shearing injuries from minor trauma, particularly in the skin over the shins.

### ACKNOWLEDGMENTS

The author is grateful to the Australian and New Zealand Dialysis and Transplantation Registry for permission to reproduce the data in Figure 3.1 and Table 3.1. The author also wishes to acknowledge the skilled and patient assistance of Miss Christine Whyte, who prepared the manuscript for this chapter.

## COMMENTARY

### Henri Kreis

Although the majority of transplanters are eager to get rid of steroids, they probably are the only agent for which there is still no surrogate. The chapter by Rowan Walker deals perfectly with the subject of steroids in kidney transplantation, but I do wish to add a few comments on specific points.

Historically, the successful use of steroids in the treatment of acute rejection episodes was first reported in kidney transplantation in 1960 by the Boston group.

However, as early as 1951, Jean Hamburger had already used steroids in two of the very first cadaver kidney transplantations performed in the human (1). Unfortunately, the doses used were too small, which led to the erroneous conclusion that steroids were useless in kidney transplantation. For this reason they were subsequently discarded by the Paris group. Were it not for this error, transplantation would have gained about 10 years of positive experience and results.

Today, steroids are widely used, but there is no consensus concerning the innocuousness of steroid withdrawal in post-transplantation protocols. In addition, an increasing number of investigators (2,3) have suggested that steroid withdrawal may increase the risk of chronic allograft rejection. However, in some categories of patients, including recipients of an HLA-identical kidney, steroids can be avoided. In 1973, we reported that this was possible in 53% of such recipients who were on azathioprine alone. However, if an induction therapy of 2 to 4 weeks with a polyclonal, or even better, a monoclonal agent such as OKT-3 is added to the monotherapy, the proportion of patients who will never develop acute rejection episodes despite the lack of steroids can be as high as 70%.

Steroids alone can contribute to the long-term success of kidney grafts when additional immunosuppressive agents have to be discontinued because of cancer. In 1984 we reported the 10-year results for 39 kidney recipients comprising 30 cadaver kidney recipients and 9 living-related recipients on azathioprine/steroid bi-therapy who were withdrawn from azathioprine because they developed cancer (4). Their 10-year graft survival was 56.9% despite the cancer, whereas the graft survival of 79 matched control kidney recipients maintained on bi-therapy was 63.2% at the same end point. Thus, at least in cancer patients, steroids can be successfully used as the only immunosuppressive agent, which is an argument in favor of the efficacy of these drugs.

The fact that mono-agent, bi-agent, or tri-agent cyclosporine-based therapy seems to give identical 3-year graft outcome when analyzing data from the Opelz database may have a number of explanations other than the uselessness of the combination of immunosuppressive agents. It may mean, for example, that the numerous biases present in such a database can cancel out all the very real differences that exist between different groups of patients, and that only results drawn from prospectively randomized series should be considered. But it certainly does not allow the conclusion that steroids combined with cyclosporine are useless (5).

The overall power of the immunosuppressive regimen probably affects graft outcome (i.e., the occurrence of chronic rejection). It is widely accepted today that the number and severity of acute rejection episodes are clearly correlated with the incidence and severity of chronic rejection. Whether steroids help to reduce the number of acute rejection episodes is more difficult to determine precisely. Before the cyclosporine era, our retrospective study compared the incidence of acute rejection episodes in cadaveric-kidney recipients who were on azathioprine only with the incidence among similar patients who had been on azathioprine plus high doses of steroids since the transplantation day (6). We were puzzled by the equal incidence of acute rejection found in both groups. However, transplant biopsies disclosed a higher incidence of inflammatory infiltrates in the transplants of patients who did not receive steroids. It was then suggested that steroids probably act more through their anti-inflammatory mechanisms than through their immunosuppressive properties. For this reason, we further compared patients receiving antithymocyte immunoglobulin (Atgam) induction combined with azathioprine and steroids to patients who received Atgam induction, azathioprine, and the nonsteroidal anti-inflammatory agent Brufen (ibuprofen) (7). The frequency of rejection was higher in the Brufen group (2.18 episodes per patient) than in the steroids group (1.44 episodes per patient).

Since the advent of the cyclosporine era, the role of steroids has become more difficult to assess, as the cyclosporine dose is often lower when it is combined with steroids than when it is used as monotherapy. Nevertheless, three publications reported results observed in controlled studies in which steroids were avoided (8–10). They all showed that the incidence or severity of acute rejection episodes was lower when steroids were used.

Whatever the effect of steroids on acute rejection, they might also play a more direct role in the permanent prevention of chronic rejection by reducing inflammation within the transplant. In fact, studies based on histologic findings suggest that both the rate of sclerosing arteriopathy (11) and that of interstitial fibrosis (12) are higher in patients withdrawn from steroids compared to steroid-treated controls. These findings both correlate closely with chronic rejection. Were this to be confirmed, it would mean that not only the weight of immunosuppression is important for the prevention of chronic rejection but also the presence of other specific agents, including those with anti-inflammatory properties such as steroids.

## STEROIDS AND TREATMENT OF REJECTION EPISODES

When used for the prevention of an acute rejection episode, steroids appear more effective in the prevention of the inflammatory changes made of cellular infiltrates and interstitial edema than of the vascular component. Similarly, it is probable that the main target of steroids, when they are used to treat acute rejection, is the inflammatory reaction present in the majority of cases. Their effect on the vascular lesions remains to be proven.

Although steroids continue to be the most important first-line treatment of acute rejection, the way they are used varies greatly from one group to another. Some groups use the intravenous route (with different protocols), while others prefer an oral regime (again, according to different protocols). There is no agreement on the most effective steroid protocol to treat acute rejection. In our group, we have observed a higher number of re-rejection episodes when intravenous boluses were used as compared to high-dose oral administration followed by a slow decrease over weeks.

Because of the variety of approaches used in the treatment of an acute rejection episode, a widely accepted definition of steroid-resistant rejection appears unlikely. Thus, one must be cautious when an immunosuppressive agent is said to be efficient in the treatment of steroid-resistant rejection on the basis of compassionate use. A correct definition of steroid resistance must include the daily dose of steroids, the exact timing of administration, the duration of treatment, and the number of follow-up days required after treatment withdrawal. For multicenter trials, these data must be identical for all the participating centers.

## STEROIDS AND AVASCULAR BONE NECROSIS

It is clear that steroids are closely related to the incidence of avascular bone necrosis. In our group, for example, such necrosis has never been observed in recipients of an HLA-identical kidney who did not receive steroids. We have never found an obvious relationship between avascular bone necrosis and the duration or the level of maintenance steroid, but patients who received short courses of high doses for rejection had a higher incidence of bone lesions. This may explain why the incidence of avascular bone necrosis has tremendously decreased today, along with steroid-treated acute rejection episodes.

## STEROIDS AND SKIN DISORDERS

That long-term corticosteroid treatment is responsible for atrophy of the skin by loss of collagen is widely accepted today. The deterioration, which is present from the sixth month onward (13), gives the skin an appearance of aging. Up to now, the only way to deal with this complication was for the patient to wear protective apparel or use a protective cosmetic preparation. Seeking a treatment, we studied the effect of topical all-*trans* retinoic acid (0.05%; Galderma Labs) over a 6-month period (14). Clinically, an increase in skin thickness was observed, which was confirmed by noninvasive techniques showing an increase in skin thickness, skin elasticity, skin conductance, and a reduction in the size of the corneocytes. Thus, it appears possible to obtain an improvement in skin atrophy when prevention has not been successful.

# CHAPTER REFERENCES

1. Ackerman GL, Nolan CM. Adrenocortical responsiveness after alternate-day corticosteroid therapy. N Engl J Med 1968;278:405–409.
2. Elion GB, Callahan S, Bieber S, et al. A summary of investigations with 6-(1-methyl-4-nitro-r-imidazolyl) thio purine (BW 57-322) Cancer Chemother Rep 1961;14:93–98.
3. Calne RY, Alexandre GPJ, Murray JE. A study of the effects of drugs in prolonging survival of homologous renal transplants in dogs. Ann NY Acad Sci 1962;99:743–761.
4. Murray JE, Merrill JP, Damin GJ, et al. Kidney transplantation in modified recipients. Ann Surg 1962;156:337–355.
5. Murray JE, Merrill JP, Harrison JH, et al. Prolonged survival of human-kidney homograft by immunosuppressive drug therapy. N Engl J Med 1963;268:1315–1323.
6. Starzl TE, Marchioro TL, Waddell WR. The reversal of rejection in human renal homografts with subsequent development of monograft. Surg Gynecol Obstet 1963;117:385–390.
7. Goodwin WE, Mims MM, Kaufman JJ. Human renal transplantation. III. Technical problems encountered in 6 cases of homotransplantation. Trans Am Assoc Genitorin Surg 1985;54:116–125.
8. Kreis H, Lacombe M, Noel LH, et al. Kidney-graft rejection: has the need for steroids to be re-evaluated? Lancet 1978;ii:1169–1172.
9. Cupps TR, Fauci AS. Corticosteroid-mediated immunoregulation in man. Immunol Rev 1982;65:132–155.
10. Dupont E, Schandene L, Denys C, Wybran J. Differential in-vitro actions of cyclosporin, methyl-prednisolone, and 6-metacaptopurine: implications for drugs' influence on lymphocyte activation mechanisms. Clin Immunol Immunopathol 1986;40:422.
11. Metcalfe S. Cyclosporine does not prevent cytoplasmic calcium changes associated with lymphocyte activation. Transplantation 1984;38:161.
12. Gerrard TL, Cupps TR, Jurgensen CH, Fauci AS. Hydrocortisone-mediated inhibition of monocyte antigen presentation: dissociation of inhibitory effect and expression of DR antigens. Cell Immunol 1984;85:330.
13. Crabtree GR. Contingent genetic events in T-cell activation. Science 1989;243:355–363.
14. Knudsen PJ, Dinarello CA, Strom TB. Glucocorticoids inhibit transcription and post-transcriptional expression of interleukin-1. J Immunol 1987;139:4129–4134.
15. Zanker B, et al. Glucocorticoids block transcription of human interleukin-6 gene by accessory cells. Transplantation 1990;49:183–185.
16. Kauffman HM, Sampson D, Fox PS, Stawicki BS. High-dose (bolus) intravenous methylprednisolone at the time of kidney homotransplantation. Ann Surg 1977;186:631–634.
17. McGeown MG, Kennedy JA, Loughridge WGG, et al. One hundred kidney transplants in the Belfast City Hospital. Lancet 1977;ii:648–651.
18. McGeown MG, Douglas JF, Brown WA, et al. Advantages of low-dose steroid from the day after renal transplantation. Transplantation 1980;29:287–289.
19. Descamps B, Huiglais N, Crosnier J. Renal transplantation between 33 HLA-identical siblings. Transplant Proc 1973;5:231.
20. Chan L, French ME, Beare J, et al. Prospective trial of high-dose versus low-dose prednisolone in renal transplant patients. Transplant Proc 1980;12:323–326.
21. Chan L, French ME, Oliver DO, Morris PJ. High- and low-dose prednisolone. Transplant Proc 1981;13:336–338.
22. Morris PJ, Chan L, French ME, Ting A. Low-dose oral prednisolone in renal transplantation. Lancet 1982;i:525–527.
23. Buckles JAC, Mackintosh P, Barnes AD. Controlled trial of low-versus high-dose oral steroid therapy in 100 cadaveric renal transplants. Proc EDTA 1981;18:394–399.
24. Papadakis JT, Bewick M, Brown CM, et al. Low-dose steroids in renal transplantation (letter). Lancet 1982;i:916–917.
25. Glass NR, Miller DT, Sollinger HW, Belzer FO. A comparative study of steroids and heterologous antiserum in the treatment of renal allograft rejection. Transplant Proc 1983;15:617.
26. Hricik DE, Almawi WY, Strom TB. Trends in the use of glucocorticoids in renal transplantation. Transplantation 1994;57:979–989.
27. d'Apice AJF, Becker GJ, Kincaid-Smith P, et al. A prospective randomized trial of low-dose versus high-dose steroids in cadaveric renal transplantation. Transplantation 1984;37(4):373–377.
28. Walker RG, d'Apice AJF, Mathew TH, et al. Long-term follow-up of a prospective trial of low-dose versus high-dose steroids in renal transplantation. Transplant Proc 1987;19:2825–2828.
29. Walker RG, d'Apice AJF. Non-specific immunosuppression: azathioprine and steroids. In: Morris PJ, ed. Kidney transplantation: principles and practice. 4th ed. Philadelphia: WB Saunders, 1984:202–204.
30. Opelz G. Comparison of immunosuppressive protocols in renal transplantation: a multi-center view. Transplant Proc 1988;20:31–36.
31. Canafax CM, Sutherland DER, Simmons RL, et al. Combination immunosuppression: three drugs (azathioprine, cyclosporine, prednisolone) for mismatched related and four drugs (antilymphocyte globulin, azathioprine, cyclosporine, prednisolone) for cadaver renal allograft recipients. Transplant Proc 1985;17:2671–2672.
32. Hiesse C, Charpentier B, Fries D. Safety of triple immunosuppressive treatment (cyclosporine, azathioprine and prednisolone). Lancet 1985;2:1355.
33. Schareck WD, Hopt UT, Muller GH, et al. Reduction of nephrotoxicity and improvement of immuno-suppression by combination of cyclosporine A and azathioprine. Transplant Proc 1987;19:1937–1939.
34. O'Connell PJ, d'Apice AJF, Walker RG, et al. Results of steroid withdrawal in renal allograft recipients on low dose cyclosporine A, azathioprine and prednisolone. Clin Transplant 1988;2:102–106.
35. Slapak M, Digard N, Wise M, Setakis N. Triple therapy. Transplant Proc 1991;23:2186–2188.
36. Sollinger HW for the US Renal Transplant Mycophenolate Mofetil Study Group. Mycophenolate mofetil for the prevention of acute rejection in primary cadaveric renal allograft recipients. Transplantation 1995;60:225–232.
37. European Mycophenolate Mofetil Cooperative Study Group. Placebo-controlled study of mycophenolate mofetil combined with cyclosporin and corticosteroids for prevention of acute rejection. Lancet 1995;345:1321–1325.
38. Tricontinental Mycophenolate Mofetil Renal Transplantation Study Group. A blinded, randomised clinical trial of mycophenolate mofetil for the prevention of acute rejection in cadaveric renal transplantation. Transplantation 1996;61:1029–1037.
39. Davis M, Williams R, Chakraborty J, et al. Prednisone or prednisolone for the treatment of chronic active hepatitis? a comparison of plasma availability. Brit J Clin Pharmacol 1978;5:501–505.
40. Pickup ME. Clinical pharmacokinetics of prednisone and prednisolone. Clin Pharmacokinet 1979;4:111–128.
41. Lewis GP, Jusko WJ, Burke CW, Graves L. Prednisone side-effects and serum-protein levels. A collaborative study. Lancet 1971;ii:778–780.
42. Baxter JD, Forsham PH. Tissue effects of glucocorticoids. Am J Med 1972;53:573–589.
43. Grant SD, Forsham PH, Di Raimondo VC. Suppression of 17-hydroxycorticosteroids in plasma and urine by single and divided doses of triamcinolone. N Engl J Med 1985;273:1115–1118.
44. Nichols T, Nugent CA, Tyler FH. Diurnal variation in suppression of adrenal function by glucocorticoids. J Clin Endocrinol Metab 1965;25:343–349.
45. Harter JC, Reddy WJ, Thorn GW. Studies on an intermittent corticosteroid dosage regimen. N Engl J Med 1963;269:591–596.
46. Soyka LF, Saxena KM. Alternate-day steroid therapy for nephrotic children. J Am Med Assoc 1965;192:225–230.
47. Fleisher DS. Pituitary-adrenal responsiveness after corticosteroid therapy in children with nephrosis. J Paediatr 1967;70:54–59.
48. Dumler F, Levin NW, Szego G, et al. Long-term alternate day steroid therapy in renal transplantation: a controlled study. Transplantation 1982;34:78–82.
49. MacGregor RR, Sheagren JN, Lipsett MB, Wolff SM. Alternate-day prednisone therapy: evaluation of delayed hypersensitivity responses, control of disease, and steroid side effects. N Engl J Med 1969;280:1427–1431.
50. Diethelm AG, Sterling WA, Hartley MW, Morgan JM. Alternate-day prednisone therapy in recipients of renal allografts. Risk and benefits. Arch Surg 1976;111:867–870.
51. Leb DE. Alternate-day prednisone treatment may increase kidney transplant rejection. Proc Dial Transplant Forum 1979;6:136.
52. Breitenfield RV, Herbert LA, Lemann J Jr, et al. Stability of renal transplant function with alternate-day corticosteroid therapy. J Am Med Assoc 1980;244:151–156.
53. McDonald FD, Horensten ML, Mayor GB, et al. Effect of alternate-day steroids on renal transplant function. A controlled study. Nephron 1976;17:415–429.
54. Potter DE, Holliday MA, Wilson CJ, et al. Alternate-day steroids in children after renal transplantation. Transplant Proc 1975;7:79–82.
55. Van Dieman-Steenvorde R, Donckerwoicke RA, Brack DH, et al. Growth and sexual maturation in children after kidney transplantation. J Pediatr 1987;110:351–356.
56. Briggs JD. A critical review of immunosuppressive therapy. Immunol Lett 1991;29:89–94.
57. Hussey JL. Letter. Discontinuance of immuno-suppression. Arch Surg 1976;111:614.
58. Calne RY, Thiru S, McMaster P, et al. Cyclosporin A in patients receiving renal allografts from cadaver donors. Lancet 1978;2:1323–1327.
59. Kahan BD, Flechner SM, Lorber MI, et al. Complications of cyclosporine-prednisolone immunosuppression in 402 renal allograft recipients exclusively

followed at a single center for from one to five years. Transplantation 1987;43:197–204.

60. Sutherland DER, Fryd DS, Strand MH, et al. Results of the Minnesota randomized prospective trial of cyclosporine versus azathioprine-antilymphocyte globulin for immunosuppression in renal allograft recipients. Am J Kidney Dis 1985;5:318–327.

61. Kupin WL, Venkat KK, Norris C, et al. Effective long-term immunosuppression maintained by low cyclosporine levels in primary cadaveric renal transplant recipients. Transplantation 1987;43:214–218.

62. Wood RFM, Thompson JE, Allen NH, et al. The consequences of conversion from cyclosporine to azathioprine and prednisolone in renal allograft recipients. Transplant Proc 1983;15:2862–2868.

63. Thiel G, Harder F, Loertscher R, et al. Cyclosporine alone or in combination with prednisolone in cadaveric renal transplantation. Transplant Proc 1984;16:1187–1190.

64. Starzl IE, Weil R, Iwatsuki S. The use of cyclosporin A and prednisolone in cadaver kidney transplantation. Surg Gynecol Obstet 1980;151:17–26.

65. Brown MW, Forwell MA. Rejection reaction after stopping prednisolone in kidney-transplant recipients taking cyclosporine. N Engl J Med 1986;314:183.

66. Cristinelli L, Brunori G, Setti G, et al. Withdrawal of methylprednisolone at the sixth month in renal transplant recipients treated with cyclosporine. Transplant Proc 1987;19:2021–2023.

67. Squifflet JP, Sutherland DER, Rynasiewicz JJ, et al. Combined immunosuppressive therapy with cyclosporine A and azathioprine. Transplantation 1982;34:315–318.

68. Chao S-H, Tsai K-S, Chieng P-U, et al. Bone mineral density profile in uremic and renal transplant patients. Transplant Proc 1994;26:2009–2011.

69. Stegall MD, Wachs ME, Everson G, et al. Prednisone withdrawal 14 days after liver transplantation with mycophenolate. Transplantation 1997;64:1755–1760.

70. Russ GR, May S, Jacob CK, et al. Experience with cyclosporine A and azathioprine double therapy in low-risk recipients of first cadaveric renal allografts. Clin Transplant 1990;4:26–31.

71. Thistlethwaite JR Jr, Gaber AO, Haag BW, et al. OKT3 treatment of steroid-resistant renal allograft rejection. Transplantation 1987;43(2):176–184.

72. Barry JM. Immunosuppressive drugs in renal transplantation. Drugs 1992;48(4):554–566.

73. Orta-Sibu N, Chantler C, Bewick M, Haycock G. Comparison of high-dose intravenous methylprednisolone with low-dose oral prednisolone in acute renal allograft rejection in children. BMJ 1982;285:258–260.

74. Kauffman HM Jr, Stromstad SA, Sampson D, Stawicki AT. Randomized steroid therapy of human kidney transplant rejection. Transplant Proc 1979;11:36–38.

75. Gray D, Shepherd H, Daar A, et al. Oral versus intravenous high-dose steroid treatment of renal allograft rejection: the big shot or not? Lancet 1978;i:117–118.

76. Mussche MM, Ringoir SGM, Lameire NN. High intravenous doses of methylprednisolone for acute cadaveric renal allograft rejection. Nephron 1976;16:289–291.

77. Sollinger HW, Deierho MH, Belzer FO, et al. RS-61443—a phase I clinical trial and pilot rescue study. Transplantation 1992;53:428.

78. Mycophenolate Mofetil Renal Refractory Rejection Study Group. Mycophenolate mofetil for the treatment of refractory, acute, cellular renal transplant rejection. Transplantation 1996;61:722–729.

79. Dumble LJ, Clunie GJA, Macdonald IM, et al. Prediction of renal allograft rejection response to steroids from aDCC response to in vitro steroids. Transplant Proc 1983;15:1145–1147.

80. Francis DMA, Dumble LJ, Bowes LG, et al. Adverse influence of recipient lymphoid resistance to in vitro immunosuppression on the outcome of kidney transplants. Transplantation 1988;46:853–857.

81. Ratcliffe PJ, Dudley CRK, Higgins RM, et al. Randomised controlled trial of steroid withdrawal in renal transplant recipients receiving immunosuppression. Lancet 1996;348:643–648.

82. Rizzoni G, Broyer M, Guest G, et al. Growth retardation in children with chronic renal disease: scope of the problem. Am J Kidney Dis 1986;7:256–261.

83. Watson AR. Safety of growth hormone. Lancet 1991;337:108–109.

84. Fine RN, Yadin O, Nelson PA, et al. Recombinant human growth hormone treatment of children following renal transplantation. Paediatr Nephrol 1991;5:147–151.

85. Woo KT, Junor BJR, Vikraman P, d'Apice AJF. Serum-alkaline-phosphatase as predictor of avascular necrosis of bone in renal-transplant recipients (letter). Lancet 1979;i:620.

86. Horber FF, Casez JP, Steiger U, et al. Changes in bone mass early after kidney transplantation. J Bone Miner Res 1994;9:1–9.

87. Almond MK, Kwan JT, Evans K, Cunningham J. Loss of regional bone mineral density in the first 12 months following renal transplantation. Nephron 1994;66(1):52–57.

88. Julian BA, Laskow DA, Dubovsky J, et al. Rapid loss of vertebral mineral density after renal transplantation. N Engl J Med 1991;325:544–550.

89. Grotz WH, Mundinger FA, Gugel B, et al. Bone mineral density after kidney transplantation. A cross-sectional study in 190 graft recipients up to 20 years after transplantation. Transplantation 1995;59(7):982–986.

90. Wolpaw T, Deal CL, Fleming-Brooks S, et al. Factors influencing vertebral bone density after renal transplantation. Transplantation 1994;58:1186–1189.

91. Grotz WH, Mundinger FA, Gugel B, et al. Bone fracture and osteodensitometry with dual energy X-ray absorptiometry in kidney transplant recipients. Transplantation 1994;58(8):912–915.

92. Shun-Shin GA, Ratcliffe P, Bron AJ, et al. The lens after renal transplantation. Brit J Ophthalmol 1990;74:261–271.

93 d'Apice AJF, Mathews JD, Tait BD, Kincaid-Smith P. Association of HLA antigens with glucose intolerance following renal transplantation. Tissue Antigens 1978;11:423–426.

94. Drueke TB, Abdulmassih Z, Lacour B, et al. Atherosclerosis and lipid disorders after renal transplantation. Kidney Int 1991;39:(suppl 31):S24–S28.

95. Kasiske BL, Umen AJ. Persistent hyerlipidaemia in renal transplant patients. Medicine 1987;66:309–316.

96. Markell MS, Friedman EA. Hyperlipidemia after organ transplantation. Am J Med 1989;87(5N):61N–67N.

97. Sheil AGR, Disney APS, Mathew TH, et al. Cancer development in cadaveric donor renal allograft recipients treated with azathioprine (AZA) or cyclosporine (CyA) or AZA/CyA. Transplant Proc 1991;23:1111–1112.

98. Venning VA. Nonmalignant skin lesion in renal transplant patients. In: Morris PJ, ed. Kidney transplantation: principles and practice. 4th ed. Philadelphia: WB Saunders, 1984:401–411.

## COMMENTARY REFERENCES

1. Dubost C, Oeconomos N, Vaysse J, et al. Note préliminaire sur l'étude des fonctions rénales de reins greffés chez l'homme. Bull et Mém Soc Med Hôp de Paris 1951;67:105–106.

2. Almond P, Matas A, Gillingham K. Risk factors for chronic rejection in renal allograft recipients. Transplantation 1993;55:752–757.

3. Basadonna G, Matas A, Gillingham K, et al. Early versus late acute renal allograft rejection: impact on chronic rejection. Transplantation 1993;55(5):993–995.

4. Campos H, Kreis H, Rioux P, Crosnier J. Azathioprine withdrawal in renal transplant recipients. A long-term follow-up. Transplantation 1984;38(1):29–31.

5. Fries D, Hiesse C, Santelli G, et al. Triple therapy with low-dose cyclosporine, azathioprine, and steroids: long-term results of a randomized study in cadaver donor renal transplantation. Transplant Proc 1988;20(suppl 3):130–135.

6. Kreis H, Lacombe M, Noel L, et al. Kidney-graft rejection: has the need for steroids to be re-evaluated? Lancet 1978;2(8101):1169–1172.

7. Kreis H, Chkoff N, Droz D, et al. Nonsteroid antiinflammatory agents as a substitute treatment for steroids in ATGAM-treated cadaver kidney recipients. Transplantation 1984;37(2):139–145.

8. Johnson R, Mallick N, Bakran A, et al. Cadaver renal transplantation without maintenance steroids. Transplant Proc 1989;21:1581–1582.

9. Salaman J. Cyclosporine mono-drug therapy. Transplant Proc 1988;20(suppl 3):117–120.

10. Tarantino A, Aroldi A, Stucchi L, et al. A randomized prospective trial comparing cyclosporine monotherapy with triple-drug therapy in renal transplantation. Transplantation 1991;52(1):53–57.

11. Offermann G, Schwarz A, Krause P. Long-term effects of steroid withdrawal in kidney transplantation. Transplant Int 1993;6(5):290–292.

12. Isoniemi H, Krogerus L, von Willebrand E, et al. Histopathological findings in well-functioning, long-term renal allografts. Kidney Int 1992;41(1):155–160.

13. Teillac D, Prost Y, Debure A, et al. Clinical and biophysical studies of the skin in renal allograft patients. Clin Transplant 1987;1:1–3.

14. Lacharriere OD, Escoffier C, Gracia A, et al. Reversal effects of topical retinoic acid on the skin of kidney transplant recipients under systemic corticotherapy. J Invest Dermatol 1990;95(5):516–522.

# Tacrolimus

Goran B. Klintmalm

## HISTORY

Tacrolimus (FK506, Prograf; Fujisawa, Deerfield, IL, USA) is a macrolide compound isolated from *Streptomyces tsukubaensis*, a soil fungus that can be found in Northern Japan (1). Its immunosuppressive properties were first recognized in 1984 during a screening program directed at identifying new immunosuppressive agents. Subsequent in vitro and animal experiments in Japan and at the University of Pittsburgh helped to characterize the mechanism of action of tacrolimus and demonstrated its potent immunosuppressive properties in transplantation (1–6).

## IMMUNOLOGY

Most clinically useful immunosuppressive drugs either inhibit the proliferation of T lymphocytes or destroy them. Cyclosporine inhibits cytokine synthesis by binding to cytoplasmic proteins (cyclophylins) in T lymphocytes (see Chapter 1). Tacrolimus functions in a similar fashion, binding to FK-binding proteins (FKBP) in the cytoplasm; however, tacrolimus has a greater binding affinity to FKBP than does cyclosporine to cyclophilin. Rapamycin, which is structurally similar to tacrolimus, does not inhibit cytokine synthesis but rather inhibits the response of T cells to interleukin 2 (IL-2) and other cytokines (see Chapters 1 and 6).

The complex formed by the binding of tacrolimus to FKBP-12 associates with calcium-dependent calcineurin/calmodulin complexes to impede calcium-dependent signal transduction subsequent to stimulation of calcium influx in lymphocytes. Transcription factors that promote cytokine gene activation are direct or indirect substrates for calcineurin, and their activity is reduced by association with the tacrolimus complex. Tacrolimus inhibits the mixed lymphocyte reaction assay, the formation of IL-2 by T lymphocytes, and formation of other soluble mediators including IL-3, IL-4, IL-5, tumor necrosis factor alpha (TNF-$\alpha$), and granulocyte-macrophage-colony stimulating factor (7). Tacrolimus also inhibits the expression of IL-2 and IL-7 receptors. As an immunosuppressive agent, tacrolimus is approximately 100 times more potent than cyclosporine (8).

## PHARMACOKINETICS AND MONITORING

Tacrolimus achieves adequate absorption from the upper small intestine following oral administration, but the extent of absorption is widely variable (range = 5% to 67%) among patients. Administration with food generally does not affect the oral absorption of tacrolimus, although fatty meals may reduce bioavailability (9). Because absorption is bile independent, intravenous administration is not required in most patients (as is often required with cyclosporine [Sandimmune], particularly during the early postoperative period), and dosage changes are not required when clamping a T-tube following liver transplantation (10).

During liver graft failure or hepatic dysfunction, especially with cholestasis, tacrolimus bioavailability increases and clearance decreases owing to its extensive hepatic metabolism. The result is markedly elevated tacrolimus levels with related toxicity necessitating a rapid reduction in dosage (10,11). In contrast, initial dosing reductions usually are not required in patients with renal impairment (10).

Tacrolimus concentrations can be measured either in whole blood or plasma using an enzyme-linked immunosorbent assay (ELISA) (12) or in whole blood with a microparticle enzyme immunoassay (13). Measurement of plasma tacrolimus concentrations may be less desirable both because of the complexity of the methodology and because plasma must be separated at 37°C due to temperature-dependent distribution of tacrolimus into erythrocytes, similar to that of cyclosporine (14). Importantly, plasma levels of tacrolimus measured by ELISA were found to correlate poorly with rejection and toxicity (15), whereas whole blood tacrolimus levels were well correlated with rejection and toxicity (16). Other studies indicated a higher correlation of plasma tacrolimus levels with clinical events (17). As with cyclosporine, plasma level monitoring can be used if samples are handled carefully. However, because of the technical difficulties inherent in plasma level monitoring, whole blood levels are usually considered the standard of care.

During oral therapy with tacrolimus, concentrations should be monitored to maintain 12-hour trough levels in the range of 5 to 15 ng/mL for whole blood or 0.5 to 1.5 ng/mL for plasma to optimize efficacy and minimize toxicity. Clinical experience has shown that high trough tacrolimus levels correlate with a lower incidence of rejection, and high peak levels correlate with increased toxicity

(18,19). A definite correlation between tacrolimus levels and nephrotoxicity has not been recognized, but a reduction in serum creatinine levels was reported in liver transplant recipients when tacrolimus levels were reduced (17).

## PRECLINICAL EXPERIENCE WITH TACROLIMUS

Numerous animal studies have been conducted demonstrating the in vitro and in vivo effects of tacrolimus (Table 4.1) (20). Although many studies have evaluated the use of tacrolimus in preventing graft rejection, the published literature has also described the effects of tacrolimus on the inhibition of cell-mediated responses, proliferative responses, cytotoxic responses, and humoral responses, as well as its effect on various autoimmune disorders.

An in vitro study evaluated the effect of tacrolimus compared to cyclosporine and prednisolone on the mixed lym-

**Table 4.1.**     Experimental Autoimmune Diseases Suppressed by Tacrolimus

| Disease | Species | Tacrolimus Dose (mg/kg/day unless specified) | Reference |
|---|---|---|---|
| Arthritis (Type II collagen-induced) | Rat (Lewis) | 0.32[a,b] | Inamura et al, 1988 (21) |
| | Rat (Outbred) | 2.5[c] | Arita et al, 1990 (22) |
| | Mouse (DBA/1) | 2.0 | Takagishi et al, 1989 (23) |
| Type 1 diabetes | NOD mouse | 2.0 mg/kg/48 h[a] | Miyagawa et al, 1990 (24) |
| | Cyclophosphamide-treated NOD mouse | 0.2, 1.0, 2.0 | Carroll et al, 1991 (25) |
| | BB rat | 1.0[a] | Murase et al, 1990 (26) |
| | BB rat | 25 μg IM[d] | Nicoletti et al, 1991 (27) |
| Uveoretinitis | Rat (Lewis) | 1.0[a,e] | Kawashima et al, 1990 (28) |
| | Rhesus and cynomolgus monkeys | 0.5[f] | Fujino et al, 1990 (29) |
| Thyroiditis | Rat (PVG) | 2.0[g] | Tamura et al, 1992 (30) |
| Lupus (SLE) | MRL-lpr/lpr mouse | 2 mg[h] | Yamamoto et al, 1988 (31) |
| | NZB/NZW F[1] mouse | 2.5 mg/kg/48 h[i] | Takabayashi et al, 1989 (32) |
| Glomerulonephritis | Rat (Wistar) | 0.3 mg[j] | Hara et al, 1990 (33) |
| (Nephrotoxic antiserum nephritis) | Rat (Wistar) | 0.64 | Okuba et al, 1990 (34) |
| Heymann nephritis | Rat (Wistar) | 0.64 | Okuba et al, 1990 (34) |
| | Rat (Lewis) | 1.0 | Matsukawa et al, 1992 (35) |
| Allergic encephalomyelitis | Rat (Lewis) | 1.0 | Inamura et al, 1988 (36) |
| Autoimmune myocarditis | Rat (Lewis) | 1.0, 0.32, 1.0 | Hanawa et al, 1992 (37) |
| Experimental allergic contact dermatitis | Farm pig | 0.04, 0.4% topical | Meingassner and Stutz, 1992 (38) |
| Murine (coxsackie B[3]) myocarditis | Mice (C3H/He) | 2.5 | Hiraoka et al, 1992 (39) |

[a]   Suppresses induction of disease.
[b]   Partially effective during efferent phase of response.
[c]   On day of immunization.
[d]   Administered daily from 27–120 days of age.
[e]   Effective only in induction phase.
[f]   Administered from 3 weeks after immunization.
[g]   Administered for 3 weeks following induction of disease.
[h]   Administered from 8 weeks of age.
[i]   From time of immunization.
[j]   Administered 5 days per week after immunization.
[k]   Administered from day 0–13 or 56–69.
Adapted from Thomson AW, Murase N, Nalesnik MA, Starzl TE. The influence of tacrolimus on experimental autoimmune disease. In: Lieberman R, Mukherjee A, eds. Principles of drug development in transplantation and autoimmunity. Austin, TX: RG Landes, 1996.

phocyte reaction (MLR) (2). Tacrolimus demonstrated dose-dependent suppression of the proliferative response of human lymphocytes to alloantigen stimulation at concentrations higher than 0.1 nmol/L. The $IC_{50}$ values of tacrolimus, cyclosporine, and prednisolone were 0.22, 14.0, and 80.0 nmol/L respectively. Tacrolimus was also shown to inhibit IL-2 production almost completely at concentrations higher than 0.3 nmol/L. With an $IC_{50}$ value of approximately 0.1 nmol/L, tacrolimus was reported to be approximately 100 times more potent than cyclosporine, which had an $IC_{50}$ value of 10 nmol/L. Tacrolimus demonstrated a similar inhibitory effect on interferon (IFN)-$\gamma$ production.

In a separate study, tacrolimus inhibited the proliferation of murine spleen B lymphocytes induced by anti-mouse IgM by approximately 50% in vitro (40).

In vivo animal studies have investigated the effect of tacrolimus on humoral and cellular immunity. In one study, mice were immunized with sheep erythrocytes and received tacrolimus and cyclosporine orally for 4 days from the day of immunization (1). After 4 days, tacrolimus almost completely suppressed splenic antibody-forming cell (AFC) response at doses of 10 mg/kg or more, whereas cyclosporine almost completely suppressed AFC response at 100 mg/kg. Tacrolimus also suppressed delayed-type hypersensitivity (DTH) responses dose-dependently in mice immunized with methylated bovine serum albumin (MBSA).

The effect of tacrolimus on transplantation of the liver, kidney, heart, islet cells, and abdominal visceral organs has been widely studied in different animal models (41–46). In a liver transplantation study using beagle dogs, 8 of 10 dogs (80%) receiving tacrolimus survived longer than 30 days, providing an early in vivo demonstration that tacrolimus, 1.0 mg/kg, was as potent as cyclosporine, 20 mg/kg (42). Tacrolimus exhibited similar immunosuppressive effects in cynomolgus monkeys undergoing orthotopic liver transplantation (43).

Tacrolimus has also shown promise in animal models of cardiac transplantation. The hearts of F344 rats were heterotopically transplanted into the cervical region of WKA rat recipients receiving either tacrolimus or cyclosporine orally (4). Both agents prolonged acceptance of the cardiac allografts. Tacrolimus significantly prolonged graft survival in rats receiving a heterotopic cardiac transplantation across a strong major histocompatibility complex (MHC) barrier at a dose of 1.28 mg/kg/day (44). When a moderate histoincompatible combination was used, the animal recipients survived indefinitely.

In renal transplantation studies using tacrolimus in unrelated beagle dogs, all the animals in the control group died of renal failure due to graft rejection within 24 days; whereas, animals treated with 1.0 mg/kg/day oral dosage of tacrolimus survived over 140 days after transplantation (3). The effect of tacrolimus in kidney transplantation was also studied in baboons (46). In the tacrolimus groups, 3 of 5 (60%) and 4 of 5 (80%) animals survived longer than 80

days, depending on the dose. All of the animals in the control group died within 14 days of renal failure due to graft rejection. This preclinical trial in subhuman primates suggested that tacrolimus was a promising drug for use in humans.

Preclinical studies of tacrolimus in intestinal transplantation also have been promising (47,48). The efficacy of tacrolimus in several experimental animal models of allotransplantation is summarized in Table 4.2 (49).

## EARLY CLINICAL EXPERIENCE IN TRANSPLANTATION

Most early clinical experience with tacrolimus was gained from the pioneering work at the University of Pittsburgh in liver, renal, heart, and small bowel transplantation. Initially, tacrolimus was used as rescue therapy in patients experiencing rejection or toxicity while being treated with cyclosporine. Subsequent trials were expanded to the use of tacrolimus as primary immunosuppression (52–54). This early experience helped to identify the safety and tolerability of tacrolimus as well as its role as primary and rescue therapy following transplantation (Table 4.3).

## CLINICAL EXPERIENCE WITH TACROLIMUS FOR SOLID ORGAN TRANSPLANTATION

### Liver

Until recently, most clinical experience with tacrolimus had come from its use in liver transplantation as either primary or rescue therapy. Two prospective randomized trials conducted in the United States and Europe found that patient and graft survival were comparable with tacrolimus and cyclosporine but that the incidence of rejection, both acute and steroid refractory, was significantly lower with tacrolimus (55,56).

The US open-label, randomized, multicenter trial compared the efficacy and safety of tacrolimus to a cyclosporine (Sandimmune)-based immunosuppressant regimen in patients undergoing primary liver transplantation (55). Adult and pediatric patients were randomized at the time of transplant to tacrolimus (n = 263) or cyclosporine (n = 266) and followed for 12 months. Study end points were patient and graft survival and the incidence of acute, steroid-resistant, and refractory rejection. Patient and graft survival at 1 year were comparable for the tacrolimus and the cyclosporine groups (Fig. 4.1). Acute and steroid-resistant rejection and treatment failure due to refractory rejection were significantly lower with tacrolimus. Longer-term follow-up of these recipients now suggests a survival benefit for the tacrolimus-treated patients, compared to the Sandimmune-treated group (57). There also appears to be a significant benefit for the tacrolimus-treated liver allograft recipients with hepatitis C. Their 5-year survival rate was 78%, versus only 60% for the Sandimmune-treated HCV-positive patients.

**T a b l e  4 . 2 .**    Tacrolimus in Experimental Allotransplantation

| Animal | Organ (Reference) | Strain | | Dose (mg/kg/day) | Tacrolimus Route | Duration (Days) | Mean Survival (Days) |
|---|---|---|---|---|---|---|---|
| | | Donor | Recipient | | | | |
| Rat | Heart (50) | ACI | LEW | 0.0 | — | — | 6.0 |
| | | | | 0.6 | IM | 0–13 | 39.0 |
| | | | | 1.3 | IM | 0–13 | 87.0 |
| | | | | 1.3 | IM | 4, 5, 6 | 91.0 |
| | Liver (41) | ACI | LEW | 0.0 | — | — | 10.0 |
| | | | | 1.3 | IM | 4, 5, 6 | >100.0 |
| | Intestine (47) | BN | LEW | 0.0 | — | — | 11.7 |
| | | | | 0.6 | IM | 0–13 | >100.0 |
| | | | | 1.3 | IM | 0–13 | >100.0 |
| | | LEW | BN | 0.0 | — | — | 12.0 |
| | | | | 0.6 | IM | 0–13 | 27.3 |
| | Multivisceral (51) | BN | LEW | 0.0 | — | — | 10.6 |
| | | | | 1.3 | IM | 0–13 | >100.0 |
| Dog | Kidney (5) | Mongrel | Beagle | 0.0 | — | — | 13.0 |
| | | | | 0.5 | PO | 1–90 | 33.7 |
| | | | | 1.0 | PO | 1–90 | 31.0 |
| | | | | 1.5 | PO | 1–90 | 61.0 |
| | | | | 2.0 | PO | 1–90 | 32.1 |
| | | | | 1.0 | IM | 4, 5, 6 | 58.0 |
| | Liver (5) | Beagle | Beagle | 0.0 | — | — | 12.4 |
| | | | | 1.0 | PO | 1–90 | 66.5 |
| | | | | 1.0 | IM | 4, 5, 6 | 96.6 |
| | Intestine (42) | Mongrel | Mongrel | 0.0 | — | — | 7.8 |
| | | | | 0.1 | IV | 1–90 | 57.5 |
| | | | | 0.2 | IV | 1–90 | 23.3 |
| | | | | 1.0 | IM | 3, 4, 5 | 17.7 |
| Baboon | Kidney (46) | *Papio abunus* | *Papio abunus* | 0.0 | — | — | 9.2 |
| | | | | 6.0 | PO | 1–90 | 29.5 |
| | | | | 12.0 | PO | 1–90 | 70.8 |
| | | | | 18.0 | PO | 1–90 | 74.6 |
| | | | | 2.0 | IM | 4, 5, 6 | 53.3 |

LEW = Lewis; BN = Brown-Norway.
Adapted from Todo S and Murase N. Tacrolimus for experimental organ transplantation. In: Lieberman R, Mukherjee A, eds. Principles of drug development in transplantation and autoimmunity. New York: RG Landes, 1996.

**T a b l e  4 . 3 .**    Potential Uses for Tacrolimus

**Transplantation**
Liver
Kidney
Heart
Intestine
Bone marrow
Lung

**Autoimmune Diseases**
Psoriasis
Uveitis
Chronic inflammatory diseases of the liver
Nephrotic syndrome

Among pediatric patients, there was a trend toward less rejection and a reduced requirement for steroids with tacrolimus, although patient and graft survival were comparable (58). Major neurologic events and diarrhea were more common with tacrolimus, while hirsutism and higher serum cholesterol levels were reported with cyclosporine.

In a parallel study conducted at eight European transplant centers, 545 patients were randomized to tacrolimus or a conventional cyclosporine (Sandimmune)–based regimen (56). The primary end points were acute, refractory acute, and chronic rejection at 12 months. The rates of rejection were significantly lower with tacrolimus. Patient and graft survival rates were not different between tacrolimus and cyclosporine. The mean corticosteroid dosage

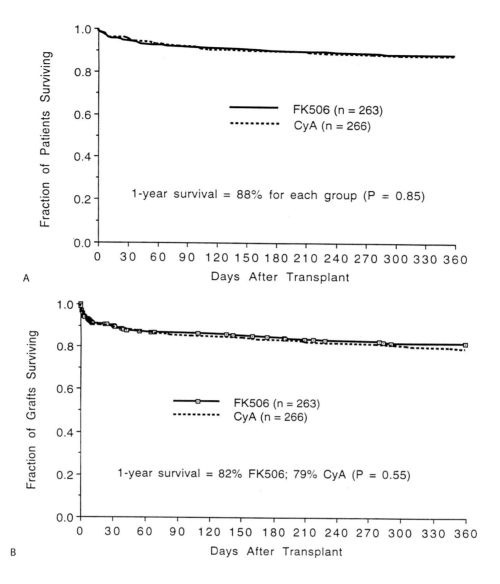

**FIGURE 4.1.** *Patient survival (**A**) and graft survival (**B**) in patients treated with FK506 or cyclosporine-based (CsA) immunosuppression (55). Kaplan-Meier estimates of 1-year patient and graft survival after liver transplantation were not significantly different between treatment groups.*

was significantly lower and almost no azathioprine or anti-lymphocyte globulin was required in the tacrolimus group compared with the cyclosporine group.

In the European experience, patients transplanted for fulminant hepatic failure had a particularly impressive response to tacrolimus (59). At 1 week, patient survival was 95.5% with tacrolimus and 82.1% with cyclosporine; by 6 months, survival was 72.7% with tacrolimus and 60.7% with cyclosporine (Fig. 4.2). Similar results were observed for graft survival. Also, the incidence of treated rejection episodes was significantly reduced with tacrolimus. This resulted in a lower mean daily corticosteroid requirement for tacrolimus- versus cyclosporine-treated patients (69 mg/day versus 150 mg/day) and was reflected in a lower incidence of infectious complications with tacrolimus.

A limitation of these studies was the comparison of tacrolimus to Sandimmune, rather than to Neoral therapy (see also Chapter 1). More recent trials suggest a lower incidence of rejection in tacrolimus-treated liver allograft recipients in comparison to those treated with Neoral, but these studies have not yet been completed.

### Rescue Therapy Following Liver Transplantation

Tacrolimus in combination with corticosteroids proved to be an effective immunosuppressant regimen for rescue therapy in patients with rejection on a cyclosporine-based regimen after liver transplantation (53). Included were 72 patients with acute rejection, 131 with chronic rejection, and 43 patients with either co-morbid disease or severe cyclosporine-related side effects. At a median follow-up of

240 days, 87% of patients were alive and 79% had functioning grafts. Graft loss was greatest among patients with chronic rejection and a serum bilirubin >2.5 mg/dL (28%) at the start of tacrolimus therapy and among those with viral hepatitis (19%).

An open-label, multicenter study evaluated the safety and efficacy of tacrolimus plus corticosteroids for rescue therapy in 300 adult and 86 pediatric liver transplant recipients experiencing refractory rejection despite conventional immunosuppression (60). All patients were followed for 1 year after conversion to tacrolimus. Of these patients, 260 completed a 1-year follow-up on tacrolimus. Patient survival at 1 year was 74.5% for adults and 79.8% for children, and

graft survival at 1 year was 64.7% for adults and 67.9% for children. When outcomes were stratified by baseline total bilirubin levels >6 or <6 mg/dL and by acute versus chronic rejection, patient and graft survival were consistently lower in patients with bilirubin levels >6 mg/dL.

### Kidney

An early multicenter, open-label trial compared various tacrolimus dosages with cyclosporine in 120 patients undergoing primary cadaveric kidney transplant (19). Patients were randomized to a cyclosporine-based regimen or to one of three tacrolimus-based regimens designed to achieve low (5 to 14 ng/mL), medium (15 to 25 ng/mL), or high (26 to 40 ng/mL) trough whole blood levels. This trial revealed that the incidence of neurotoxic and gastrointestinal events was higher among tacrolimus-treated patients during the first month after transplant and correlated with increasing maximum trough tacrolimus concentrations ($P = 0.01$). Also noted was a decreasing rate of rejection with increasing minimum trough tacrolimus concentrations at 1 month ($P = 0.021$) (Fig. 4.3). The range of tacrolimus whole blood levels that optimized efficacy and minimized toxicity was found to be 5 to 15 ng/mL corresponding to an initial oral dose of 0.2 mg/kg/day. At 1 year, patient survival was 98% for all tacrolimus-treated patients and 92% for the cyclosporine group. Graft survival was 93% and 89% in the tacrolimus and cyclosporine groups, respectively (61). The incidence of rejection episodes requiring treatment during the first year was 33% for tacrolimus and 32% for cyclosporine. Until day 42, the incidence of acute rejection was significantly lower (14% tacrolimus, 32% cyclosporine; $P = 0.048$) for the aggregate of all tacrolimus patients versus cyclosporine. In the tacrolimus group, 13 rejection episodes occurred within the first 6 weeks and 17 more were reported at 1 year. In the cyclosporine group, no new rejec-

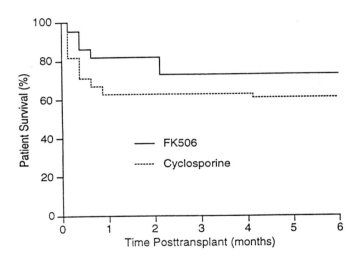

**FIGURE 4.2.** *Patient survival following liver transplantation for fulminant hepatic failure after treatment with FK506 or cyclosporine (59).*

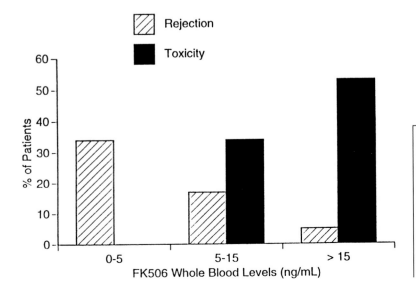

**FIGURE 4.3.** *Incidence of toxicity and rejection by whole blood FK506 levels (19). A logistic regression analysis was performed to determine the relationship between the occurrence of rejection and toxicity, and the whole blood concentrations of FK506. The occurrence of toxicity requiring a dosage reduction increased significantly with increasing levels of whole blood FK506. Conversely, the likelihood of the occurrence of rejection decreased significantly with increasing whole blood levels of FK506. These data support a recommended target whole blood FK506 level of 5 to 15 ng/mL during the first 42 days of treatment.*

tion episodes were reported beyond 42 days after transplantation. Nephrotoxicity occurred with a similar frequency with tacrolimus and cyclosporine, but the incidence of neurotoxic events and the incidence of new insulin use were higher among tacrolimus-treated patients.

A subsequent randomized, open-label US study compared the efficacy and safety of optimal dosage tacrolimus to cyclosporine (Sandimmune) immunosuppression in patients receiving cadaveric kidney transplants (62,63). A total of 412 renal transplant patients were randomized to tacrolimus (n = 205) or cyclosporine (n = 207). One-year patient survival rates were 95.6% for tacrolimus and 96.6% for cyclosporine ($P = 0.576$) and 1-year graft survival rates were 91.2% and 87.9%, respectively ($P = 0.289$). Of note, biopsy-confirmed acute rejection was significantly reduced for tacrolimus patients (30.7%) compared with cyclosporine (46.4%, $P = 0.001$), and the requirement for antilymphocyte therapy for rejection was also significantly less for tacrolimus (10.7% and 25.1%, respectively; $P < 0.001$). Impaired renal function, gastrointestinal disorders, and neurologic complications, which were rarely treatment limiting, were common in both treatment regimens. Tremor and paresthesia were more frequent for tacrolimus, and the incidence of post-transplant diabetes mellitus was 19.9% for tacrolimus patients versus 4.0% for cyclosporine ($P < 0.001$), but it was reversible in some patients. Hyperlipidemia and hypercholesterolemia were decreased in the tacrolimus group, and hirsutism and gum hypertrophy were rarely seen, resulting in a greater improvement in health-related quality of life for these patients (64).

The results of this study were very similar to those observed in the European multicenter, randomized trial that compared the 12-month efficacy and safety of tacrolimus and cyclosporine (65). In that trial, a total of 448 renal transplant recipients from 15 centers received triple-drug therapy consisting of tacrolimus (n = 303) or cyclosporine (n = 145) in conjunction with azathioprine and low-dose corticosteroids. Twelve months after transplantation, tacrolimus therapy exhibited a significant reduction in the frequency of both acute rejection (tacrolimus 25.9% versus cyclosporine 45.7%; $P < 0.001$) and corticosteroid-resistant rejection (11.3% versus 21.6%, respectively; $P = 0.001$). Actuarial 1-year patient (tacrolimus 93.0% versus cyclosporine 96.5%; $P = 0.140$) and graft survival rates (82.5% versus 86.2%, respectively; $P = 0.380$) did not differ significantly between the two treatment groups. The safety profiles of the tacrolimus- and cyclosporine-based regimens were found to be comparable. No cost comparison results of either of these randomized studies have been reported.

In another randomized, prospective, single center trial of 395 adult patients undergoing renal transplantation, the effect of adding azathioprine to tacrolimus and steroids was evaluated (66). The 2-year actuarial patient and graft survival rates were 95% and 83%, respectively, with tacrolimus-based immunosuppression. There was no significant advantage in either patient or graft survival for patients given azathio-

prine, but the incidence of acute rejection was significantly higher with double than with triple therapy (54% versus 44%; $P < 0.05$).

Tacrolimus was also evaluated as rescue therapy in 73 patients with biopsy-confirmed renal allograft rejection (67,68). The median time to tacrolimus rescue therapy was 2.5 months (range 18 days to 48 months). At least one course of antilymphocyte therapy had been used in 59 (81%) patients prior to rescue. Responses to tacrolimus therapy included improvement in 78% of patients, stabilization in 11%, and progressive deterioration in 11%. Actuarial patient and graft survival rates were 93% and 75%, respectively, 12 months after initiation of tacrolimus therapy.

In a more recent report, the results of tacrolimus rescue therapy in 169 patients experiencing biopsy-confirmed rejection were summarized (69). The median time to rescue therapy was 2 months (range 2 days to 55 months), and antilymphocyte preparations had been used in 144 (85%) patients prior to rescue. Of the 144 patients unsuccessfully treated with antilymphocyte drugs, 117 (81%) were successfully rescued with tacrolimus. Twenty-eight patients were on dialysis at the time of conversion, and of these 13 (46%) were successfully rescued. In total, 125 (74%) patients were successfully rescued with tacrolimus and had functioning grafts at a mean follow-up of 30 months. Mean prednisone doses decreased from 28.0 ± 9.0 mg/day pre-tacrolimus to 8.5 ± 4.1 mg/day post-tacrolimus.

Of note, successful renal allograft function has been achieved with the addition of tacrolimus therapy even after the patient had been returned to dialysis, sometimes for prolonged periods (70). A review of these and other trials evaluating tacrolimus in renal allograft recipients has been recently published (71).

## Kidney–Pancreas

Twenty-three recipients of kidney–pancreas transplants were studied to determine the value of tacrolimus primary immunosuppression in these patients (72). Of the evaluable patients, 10 received cyclosporine and 10 received tacrolimus therapy. The patient survival rate at 1 year was 100% for both the cyclosporine and the tacrolimus group, and the kidney graft survival rate was 90% for both groups. The pancreas graft survival rate was 80% for the tacrolimus group and 100% for the cyclosporine group (not significant). The time to the first rejection episode was significantly longer for tacrolimus compared to cyclosporine (23 versus 12 days, respectively; $P = 0.026$). There were no significant differences in the incidences of infectious complications or drug-induced nephrotoxicity.

Several other studies, with limited patient populations, have addressed the use of tacrolimus induction and rescue therapy after kidney–pancreas transplantation. In one study, the therapeutic effects of tacrolimus were documented in 61 kidney–pancreas or pancreas-only transplant patients with relapsing and resistant cellular rejection as well as chronic vascular rejection after they had been switched from cyclosporine-based immunosuppression (73). A subsequent follow-up analysis of 166 patients receiving primary tacrolimus therapy revealed a one-year graft survival rate of 88% (74). Similarly, 10 kidney–pancreas transplant patients and 1 pancreas-after-kidney patient were converted to tacrolimus following acute severe cyclosporine nephrotoxicity (75). All 11 patients were alive and 10 combined grafts were still functional 7.7 months after tacrolimus rescue therapy. All of the patients maintained stable renal function and blood glucose levels after the conversion from cyclosporine to tacrolimus. These observations have now encouraged many transplant centers to adopt tacrolimus-based primary immunosuppressive regimens for pancreas–kidney transplant recipients (76).

## Intestinal

Because of the relatively small number of procedures performed, data are more limited on the use of tacrolimus as immunosuppression following intestinal transplantation. Nevertheless, a few reports are available summarizing the results in both adults and children. In an initial report, tacrolimus was used as primary immunosuppression in 12 adults and 11 children who underwent small bowel, small bowel and liver, or multivisceral transplants (77). At a minimum follow-up of 2 months, 19 of 23 patients were alive. In a follow-up that included 15 small bowel recipients from the earlier report, patient and graft survival were 70% and 66%, respectively, at 18 months after transplant (78). This experience, now expanded to 98 consecutive recipients of intestine, liver and intestine, or multivisceral allografts, was recently updated to reveal actuarial 1- and 5-year survival rates of 72% and 48%, respectively (79). These and other reports have concluded that tacrolimus-based immunosuppression provides a higher survival rate following intestinal transplantation than any other currently available regimen.

## Heart–Lung

In an open-label study, tacrolimus was evaluated as primary immunosuppression in 62 adult heart transplant recipients and as rescue therapy in an additional 10 patients (80). At a mean follow-up of 1 year, patient survival was 92%. The mean number of rejection episodes was 0.95 per patient during the first 90 days, and recurrent rejection occurred in 28% of patients. Among the 10 patients receiving rescue therapy, 7 remained free from rejection on tacrolimus. In another study of tacrolimus rescue therapy for 16 heart and 15 lung recipients suffering acute or humoral rejection while on cyclosporine, patient survival rates of 100% in the heart recipients and 67% in the lung recipients were achieved (81).

Tacrolimus was used as primary immunosuppression in 26 pediatric heart transplant recipients (82). Patient survival was 82% at 1 and at 3 years, and 60% of patients were rejection-free at 3 and 6 months after transplantation.

Seventy-four adult patients were randomly assigned to tacrolimus or cyclosporine following single or bilateral lung transplant (83). One-year patient survival was similar between groups, but the number of patients free from acute rejection was significantly higher ($P < 0.05$) in the tacrolimus group. One patient (3%) in the cyclosporine group versus 5 of 38 (13%) in the tacrolimus group remained free from acute rejection during the first 120 days after transplant ($P < 0.05$). More patients in the cyclosporine group experienced bacterial infection, which was the major cause of late graft failure in both groups. A follow-up report of 133 patients reported similar 2-year survival rates for tacrolimus and cyclosporine but with a trend toward lower acute rejection rates with tacrolimus (84). Thirteen cyclosporine-treated patients versus 2 tacrolimus-treated patients required crossover to the alternative therapy ($P = 0.02$). The incidence of obliterative bronchiolitis was significantly lower with tacrolimus ($P = 0.025$).

Tacrolimus and cyclosporine were evaluated as primary immunosuppression in 20 pediatric lung transplant patients (85). Eight patients on each drug survived at a mean follow-up of 2 years after transplant. No differences in the incidence of rejection were reported between groups; however, 6 of 7 cyclosporine-treated patients and no tacrolimus-treated patients required antilymphocyte globulin for graft rejection. Furthermore, 4 patients on cyclosporine versus none on tacrolimus developed hypertension.

## NONTRANSPLANT USES OF TACROLIMUS

Because of its potent immunosuppressive properties, tacrolimus may have applications in the treatment of autoimmune diseases (see Table 4.3). Clinical experience with tacrolimus has been reported in patients with nephrotic syndrome, psoriasis, chronic inflammatory diseases of the liver, and uveitis (86–90). Seven patients with refractory psoriasis experienced resolution confirmed with skin biopsy following treatment with tacrolimus (87). A marked reduction in proteinuria was observed in 6 of 7 patients with nephrotic syndrome, and the response was sustained for 6 months (86).

Ten patients with primary sclerosing cholangitis were treated with tacrolimus for up to 1 year (84). Serum bilirubin, alkaline phosphatase, and transaminase levels were reduced by 70% to 86%. No adverse effects on serum creatinine or blood urea nitrogen were observed with tacrolimus. In a second trial, 21 patients with autoimmune chronic active hepatitis were treated with tacrolimus for up to 3 months (90). Transaminase levels were reduced by 70% to 80%, with minimal increases in serum creatinine and blood urea nitrogen levels.

Tacrolimus was used to treat 13 patients with refractory uveitis and produced improvement in visual acuity during 6 weeks of follow-up (91).

Tacrolimus also has been investigated for prevention of graft-versus-host disease in patients undergoing bone marrow transplantation (92). In this pilot study, 18 patients were randomized to tacrolimus alone or with methotrexate or methylprednisolone. Eight of 18 patients developed grade II–IV acute graft-versus-host disease, and 1-year disease-free survival was 39%.

## SAFETY/TOLERABILITY PROFILE OF TACROLIMUS

Much of the early toxicity reported with tacrolimus was associated with the use of unnecessarily high intravenous doses. The most frequent adverse events with tacrolimus in clinical trials have been renal impairment (highlighting the lack of correlation with blood levels), abnormalities in glucose metabolism, and neurotoxicity (Table 4.4) (55,56). In both of the liver transplant multicenter trials, the incidence of abnormal kidney function in the early post-transplant period was significantly increased with tacrolimus compared with the cyclosporine group. However, serum creatinine concentrations were not significantly different between treatment groups at the 12-month follow-up. The decrease in renal toxicity over time presumably reflected a decrease in the dose of tacrolimus and a more rapid conversion to oral therapy as experience with tacrolimus increased.

A randomized, prospective study on the effects of tacrolimus immunosuppression on lipid profiles in stable cyclosporine-treated renal transplant patients with established hyperlipidemia was undertaken by the Southeastern Organ Procurement Foundation (93). Patients with cholesterol of 240 mg/dL or greater, who were at least 1 year post-transplant with stable renal function, were randomly assigned to remain on cyclosporine (control) or be converted to tacrolimus. Renal function, glucose control, and levels of total cholesterol, triglycerides, total high-density lipoprotein (HDL), low-density lipoprotein (LDL), very-low-density lipoprotein (VLDL), and apoproteins A and B were monitored before conversion to tacrolimus. A total of 53 patients were analyzed (27 in the tacrolimus group and 26 controls) 6 months after conversion. In patients converted to tacrolimus treatment, there was a significant decrease in cholesterol (16%; $P = 0.0031$), LDL cholesterol (25%; $P = 0.0014$), and apolipoprotein B (23%; $P = 0.034$). There was no change in renal function, glycemic control, or incidence of new onset diabetes mellitus in the tacrolimus group. The authors concluded that conversion to tacrolimus from cyclosporine should be considered in the treatment of post-transplant hyperlipidemia.

New onset diabetes mellitus and hyperglycemia occurred significantly more often with tacrolimus in both the US and the European trial (55,56). Of concern is that many patients developed de novo insulin-dependent diabetes mellitus several months after transplantation, long after high-dose steroid therapy was given. However, later studies combining tacrolimus with mycophenolate mofetil (MMF) suppression indicate the incidence of insulin-dependent diabetes is reduced to 10% or less (94). The incidence of neurologic adverse events, including tremor and paresthesia, was significantly higher with tacrolimus, but the events were generally of mild or moderate severity. However, severe neurologic adverse events—such as convulsions, confusion, psychosis, encephalopathy, and even coma—were also seen, and they responded to a reduction in tacrolimus dosage. In the European trial, a decreased incidence of infection was reported with tacrolimus, while in the US study the incidence of both malignant and nonmalignant neoplasms was lower with tacrolimus. In a 2-year follow-up of the US study, a higher incidence of post-transplant hepatitis C was reported in the tacrolimus group, and the incidence of rejection was higher in this subpopulation of tacrolimus-treated patients. Whether hepatitis C is a more serious problem in those receiving tacrolimus than in those receiving cyclosporine is presently being debated (95,96).

Pediatric patients receiving tacrolimus following liver transplantation have experienced an increased incidence of neurotoxicity, diarrhea, and dyspepsia; however, the incidence of infectious complications was similar to that with cyclosporine (97). In contrast, a higher incidence of viral infections was reported in pediatric patients undergoing kidney transplantation (70). Of particular concern is the high incidence of lymphoproliferative disease, which may approach 10% in the pediatric population (98,99), and the occasional development of red cell aplasia (100) or hemolytic uremia (101). Because a large proportion of children are Epstein-Barr virus (EBV) seronegative and, thus, at risk for primary infection leading to an increased risk of post-transplant lymphoproliferative disease, a role for EBV prophylaxis needs to be clarified.

**Table 4.4.**    Common Adverse Events with Tacrolimus

**Gastrointestinal**
Anorexia
Diarrhea
Dyspepsia
Nausea

**Metabolic**
Hyperglycemia
Hyperkalemia

**Nephrotoxicity**

**Neurologic**
Confusion
Encephalopathy
Headache
Paresthesia
Psychosis
Seizure
Tremor

## DOSING AND ADMINISTRATION

Because of good intestinal absorption, intravenous administration of tacrolimus is generally not required in the immediate postoperative period, when tacrolimus can be administered through the nasogastric tube. The initial dose of tacrolimus is 0.05 mg/kg every 12 hours, with subsequent dosage adjustment depending on the measured blood levels. The targeted tacrolimus whole blood level is initially 10 to 20 ng/mL. After 4 weeks the recommended trough level is 5 to 15 ng/mL. The optimal long-term trough level has not yet been well defined. However, in many patients with stable allograft function we see tacrolimus trough levels measuring less that 5 ng/mL, which is below the reliable threshold of the current assay. With improved monitoring techniques, the therapeutic requirements should be better defined in the future.

Pediatric patients have higher clearance and larger volumes of distribution than adult patients and thus require at least two and sometimes three daily full oral doses of tacrolimus to maintain adequate whole blood concentrations (58). Also, pediatric patients are immunologically more active and often require higher drug levels to prevent rejection. Generally, intravenous administration is only required in patients who experience gut complications after transplantation. In those circumstances, the tacrolimus dose is 0.01–0.05 mg/kg per day by continuous infusion. In patients with impaired hepatic function or in patients with stage III–IV encephalopathy, tacrolimus should be initially withheld and an induction protocol using antilymphocyte antibodies considered (see Chapter 8). Also, in patients receiving suboptimal donor organs the tacrolimus starting dose should be reduced.

It should be recognized that the bioavailability of tacrolimus is highly variable, and ordinary doses can quickly make a patient profoundly toxic. Thus, careful monitoring is mandatory in all cases following initiation of therapy. Some patients require an inordinate amount of tacrolimus to produce therapeutic levels (e.g., 0.2–0.3 mg/kg twice daily). In such patients, ketoconazole, itraconazole, or diltiazem have been used effectively to inhibit the metabolism of tacrolimus and allow normalization of the dose requirements. This can be accomplished without any side effects from the antifungal medication.

During initiation of tacrolimus therapy and before stable tissue levels have been achieved, large dosage changes often are necessary. Generally, a 30% to 40% change in dosage achieves the desired results. With stable, well-maintained patients, when fine tuning is desired, small dosage adjustments of 1 mg at a time are appropriate. In patients whose tacrolimus levels are quickly escalating—for example, during periods of sudden deterioration of liver function—the tacrolimus dose should be entirely withheld until nontoxic levels have been restored. This can sometimes take several days, depending on the extent and degree of liver failure. It takes 5 half-lives of any drug before a new steady state has been achieved, and in patients with advanced liver failure, the half-life of tacrolimus could easily reach 60 hours.

The most difficult side effect to manage with tacrolimus is minor neurotoxicity, especially in elderly patients. Minor neurotoxicity can be subtle, and the physician may not notice any abnormal behavior on casual examination. At times, a detailed interview of family and friends may be necessary to identify the cause. This toxicity can occur even with low therapeutic levels of tacrolimus, and its existence may warrant a further dosage decrease, even with blood tacrolimus levels of 5 ng/mL or less. If tacrolimus is not tolerated, one can always switch to cyclosporine. Although cyclosporine also causes neurotoxicity, the signs and symptoms are often different and thus may be relieved by using the alternate drug.

The role of triple therapy in tacrolimus protocols has not been extensively investigated. However, it is clear that the addition of azathioprine and MMF to the immunosuppressive regimen can be beneficial in tacrolimus-treated patients and may limit troublesome toxicity (94). However, with potent drugs such as tacrolimus and mycophenolate mofetil, one of the most common side effects in immunosuppressed patients is overimmunosuppression, which leads to infections and malignancies. Thus, initiation of a triple drug regimen must be done with utmost care.

## COMMENTARY

*Thomas E. Starzl and John J. Fung*

Klintmalm's chapter contains useful information, the exploitation of which requires an understanding of the management principles that have guided organ transplantation since its inception. Only four drugs have been widely used as baseline immunosuppressants: azathioprine, cyclophosphamide, cyclosporine, and tacrolimus. With each agent, the dosage must be determined individually for every patient. The ceilings are imposed by toxicity, and the dose floors are revealed by breakthrough rejection. The amount of azathioprine and cyclophosphamide that can be given is limited by myelotoxicity, which can be monitored conveniently with serial white blood counts. The more complex side effects of cyclosporine and tacrolimus are shown in Table 4C.1.

## HISTORICAL PERSPECTIVE

None of the four baseline drugs can reliably prevent post-transplant rejection when used alone. However, it was learned in 1962 to 1963 that organ rejection, which previously had been considered inexorable, could be reversed and that subsequent dose requirements of immunosuppressive agents frequently declined. The same events have been observed with all treatment regimens and with all organs. Delineation of this pattern of convalescence, which was first observed with the combination of azathioprine and prednisone (1), provided the empirical launching pad for the clinical field of organ transplantation, in which dose-maneuverable prednisone has proved to be the indispensable ingredient.

The introduction of each new drug was accompanied by an easily learned trial and potential error determina-

**Table 4C.1.**   Nonimmunologic Profile (4+ = Worst), All Dose-Related

| | Tacrolimus | Cyclosporine |
|---|---|---|
| Nephrotoxicity | ++* | ++ |
| Neurotoxicity | + | + |
| Diabetogenicity | + | + |
| Growth effects | | |
|   Hirsutism | 0 | +++ |
|   Gingival hyperplasia | 0 | ++ |
|   Facial brutalization | 0 | + |
|   Hepatotrophic effects | ++++ | +++ |
|   Gynecomastia | 0 | + |
| Other metabolic effects | | |
|   Cholesterol increase | 0 | ++ |
|   Uric acid increase | +? | ++ |

\* Less hypertension.
Sources: From Starzl TE, Abu-Elmagd K, Tzakis A, et al. Selected topics on FK 506: with special references to rescue of extrahepatic whole organ grafts, transplantation of "forbidden organs," side effects, mechanisms, and practical pharmacokinetics. Transplant Proc 1991;23:914–919. (Slide presented at the Transplantation Society Congress, San Francisco, in August, 1990.)

tion of the requisite doses of the individual constituents of the cocktail. With increasingly potent baseline agents, survival of all organ grafts rose in three distinct leaps over a 33-year period. The characteristic immunologic confrontation and resolution process did not change—it merely became easier to manage.

What was being accomplished through this process remained enigmatic until it was discovered in 1992 that long-surviving organ recipients had donor leukocyte chimerism in their blood, skin, lymph nodes, and other sites as late as three decades after transplantation. It was then obvious that the prototypic post-transplant phenomena were the product of a double immune reaction: host-versus-graft (rejection) and graft-versus-host (Fig. 4C.1). Potentially tolerogenic "passenger leukocytes" of bone marrow origin, including pluripotent stem cells, had migrated from organs and engrafted peripherally. This was the seminal mechanism of organ allograft acceptance (2).

### The Tacrolimus Pilot Trials

The clinical development of tacrolimus bracketed the chimerism discoveries, beginning 3 years before and continuing for 5 years after. In 1989, we first showed that tacrolimus (FK506) could systematically reverse liver allograft rejection that had been intractable in the face of maximal cyclosporine-based conventional immunosuppression (3,4). The "rescued" patients were maintained thereafter on tacrolimus, and manifested no unique or unexpected toxicity (5). Consequently, a nonrandomized trial was begun in which tacrolimus was substituted for cyclosporine from the time of operation.

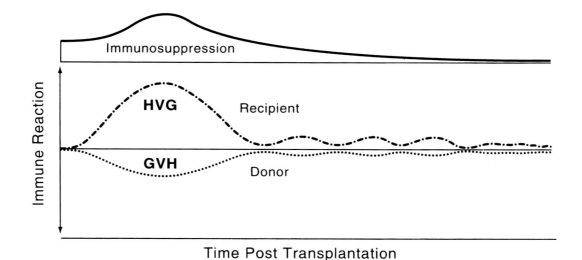

**FIGURE 4C.1.**   *Contemporaneous host-versus-graft (HVG) and graft-versus-host (GVH) reactions in the two-way paradigm of transplantation immunology (2). Following the initial interaction, the evolution of nonreactivity of each leukocyte population to the other is seen as a predominantly low-grade stimulatory state that may wax and wane, rather than as a deletional one.*

By early 1990, nearly 200 liver, kidney, and other-organ recipients who had been entered in the program had superior actuarial survival, lower requirement for prednisone, and better quality of life than we had observed in the past (6–8). Already the upgrading of outlook after liver transplantation was as obvious as it had been a decade before when cyclosporine succeeded azathioprine as the baseline immunosuppressant (Fig. 4C.2). Thus, even as the advent of cyclosporine had elevated transplantation of cadaver kidneys from a previously unacceptable level (9,10), the bar rose for liver and for kidney transplantation with the introduction of tacrolimus (Fig. 4C.3). The same was true for thoracic organs (8).

It was clear by early 1990 that the dose-limiting side effects of cyclosporine and tacrolimus were the same: nephrotoxicity, neurotoxicity, and diabetogenicity (see Table 4C.1). These manifestations could be used from the first day of treatment to determine appropriate doses (6–8,11,12). Invidious toxicity comparisons between

cyclosporine and tacrolimus were unwarranted because the scales could be tilted one way or the other by ratcheting the doses up or down. The only adverse effects observed exclusively with one drug but not the other were the dose-related cosmetic changes caused by cyclosporine (see Table 4C.1).

As had been found a decade earlier with cyclosporine (11), it was easy to relate toxic manifestations and rejection to trough plasma and blood concentrations (the plasma/blood ratio of tacrolimus was about 1:10) and promptly endow the laboratory results with clinically relevant meaning (6–8,12,13). Flexibility of dosing was important no matter what the transplanted organ, but it was especially so with the liver because the metabolism of tacrolimus is more dependent than that of cyclosporine on good hepatic function (12,14). By the beginning of 1990, doses and trough levels used for liver, kidney, heart, and lung recipients in Pittsburgh (6,7) were essentially the same as those recommended in

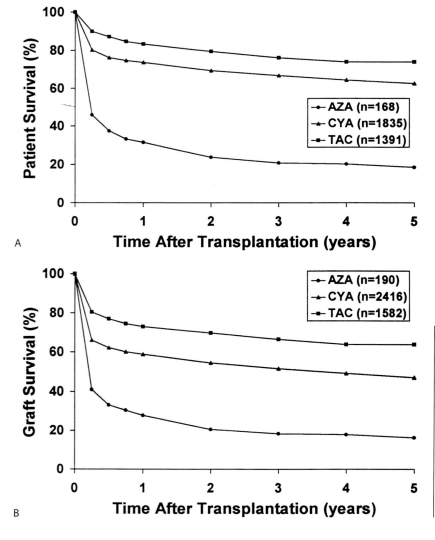

**FIGURE 4C.2.** *The three eras of orthotopic liver transplantation at the Universities of Colorado (1963–1980) and Pittsburgh (1981–1993), defined by azathioprine, cyclosporine, and tacrolimus (FK 506) immunosuppression.* **A.** *Patient survival.* **B.** *Graft survival. This was about 10% lower than patient survival in both the cyclosporine era (1980–1989) and the tacrolimus era (1989–1993), whereas patient and graft survival were essentially identical with azathioprine. The difference in later series was explained by effective retransplantation, an option that did not exist previously. AZA, azathioprine; CYA, cyclosporine; TAC, tacrolimus.*

Klintmalm's chapter. The data shown in Figure 4C.4 were presented on April 5, 1990, at the American Surgical Association, and were published 4 months later.

## The Randomized Liver Trials

Historically, new immunosuppressive drugs were evaluated in kidney recipients and then applied secondarily to transplantation of unpaired vital organs. This precedent was broken with the development of tacrolimus, largely because liver transplant surgeons demanded that the drug be released for rescue therapy of their patients. Rather than pursuing the question of rescue efficacy, it was decided at meetings with the United States Food and Drug Administration (FDA) during October and November of 1989 to proceed with randomized European and American multicenter trials comparing tacrolimus with cyclosporine as the primary immunosuppressant from the time of liver replacement. By the time these trials started the following autumn, however, a decisive trial that had started in February 1990 in Pittsburgh using the tacrolimus doses shown in Figure 4C.4 was more than half completed.

## The Pittsburgh Liver Trial

The Pittsburgh Liver Trial was a single-center, Institutional Review Board (IRB)-mandated trial. Safety and

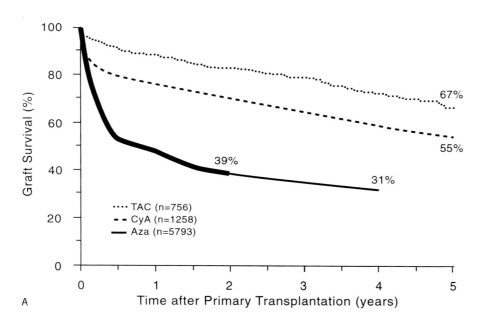

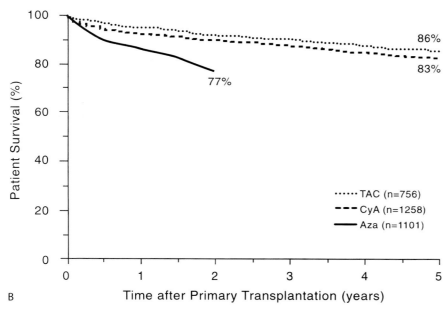

**FIGURE 4C.3.** *(A) Patient survival and (B) graft survival after primary cadaveric kidney transplantation at the University of Pittsburgh under cyclosporine (1981–1989) versus tacrolimus-based immunosuppression. These observations suggest the long-term survival of kidney allografts can also be improved by substitution of tacrolimus for cyclosporine. Graft survival curves for azathioprine in A are from Terasaki's national register. Early patient survival data are from the Southeastern Organ Procurement Foundation, to which Pittsburgh contributed. TAC, tacrolimus; CyA, cyclosporine; Aza, azathioprine.*

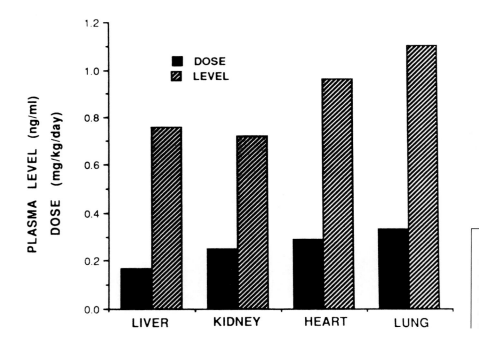

**FIGURE 4C.4.**    *The tacrolimus doses used in the Pittsburgh Liver Trial and initially recommended for recipients of other organs. Because of the dependence on good hepatic function for tacrolimus metabolism, starting doses for liver recipients are slightly lower.*

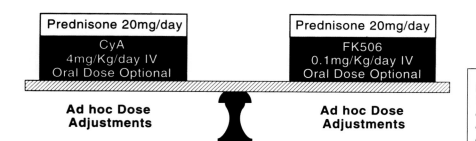

**FIGURE 4C.5.**    *The Pittsburgh Liver Trial protocol, tacrolimus (FK506) versus cyclosporine (CyA). All treatment variables except for the competing drugs were equalized.*

efficacy comparisons were ensured by equalization of all treatment variables except the competing drugs (15,16) (Fig. 4C.5). Definition of end points allowed the liver recipients early access to whichever drug had the better therapeutic margin. The trial was prematurely terminated in 1991 by a multi-institutional oversight committee, which had been insisted upon by the investigators. By the time the trial was stopped, a massive crossover from cyclosporine to tacrolimus had occurred, with only one crossover from tacrolimus to cyclosporine. Throughout the entire 5-year period of subsequent study, tacrolimus enjoyed a statistically significant greater freedom from rejection, either alone or in combination with freedom from graft loss and adverse events (16).

### The Multicenter Liver Trials

The design of the subsequent American (17) and European (18) liver transplant trials, which involved 20 insti-

tutions, was of some concern. In all 20 participating centers, the cyclosporine arm was uploaded with twice (or more) the induction doses of prednisone used for the tacrolimus patients. The cyclosporine-treated recipients also were given a third drug (azathioprine) in 95% of the centers and a fourth agent (polyclonal ALG) in a few (Fig. 4C.6). The tacrolimus doses were set higher than those concurrently used in Pittsburgh, and they remained so until the end of the study (Fig. 4C.7). The combination of excessive dosage and the sometimes delayed response to toxic events on the tacrolimus arm complicated the interpretation of some observations.

The European teams had a 5% better survival of patients on the tacrolimus arm [17% (46/270) versus 22% (61/275) mortality] and a 5% higher graft survival (18). By intent-to-treat analysis, the survival advantage was not statistically significant. However, about 10% of the surviving grafts credited to cyclosporine had been rescued from treatment failure with tacrolimus. The distorting

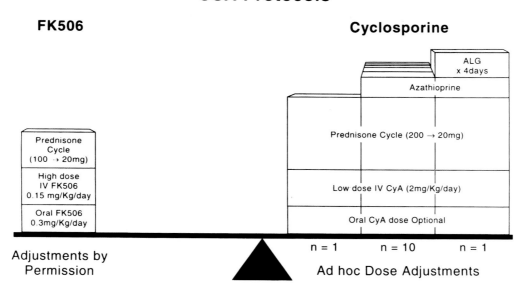

**USA Protocols**

**FK506**

**Cyclosporine**

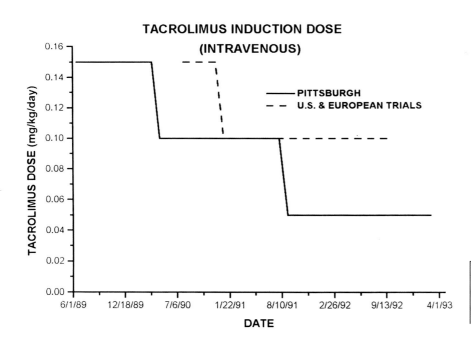

**FIGURE 4C.6.** *US protocol in the multicenter tacrolimus (FK506) trial. The cyclosporine (CyA) arm was uploaded with twice (or more) the induction doses of prednisone used for the tacrolimus patients. Cyclosporine recipients also were given a third drug (azathioprine) in 95% of the centers; polyclonal ALG was used in a few centers (n, number of centers using the regimen).*

**FIGURE 4C.7.** *Tacrolimus doses set for the Multicenter Liver Trial. The doses were higher than those used in the Pittsburgh study.*

roles of tacrolimus overdosage and the consequent high rate of toxicity were clarified by separate analyses of the early (high dose) and later (reduced dose) phases of the trial. The statistical analysis, based on the intent-to-treat approach, showed significantly greater freedom from acute rejection, intractable acute rejection, and chronic rejection. The report concluded that tacrolimus had superior therapeutic qualities (18).

In the published American report (17), use of the Kaplan-Meier and intent-to-treat methods created the impression that the better efficacy and greater toxicity of tacrolimus essentially balanced each other. An alternative analysis suggested that freedom from rejection as a single end point was accomplished more frequently with tacrolimus (19). Moreover, the superiority of tacrolimus emerged at all levels, including freedom from adverse events and, most significantly, freedom from refractory rejection. After 1 year of follow-up, 98% of the patients randomized to tacrolimus were not diagnosed with refractory rejection, compared with 87% in the competing arm. The composite freedom at 1 year from the three factors that haunt transplant recipients—refractory rejection, retransplantation, and death—was 80% for tacrolimus and 70% for cyclosporine (19).

## Randomized Trialomania

Disquieting scientific and ethical issues were exposed by the events of the 6 years following the placement of tacrolimus on the FDA fast track in November 1989. Neither the new drug's unusual rescue capability (3–5) nor its superiority as a baseline agent (6,7) were in doubt from late 1989 onward. The evidence for this as well as management recommendations had been published by the summer of 1990 (3,6–8,12), although, as with all new therapies, independent confirmation was needed from other centers. The FDA has a range of options for confirmation, as shown in Table 4C.2. However, the agency has increasingly insisted on multicenter, controlled, randomized trials as a prerequisite for marketing new drugs, and tacrolimus would be no different.

The FDA feared that pilot studies might suggest superiority of tacrolimus to potential multicenter participants, making them as reluctant as the Pittsburgh investigators had been to participate in a randomized trial. Therefore, no familiarization cases that used the drug from the time of transplantation were allowed. Also, by the nature of transplantation biology, cocktail regimens can never be applied in exactly the same way to any two recipients. In spite of this, the multicenter trial design insisted on rigidity of therapeutic protocols for tacrolimus (but not for the competing drug).

Although the design and dosing errors of the multicenter liver trials were ascribed to the investigators, the protocols and the trials themselves were efforts to comply with regulatory requirements. The FDA does not ostensibly engage in human experimentation; however, when

**Table 4C.2.**    Spectrum of Most to Least "Adequate" Controls

1. Placebo concurrent control (randomized, double-blinded).
2. Dose-comparison concurrent control (randomized, 2 doses, often with placebo or active treatment arm [competing drug]).
3. No treatment concurrent control (randomized, with no treatment arm).
4. Active treatment concurrent control (randomized versus competing agent).
5. Historical control versus concurrent treatment (special situations, when outcome is self-evident or in absence of equipoise).

Code of Federal Regulations (CFR 314.126). Revised by FDA, April 1, 1994.

the agency imposed a learning curve for tacrolimus on 20 different centers as a condition for the sale of a new drug that was urgently needed for rescue purposes, the agency became the de facto instigator of a human experiment. It is not possible to pull this switch and disavow responsibility for what followed.

Ill-advised or poorly designed randomized trials achieve the opposite objectives of their intent: improved and less expensive patient care. The lack of familiarization studies, together with the inexplicable error in dosing and the disadvantage of no on-site assays for drug monitoring, resulted in the muddled picture of the new drug's potential that emerged in the published literature between 1992 and 1995. Nevertheless, tacrolimus survived the irrational gauntlet not only because it was user friendly, but also because the talented group of multicenter clinical investigators rebelled against the protocol and introduced treatment flexibility. This confirmed our earlier experience, that throughout the entire history of liver transplantation only two key developments have upgraded graft and patient survival: Calne's introduction of cyclosporine in 1979 (21) and its use in combination with prednisone (22), and the arrival of tacrolimus (see Fig. 4C.2).

## Other-Organ Uses

Following the uneven literature that came out of the American multicenter liver trials, an avalanche of articles involving organ after organ, and eventually bone marrow transplantation, would confirm essentially every detail of the original Pittsburgh experience (20).

The same developmental leaps were seen in renal transplantation, for example. The 1-year cadaver kidney survival rate in the United States had remained fixed at less than 50% until the advent of cyclosporine, after which it rose to 77% at the University of Pittsburgh. A second abrupt increase to nearly 90% followed the routine use of tacrolimus (see Fig. 4C.3). The maintenance of the gap between cyclosporine and tacrolimus after 1 year was congruent with the report of Gjertson, Cecka, and Terasaki, based on the cadaver kidney half-life projections from 24 American kidney transplant centers with access to tacrolimus. Their suggestion was: "FK 506 (tacrolimus) appears to be the first therapeutic agent to significantly improve long-term kidney graft survival rates" (23). A thorough review of the use of tacrolimus following kidney transplantation has been provided by Laskow et al (24).

## POST-TRANSPLANT LYMPHOPROLIFERATIVE DISORDERS

It has not been surprising to observe an incremental increase in post-transplant lymphoproliferative disorders (PTLDs) with the successively more potent baseline immunosuppressants (21,25–27). This risk can be reduced at the outset by avoiding the joint use of the biologic antilymphoid agents (e.g., ALG and OKT-3) in conjunction with cyclosporine and tacrolimus except as a last resort, and then only with extreme caution.

When PTLD is diagnosed early in development, it usually is a trivial problem requiring only drug dose reduction. At the Children's Hospital of Pittsburgh, 9 (13.2%) of 68 recipients (of 69 kidney allografts) treated with tacrolimus-based immunosuppression between 1989 and 1995 developed histopathologically verified PTLD (28). No deaths resulted, nor did any graft losses. All kidneys are still functioning (at the time of this writing) except one that was chronically rejected 3 years later.

At the same institution, histopathologically verified PTLD was diagnosed in 28 (12.1%) of the 232 consecutive primary pediatric liver recipients treated with tacrolimus between 1989 and 1995. Although 5 of the 28 died of potentially PTLD-related complications, the 4-year patient and graft survival rate (82.2%) was essentially the same as in the 204 non-PTLD patients (Table 4C.3) (27). Management was facilitated by the policies of gradual tacrolimus dose reduction with acceptance of lower blood levels as time passes (see Table 4C.3), early discontinuance of prednisone, avoidance of adjunct agents including OKT-3 and azathioprine, and surveillance for Epstein-Barr virus (EBV) infection.

Except for their frequent EBV association, human B-cell lymphomas are indistinguishable from those induced by Robert S. Schwartz in a mouse chimerism model (29) 3 years before they were reported in human kidney recipients (30). Schwartz attributed the experimental tumors to an active lymphoproliferative response by the dominant immune apparatus to the persistent subclinical graft-versus-host counterattack of the minority donor leukocyte population. The relevance of his observations to clinical PTLD would only be appreciated 30 years later (27), after the discovery that similar microchimerism was a characteristic feature of successful organ transplantation (2). This fresh insight about PTLD has been used to map treatment strategies of cellular immune modulation as discussed elsewhere (27).

## CHAPTER REFERENCES

1. Kino T, Hatanaka H, Miyata S, et al. FK-506, A novel immunosuppressant isolated from a *Streptomyces*. II. Immunosuppressive effect of FK-506 in vitro. J Antibiotics 1987;40:1256–1265.
2. Kino T, Inamura N, Sakai F, et al. Effect of FK506 on human mixed lymphocyte reaction in vitro. Transplant Proc 1987;19:36–39.
3. Ochiai T, Nagata M, Nakajima K, et al. Studies of the effects of FK506 on renal allografting in the beagle dog. Transplantation 1987;44:729–733.
4. Ochiai T, Nakajima K, Nagata M, et al. Studies of the induction and maintenance of long-term graft acceptance by treatment with FK506 in heterotopic cardiac allotransplantation in rats. Transplantation 1987;44:734–738.
5. Todo S, Ueda Y, Demetris JA, et al. Immunosuppression of canine, monkey, and baboon allografts by FK 506: with special reference to synergism with other drugs and to tolerance induction. Surgery 1988;104:239–249.
6. Tsuchimoto S, Kusumoto K, Nakajiwa Y, et al. Orthotopic liver transplantation in rats receiving FK506. Transplant Proc 1989;21:1064–1065.
7. Jiang H, Suguo H, Takahara S, et al. Combined immunosuppressive effect of FK506 and other immunosuppressive agents on PHA- and CD3-stimulated human lymphocyte proliferation in vitro. Transplant Proc 1991;23:2933–2936.
8. Sigal NH, Dumont FJ. Cyclosporin A, FK506, and rapamycin: pharmacologic probes of lymphocyte signal transduction. Ann Rev Immunol 1992;10:519–560.
9. Mekki Q, Lee C, Carrier S, et al. The effect of food on oral bioavailability of tacrolimus (FK506) in liver transplant patients. Clin Pharmacol Ther 1993;53:229.
10. Lee C, Jusko W, Shaefer M, et al. Pharmacokinetics of tacrolimus (FK506) in liver transplant patients. Clin Pharmacol Ther 1993;53:181–190.
11. Abu-Elmagd K, Fung JJ, Alessiani M, et al. The effect of graft function on FK506 plasma levels, dosages, and renal function, with particular reference to the liver. Transplantation 1991;52:71–77.
12. Jusko WJ, D'Ambrosio R. Monitoring FK 506 concentrations in plasma and whole blood. Transplant Proc 1991;23:2732–2735.
13. Kershner RP, Fitzsimmons WE. Relationship of FK506 whole blood concentrations and efficacy and toxicity after liver and kidney transplantation. Transplantation 1996;62:920–926.
14. Machida M, Takahara S, Ishibashi M, et al. Effect of temperature and hematocrit on plasma concentration of FK 506. Transplant Proc 1991;6:2753–2754.
15. Winkler M, Ringe B, Rodeck B, et al. The use of plasma levels for FK 506 dosing in liver-grafted patients. Transplant Int 1994;7:329–333.
16. Winkler M, Ringe B, Baumann J, et al. Plasma vs whole blood for therapeutic drug monitoring of patients receiving FK 506 for immunosuppression. Clin Chem 1994;40:2247–2253.
17. Backman L, Nicar M, Levy M, et al. FK506 trough levels in whole blood and plasma in liver transplant recipients: correlation to clinical events and side effects. Transplantation 1994;57:519–524.
18. Christians U, Braun F, Schmidt M, et al. Specific and sensitive measurement of FK506 and its metabolites in blood and urine of liver-graft recipients. Clin Chem 1992;38:2025–2032.
19. Laskow DA, Vincenti F, Neylan JF, et al. An open-label, concentration-ranging trial of FK506 in primary kidney transplantation: a report of the United

**Table 4C.3.** Primary Liver Transplantation in Children Under Tacrolimus (n = 232)[a,b]

| | Months' Follow-Up | | | | |
|---|---|---|---|---|---|
| | 3 | 12 | 24 | 36 | 48 |
| **Survival (%)** | | | | | |
| Patient | 90.2 | 86 | 85 | 84 | 84 |
| Graft | 83 | 79.2 | 78.2 | 77.3 | 77.3 |
| **Tacrolimus (mean)** | | | | | |
| Dose (mg/day) | 5.6 | 3.3 | 2.9 | 2.9 | 2.4 |
| Plasma concentration (trough ng/mL)[c] | 0.84 | 0.56 | 0.43 | 0.4 | 0.24 |
| **Prednisone (%)** | | | | | |
| None | 79 | 82 | 88 | 93 | 91 |
| ≤5 mg/day | 9 | 13 | 7 | 5 | 7 |
| >5 mg/day | 12 | 5 | 5 | 2 | 2 |

[a] September 1989–January 1995. Age 5.0 ± 5.2 (SD) years (medium 2.7). Mean follow-up 44 ± 14.6 months.
[b] 28 patients developed PTLD. Principal sites were the gastrointestinal system (n = 9), lymph nodes (n = 8), liver (n = 6), spleen (n = 2), and tonsils, skin, and blood (leukemia) (n = 1 each).
[c] For approximate whole blood values, multiply by 10.
Data from Dr. Jorge Reyes. Presented at the 2nd International Congress on Pediatric Transplantation, Paris, France, August 23–24, 1996.

States Multicenter FK506 Kidney Transplant Group. Transplantation 1996;62: 900–905.

20. Thomson AW, Murase N, Nalesnik MA, Starzl TE. The influence of tacrolimus on experimental autoimmune disease. In: Lieberman R, Mukherjee A, eds. Principles of drug development in transplantation and autoimmunity. Austin, TX: RG Landes, 1996.

21. Inamura N, Hashimoto M, Nakahara K, et al. Immunosuppressive effect of FK506 on collagen-induced arthritis in rats. Clin Immunol Immunopathol 1988;46:82–90.

22. Arita C, Hotokebuchi T, Miyahara H, et al. Inhibition by FK506 of established lesions of collagen-induced arthritis in rats. Clin Exp Immunol 1990;82:456–461.

23. Takagishi K, Yamamoto M, Nishimura A, et al. Effects of FK-506 on collagen arthritis in mice. Transplant Proc 1989;21(pt1):1053–1055.

24. Miyagawa J, Yamamoto K, Hanafusa T, et al. Preventive effect of a new immunosuppressant FK-506 on insulitis and diabetes in non-obese diabetic mice. Diabetologia 1990;33:503–505.

25. Carroll PB, Strasser S, Alejandro R. The effect of FK 506 on cyclophosphamide-induced diabetes in the NOD mouse model. Transplant Proc 1991;23:3348–3350.

26. Murase N, Lieberman I, Nalesnik M, et al. FK-506 prevents spontaneous diabetes in the BB rat. Lancet 1990;ii:373–374.

27. Nicoletti F, Meroni PL, Barcellini W, et al. FK-506 prevents diabetes in diabetes-prone BB/Wor rats. Int J Immunopharmacol 1991;13:1027–1030.

28. Kawashima H, Mochizuki M. Effects of a new immunosuppressive agent, FK 506, on the efferent limb of the immune responses. Exp Eye Res 1990;51:565–572.

29. Fujino Y, Mochizuki M, Raber J, et al. Treatment of S-antigen induced uveitis in primates. Invest Ophthalmol Vis Sci 1990;31:61.

30. Tamura K, Woo J, Murase N, et al. Suppression of autoimmune thyroid disease by FK 506: influence on thyroid-infiltrating cells, adhesion molecule expression and anti-thyroglobulin antibody production. Clin Exp Immunol 1993;91:368–375.

31. Yamamoto K, Mori A, Nakahama T, et al. Experimental treatment of autoimmune MRL-lpr/lpr with immunosuppressive compound FK506. Immunology 1988;69:222–227.

32. Takabayashi K, Koike T, Kurasawa K, et al. Effect of FK-506, a novel immunosuppressive drug on murine systemic lupus erythematosus. Clin Immunol Immunopathol 1989;51:110–117.

33. Hara S, Fukatsu A, Suzuki N, et al. The effects of a new immunosuppressive agent, FK506, on the glomerular injury in rats with accelerated nephrotoxic serum glomerulonephritis. Clin Immunol Immunopathol 1990;57:351–362.

34. Okuba Y, Tsukada Y, Maezawa A, et al. FK-506, a novel immunosuppressive agent, induces antigen-specific immunotolerance in active Heymann's nephritis and in the autologous phase of Masugi nephritis. Clin Exp Immunol 1990;82:450–455.

35. Matsukawa W, Hara S, Yoshida F, et al. Effects of a new immunosuppressive agent, FK506, in rats with active Heymann nephritis. J Lab Clin Med 1992;119:116–123.

36. Inamura N, Hashimoto M, Nakahara K, et al. Immunosuppressive effect of FK506 on experimental allergic encephalomyelitis in rats. Int J Immunopharmacol 1988;10:991–995.

37. Hanawa H, Kodama M, Zhang S, et al. An immunosuppressant compound, FK-506, prevents the progression of autoimmune myocarditis in rats. Clin Immunol Immunopathol 1992;62:321–326.

38. Meingassner JG, Stutz A. Immunosuppressive macrolides of the type FK 506: a novel class of topical agents for treatment of skin diseases? J Invest Dermatol 1992;98:851–855.

39. Hiraoka Y, Kishimoto C, Kurokawa M, et al. The effects of FK-506, a novel and potent immunosuppressant, upon murine Coxsackie virus B3 myocarditis. J Pharmacol Exp Ther 1992;260:1386–1391.

40. Walliser P, et al. Inhibition of murine B lymphocyte proliferation by the novel immunosuppressive drug FK506. Immunology 1989;68:434–435.

41. Murase N, Kim DG, Todo S, et al. Suppression of allograft rejection with FK-506. I. Prolonged cardiac and liver survival in rats following short-course therapy. Transplantation 1990;50:186–189.

42. Todo S, Podesta L, ChapChap P, et al. Orthotopic liver transplantation in dogs receiving FK-506. Transplant Proc 1987;19(suppl 6):64–67.

43. Monden M, Gotoh M, Kanai T, et al. A potent immunosuppressive effect of FK506 in orthotopic liver transplantation in primates. Transplant Proc 1990;22(suppl 1):66.

44. Murase N, Todo S, Lee PH, et al. Heterotopic heart transplantation in the rat receiving FK-506 alone or with cyclosporine. Transplant Proc 1987;5:71–75.

45. Yasunami Y, Ryu S, Kamei T. FK506 as the sole immunosuppressive agent for prolongation of islet allograft survival in the rat. Transplantation 1990;49: 682–686.

46. Todo S, Demetris A, Ueda Y, et al. Renal transplantation in baboons under FK 506. Surgery 1989;106:444–450.

47. Hoffman AL, Makoka L, Banner B, et al. The use of FK506 for small intestine allotransplantation. Transplantation 1990;49:483–490.

48. Yoshimi F, Nakamura K, Zhu Y, et al. Canine total orthotopic small bowel transplantation under FK-506. Transplant Proc 1991;23:3240–3242.

49. Todo S, Murase N. Tacrolimus for experimental organ transplantation. In: Lieberman R, Mukherjee A, eds. Principles of drug development in transplantation and autoimmunity. Austin, TX: RG Landes, 1996.

50. Eiras G, Inventarza O, Murase N, et al. Species differences in sensitivity of T lymphocytes to immunosuppressive effects of FK 506. Transplantation 1990;49:1170–1172.

51. Murase N, Demetris AJ, Matsuzaki T, et al. Long survival in rats after multivisceral versus isolated small-bowel allotransplantation under FK 506. Surgery 1991;110:87–98.

52. Fung J, Abu-Elmagd K, Jain A, et al. A randomized trial of primary liver transplantation under immunosuppression with FK506 vs cyclosporine. Transplant Proc 1991;23:2977–2983.

53. Fung JJ, Todo S, Tzakis A, et al. Conversion of liver allograft recipients from cyclosporine to FK506-based immunosuppression. Benefits and pitfalls. Transplant Proc 1991;23:14–21.

54. Todo S, Fung JJ, Starzl TEA, et al. Liver, kidney, and thoracic organ transplantation under FK506. Ann Surg 1990;212:295–307.

55. U.S. Multicenter FK506 Liver Transplant Study Group. A comparison of tacrolimus (FK506) and cyclosporine for immunosuppression in liver transplantation. N Engl J Med 1994;331:1110–1115.

56. European FK506 Multicentre Liver Study Group. Randomised trial comparing tacrolimus (FK506) and cyclosporin in prevention of liver allograft rejection. Lancet 1994;344:423–428.

57. Wiesner RH. A long-term comparison of tacrolimus versus cyclosporine in liver transplantation: a report of the U.S. FK506 study group. Transplantation 1998;66:493–499.

58. McDiarmid SV, Busuttil RW, Ascher NL, et al. FK506 (tacrolimus) compared with cyclosporine for primary immunosuppression after pediatric liver transplantation. Results from the U.S. Multicenter Trial. Transplantation 1995;59:530–536.

59. Devlin J, Wong P, Williams R, et al. FK506 primary immunosuppression following emergency liver transplantation for fulminant hepatic failure. Transplant International 1994;7:64–69.

60. Klintmalm GB, Goldstein R, Gonwa T, et al. Use of Prograf (FK506) as rescue therapy for refractory rejection after liver transplantation. U.S. Multicenter FK506 Liver Transplant Study Group. Transplant Proc 1993;25:679–688.

61. Vincenti F, Laskow DA, Neylan JF, et al. One-year follow-up of an open-label trial of FK506 for primary kidney transplantation. A report of the U.S. Multicenter FK506 Kidney Transplant Group. Transplantation 1996;61: 1576–1581.

62. Pirsch JD, Miller J, Deierhoi MH, et al. A comparison of tacrolimus (FK506) and cyclosporine for immunosuppression after cadaveric renal transplantation. FK506 Kidney Transplant Study Group. Transplantation 1997;63:977–983.

63. Cavaille-Coll MW, Elashoff MR. Commentary on a comparison of tacrolimus and cyclosporine for immunosuppression after cadaveric renal transplantation. Transplantation 1998;65:142–145.

64. Shield CF, McGrath MM, Goss TF. Assessment of health-related quality of life in kidney transplant patients receiving tacrolimus-based versus cyclosporine-based immunosuppression. Transplantation 1997;64:1738–1743.

65. Mayer AD, Dmitrewski J, Squifflet JP, et al. Multicenter randomized trial comparing tacrolimus (FK506) and cyclosporine in the prevention of renal allograft rejection: a report of the European Tacrolimus Multicenter Renal Study Group. Transplantation 1997;64:436–443.

66. Shapiro R, Jordan ML, Scantlebury VP, et al. A prospective, randomized trial of FK 506/prednisone vs FK506/azathioprine/prednisone in renal transplant patients. Transplant Proc 1995;27:814–817.

67. Woodle SE, Thistlethwaite JR, Gordon JH, et al. A multicenter trial of FK506 (tacrolimus) therapy in refractory acute renal allograft rejection. Transplantation 1996;62:594–599.

68. Woodle SE, Cronin D, Newell KA, et al. Tacrolimus therapy for refractory acute renal allograft rejection. Definition of the histologic response by protocol biopsies. Transplantation 1996;62:906–910.

69. Jordan ML, Naraghi R, Shapiro R, et al. Tacrolimus rescue therapy for renal allograft rejection—five-year experience. Transplantation 1997;63:223–228.

70. Witzke O, Becker G, Erhard J, et al. Tacrolimus rescue therapy in patients with rejection and long-term dialysis after kidney transplantation. Clin Nephrol 1998;49:24–27.

71. Laskow DA, Neylan JF, Shapiro RS, et al. The role of tacrolimus in adult kidney transplantation: a review. Clin Transplantation 1998;12:489–503.

72. Ketel BL, Turton-Weeks S, Reed K, Barone GW. Tacrolimus-based vs cyclosporine-based immunotherapy in combined kidney-pancreas transplantation. Transplant Proc 1996;28:899.

73. Gruessner RWG, Burke GW, Stratta R, et al. A multicenter analysis of the first experience with FK506 for induction and rescue therapy after pancreas transplantation. Transplantation 1996;61:261–273.

74. Gruessner RWG. Tacrolimus in pancreas transplantation: a multi-center analysis. Clin Transplantation 1997;11:299–312.

75. Hariharan S, Munda R, Cavallo T, et al. Rescue therapy with tacrolimus after combined kidney/pancreas and isolated pancreas transplantation in patients with severe cyclosporine nephrotoxicity. Transplantation 1996;61:1161–1165.

76. Gruessner RW, Bartlett ST, Burke GW, Stock PG. Suggested guidelines for the use of tacrolimus in pancreas/kidney transplantation. Clin Transplant 1998;12:260–262.

77. Todo S, Tzakis A, Reyes J, et al. Intestinal transplantation in humans under FK-506. Transplant Proc 1993;25:1198–1199.

78. Todo S, Tzakis A, Reyes J, et al. Small intestinal transplantation in humans with or without the colon. Transplantation 1994;57:840–848.

79. Abu-Elmagd K, Reyes J, Todo S, et al. Clinical intestinal transplantation: new perspectives and immunologic considerations. J Am Coll Surg 1998;186:512–525.

80. Armitage JM, Kormos RL, Morita S, et al. Clinical trial of FK-506 immunosuppression in adult cardiac transplantation. Ann Thorac Surg 1992;54:205–210.

81. Mentzer RM Jr, Jahania MS, Lasley RD. Tacrolimus as a rescue immunosuppressant after heart and lung transplantation. The U.S. Multicenter FK506 Study Group. Transplantation 1998;65:109–113.

82. Armitage JM, Fricker FJ, del Nido P, et al. A decade (1982 to 1992) of pediatric cardiac transplantation and the impact of FK-506 immunosuppression. J Thorac Cardiovasc Surg 1993;105:464–473.

83. Griffith BP, Bando K, Hardesty RL, et al. A prospective randomized trial of FK506 versus cyclosporine after human pulmonary transplantation. Transplantation 1994;57:848–851.

84. Keenan RJ, Konishi H, Kawai A, et al. Clinical trial of tacrolimus versus cyclosporine in lung transplantation. Ann Thorac Surg 1995;60:580–584.

85. Armitage JM, Fricker FJ, Kurland G, et al. Pediatric lung transplantation: the years 1985 to 1992 and the clinical trial of FK506. J Thorac Cardiovasc Surg 1993;105:337–346.

86. McCauley J, Shapiro R, Scantlebury V, et al. FK 506 in the management of transplant-related nephrotic syndrome and steroid-resistant nephrotic syndrome. Transplant Proc 1991;23:3354–3356.

87. Jegasothy BV, Ackerman CD, Todo S, et al. Tacrolimus (FK 506)—a new therapeutic agent for severe recalcitrant psoriasis. Arch Dermatol 1992;128:781–785.

88. Japanese FK 506 Study Group on Refractory Uveitis. A multicenter clinical open trial of FK506 in refractory uveitis, including Behcet's disease. Transplant Proc 1991;23:3343–3346.

89. van Thiel DH, Carroll P, Abu-Elmagd K, et al. Tacrolimus (FK506), a treatment for primary sclerosing cholangitis: results of an open-label preliminary trial. Am J Gastroenterol 1995;90:455–459.

90. van Thiel DH, Wright H, Carroll P, et al. Tacrolimus: a potential new treatment for autoimmune chronic active hepatitis: results of an open-label preliminary trial. Am J Gastroenterol 1995;90:771–776.

91. Ishioka M, Ohno S, Nakamura S, et al. FK506 treatment of noninfectious uveitis. Am J Ophthalmol 1994;118:723–729.

92. Nash RA, Etzioni R, Storb R, et al. Tacrolimus (FK506) alone or in combination with methotrexate or methylprednisolone for the prevention of acute graft-versus-host disease after marrow transplantation from HLA-matched siblings: a single-center study. Blood 1995;85:3746–3753.

93. McCune TR, Thacker LR II, Peters TG, et al. Effects of tacrolimus on hyperlipidemia after successful renal transplantation: a Southeastern Organ Procurement Foundation multicenter clinical study. Transplantation 1998;65:87–92.

94. Eckhoff DE, McGuire BM, Frenette LR, et al. Tacrolimus and mycophenolate mofetil combination therapy versus tacrolimus in adult liver transplantation. Transplantation 1998;65:180–187.

95. Mueller AR, Platz KP, Blumhardt G, et al. The optimal immunosuppressant after liver transplantation according to diagnosis: cyclosporine A or FK506? Clin Transplant 1995;9:176–184.

96. Zervos XA, Weppler D, Fragulidis GP, et al. Comparison of tacrolimus with microemulsion cyclosporine as primary immunosuppression in hepatitis C patients after liver transplantation. Transplantation 1998;65:1044–1046.

97. McDiarmid SV, Colonna JO, Shaked A, et al. Differences in oral FK506 dose requirements between adult and pediatric liver transplant patients. Transplantation 1993;55:1328–1332.

98. Cox KL, Lawrence-Miyasaki LS, Garcia-Kennedy R, et al. An increased incidence of Epstein-Barr virus infection and lymphoproliferative disorder in young children on FK506 after liver transplantation. Transplantation 1995;59:524–529.

99. Cacciarelli TV, Green M, Jaffe R, et al. Management of post-transplant lymphoproliferative disease in pediatric liver transplant recipients receiving primary tacrolimus therapy. Transplantation 1998;66:1047–1052.

100. Misra S, Moore TB, Ament ME, et al. Red cell aplasia in children on tacrolimus after liver transplantation. Transplantation 1998;65:575–577.

101. Walder B, Ricou B, Suter PM. Tacrolimus-induced hemolytic uremic syndrome after heart transplantation. J Heart Lung Transplant 1998;17:1004–1006.

## COMMENTARY REFERENCES

1. Starzl TE, Marchioro TL, Waddell WR. The reversal of homografts with subsequent rejection in human renal development of homograft tolerance. Surg Gynecol Obstet 1963;117:385–395.

2. Starzl TE, Demetris AJ, Murase N, et al. The lost chord: microchimerism. Immunol Today 1996;17:577–584.

3. Starzl TE, Todo S, Fung J, et al. FK 506 for human liver, kidney and pancreas transplantation. Lancet 1989;2:1000–1004.

4. Fung JJ, Todo S, Jain A, et al. Conversion of liver allograft recipients with cyclosporine related complications cyclosporine to FK 506. Transplant Proc 1990;22:6–12.

5. Fung JJ, Todo S, Tzakis A, et al. Conversion of liver allograft recipients from cyclosporine to FK506-based immunosuppression: benefits and pitfalls. Transplant Proc 1991;23:14–21.

6. Todo S, Fung JJ, Starzl TE, et al. Liver, kidney, and thoracic organ transplantation under FK 506. Ann Surg 1990;212:295–305.

7. Starzl TE, Fung J, Jordan M, et al. Kidney transplantation under FK 506. JAMA 1990;264:63–67.

8. Armitage JM, Kormos RL, Fung J, et al. Preliminary experience with FK 506 in thoracic transplantation. Transplantation 1991;52:154–167.

9. McDonald JC, Vaughn W, File RS, et al. Cadaver donor renal transplantation by centers of the Southeastern Organ Procurement Foundation. Ann Surg 1981;193:1–8.

10. Opelz G, Mickey MR, Terasaki PI. HLA matching and cadaver kidney transplant survival in North America. Transplantation 1977;23:490–497.

11. Starzl TE, Hakala TR, Rosenthal JT, et al. Variable convalescence and therapy after cadaveric renal transplantation under cyclosporin A and steroids. Surg Gynecol Obstet 1982;154:819–825.

12. Starzl TE, Abu-Elmagd K, Tzakis A, et al. Selected topics on FK 506: with special references to rescue of extrahepatic whole organ grafts, transplantation of "forbidden organs," side effects, mechanisms, and practical pharmacokinetics. Transplant Proc 1991;23:914–919.

13. Starzl TE, Fung JJ. Contempo 90: transplantation. JAMA 1990;263:2686–2687.

14. Abu-Elmagd K, Fung JJ, Alessiani M, et al. The effect of graft function on FK506 plasma levels, doses, and renal function, with particular reference to the liver. Transplantation 1991;52:71–77.

15. Fung J, Abu-Elmagd K, Jain A, et al. A randomized trial of primary liver transplantation under immunosuppression with FK 506 vs cyclosporine. Transplant Proc 1991;23:2977–2983.

16. Starzl TE, Fung JJ, Todo S, et al. The Pittsburgh randomized trial of tacrolimus versus cyclosporine for liver transplantation. J Am Coll Surg 1996;183:117–125.

17. Klintmalm A for the U.S. Multicenter FK 506 Liver Study Group. A comparison of tacrolimus (FK 506) and cyclosporine for immunosuppression in liver transplantation. N Engl J Med 1994;331:1110–1115.

18. Neuhaus P, Pichlmayr R, Williams R for the European FK 506 Multicentre Liver Study Group. Randomised trial comparing tacrolimus (FK 506) and cyclosporin in prevention of liver allograft rejection. Lancet 1994;344:423–428.

19. Starzl TE, Donner A, Eliasziw M, et al. Randomised trialomania? The multicenter liver transplant trials. Lancet 1995;346:1346–1350.

20. Transplantation Society in Transplantation Proceedings. Vol. 29. March 1997.

21. Calne RY, Rolles K, White DJG, et al. Cyclosporin A initially as the only immunosuppressant in 34 recipients of cadaveric organs: kidneys, 2 pancreases, and 2 livers. Lancet 1979;2:1033–1036.

22. Starzl TE, Klintmalm GBG, Porter KA, et al. Liver transplantation with use of cyclosporin A and prednisone. N Engl J Med 1981;305:266–269.

23. Gjertson DW, Cecka JM, Terasaki PI. The relative effects of FK 506 and cyclosporine on short- and long-term kidney graft survival. Transplantation 1995;60:1384–1388.

24. Laskow DA, Neylan JF, Shapiro RS, et al. The role of tacrolimus in adult kidney transplantation: a review. Clin Transplantation 1998;12:489–503.

25. Starzl TE, Nalesnik MA, Porter KA, et al. Reversibility of lymphomas and lymphoproliferative lesions developing under cyclosporine-steroid therapy. Lancet 1984;1:583–587.

26. Cox KL, Lawrence-Miyasaki LS, Garcia-Kennedy R, et al. An increased incidence of Epstein-Barr virus infection and lymphoproliferative disorder in young children on FK506 after liver transplantation. Transplantation 1995;59:524–529.

27. Starzl TE. The mother lode of liver transplantation, with particular reference to our new journal. Liver Transpl Surg 1998;4:1–14.

28. Shapiro R, Scantlebury VP, Jordan ML, et al. Tacrolimus in pediatric renal transplantation. Transplantation 1996;62:1752-1758.

29. Schwartz R, Andre-Schwartz J, Armstrong MYK, Beldotti L. Neoplastic sequelae of allogenic disease. Theoretical considerations and experimental design. Ann NY Acad Sci 1966;129:804–821.

30. Penn I, Hammond W, Brettschneider L, Starzl TE. Malignant lymphomas in transplantation patients. Transplant Proc 1969;1:106–112.

# Mycophenolate Mofetil: Experimental and Clinical Experience

STEPHEN C. RAYHILL    HANS W. SOLLINGER

The clinical success of solid organ transplantation took a great leap forward in the early 1980s with the development of cyclosporine (see Chapter 1). In synergy with corticosteroids and the antimetabolite azathioprine, cyclosporine significantly reduced cell-mediated graft rejection and allowed for successful organ transplantation. However, despite the improved clinical success produced by this triple drug regimen, enthusiasm was tempered for two reasons: 1) the particular toxicities of the agents; and 2) the nonspecific immunosuppression produced by the regimen, which resulted in opportunistic infections and increased incidence of malignancies. Thus, efforts in developing new immunosuppressive treatments for transplantation have focused on the development of specific immunomodulation and on agents that might additionally produce attenuation of the antibody response, which is felt to be important in the development of chronic rejection (1).

Mycophenolate mofetil (MMF) is the first drug approved for the prevention of allograft rejection in the United States since the development of the calcineurin inhibitors in the 1980s. Like azathioprine, it is an antimetabolite, but it has several advantages. First and foremost, it is more potent and more selective than azathioprine. Because it is a relatively specific inhibitor of lymphocyte proliferation, doses that are strongly inhibitory can be used without major side effects on other proliferating tissues. This represents its major advantage over other antimetabolites. In addition, because it is a strong inhibitor of lymphocyte proliferation, it inhibits both cell-mediated immunity and humoral immunity. As noted, the inhibition of B cells is felt to be important in the attenuation of the development of chronic rejection. Thus, the development of MMF to replace azathioprine in the triple immunosuppression regimen is a major advance in immunosuppressive therapy.

MMF was developed by Nelson, Allison, and Eugui of Roche Laboratories (previously Syntex Research) (1). It is

a more orally bioavailable prodrug of mycophenolic acid (MPA), its active form, to which it is converted in the gastrointestinal tract. Its development was based on the observation that a deficiency in de novo purine synthesis in lymphocytes results in a general state of immunosuppression. Specifically, they noted that a genetic deficiency in the production of adenine deaminase, an enzyme critical to de novo purine synthesis, resulted in reduced numbers and reduced function of B and T lymphocytes, while producing no other clinical abnormalities (2). In contrast, children with a defect in the salvage pathway for purine synthesis maintain normal lymphocyte responses, despite being unable to recycle purines, a defect that produces significant abnormalities in other systems (3). Thus, they reasoned that human lymphocytes depend almost exclusively on the de novo pathway of purine synthesis, while other cells can fall back on the salvage pathway in the absence of effective de novo purine synthesis. With this in mind, they sought to develop a vector to block de novo purine synthesis and thereby produce a selective inhibitor of lymphocytes.

The purines guanosine and adenosine are produced from inosine via the de novo pathway (Fig. 5.1). Adenosine deaminase converts inosine to adenosine, while inosine monophosphate dehydrogenase (IMPDH) affects the conversion of inosine to guanosine. Inhibition of either enzyme results in decreased production of these nucleotides, and therefore, cell proliferation as the cell becomes deficient in these substrates. In addition, because guanosine nucleotides are important regulatory stimulators of the rate-limiting enzymes catalyzing inosine synthesis, the reduction in intracellular concentration of guanosine has an indirect inhibitory effect. This is in contrast to the adenosine nucleotides, which allosterically inhibit inosine synthesis. Thus, an inhibitor of de novo guanosine synthesis is a particularly effective inhibitor of de novo purine synthesis—both directly, by depleting the levels of guanosine, and

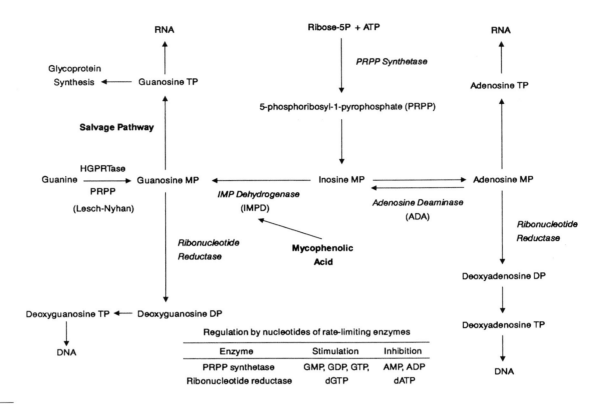

**FIGURE 5.1.**    *The de novo pathway of purine biosynthesis, showing the central position of IMP. MPA inhibits IMP dehydrogenase, thereby depleting GMP, GTP, and dGTP. Two rate-limiting enzymes in the purine synthesis pathway are activated by guanosine ribonucleotides and dGTP, and inhibited by adenosine ribonucleotides and dATP.*

indirectly, by downregulation of enzymes critical to synthesis. Allison, Eugui, and Nelson sought a specific inhibitor of guanosine production. Of the several possible inhibitors of IMPDH available, they selected mycophenolic acid, a fermentation product of several *Penicillium* species, because it is a specific, potent, noncompetitive, and reversible inhibitor of eukaryotic inosine monophosphate dehydrogenases (4,5). It has the additional benefit of not being a nucleoside analog, which, although also inhibitory, could produce undesirable mutagenic effects such as inhibition of DNA repair enzymes and production of chromosomal breaks, which can lead to lymphomas (6). Thus, by defining a specific biochemical pathway critical for the proliferation of human T and B lymphocytes, the development of an organ-specific immunosuppressive was begun.

## MECHANISMS OF ACTION

The major advantage of MPA over other antimetabolite immunosuppressants is its relatively selective effect on lymphocyte activation. This is due to two aspects of the drug's mechanism of action. The first is inhibition of purine synthesis. Guanosine and adenosine, the two purine nucleosides, are synthesized via the de novo pathway (see Fig. 5.1). The initial step is the conversion of ribose-5-phosphate and ATP

into the amino sugar phosphate 5-phosphoribosyl-amine by 5-phosphoribosyl-1-pyrophosphate synthetase. This step, in which the amide amino group of glutamine replaces the pyrophosphate group of PRPP, is the rate-controlling process of purine synthesis. The 5-phosphoribosyl-1-pyrophosphate synthetase is allosterically inhibited by adeninal nucleotides, and is stimulated by guanosine nucleotides. Via a subsequent series of steps, including the addition of an entire glycene molecule, the pentose sugar is converted into an imidazole ring and then a purine ring, resulting in inosine monophosphate. Inosine monophosphate is the precursor for both adenosine monophosphate and guanosine monophosphate. Inosine monophosphate is converted to adenosine monophosphate by adenosine deaminase and into guanosine monophosphate via inosine monophosphate dehydrogenase. It is the conversion of inosine monophosphate into guanosine monophosphate by IMPDH that is blocked by mycophenolic acid. This competitive inhibition of IMPDH results in the reduction of guanosine monophosphate via decreased synthesis of the molecule and, indirectly, by the loss of its stimulatory effect on the inosine monophosphate synthesis pathway. Thus, the synthesis of both adenosine monophosphate and guanosine monophosphate is inhibited. With these vital DNA substrates depleted, lymphocytes are unable to proliferate. In contrast, cells other than lymphocytes can use the salvage pathway to produce adequate quantities of guanosine monophosphate and adenosine monophosphate by recycling guanine and adenine already present in the cell.

The second mechanism for the selective inhibition of lymphocytes by MPA is based on the unique isoforms of IMPDH employed by lymphocytes. Natsumeda et al have isolated two cDNA clones for two distinct isoforms of IMPDH (7,8). A constitutive form, type I, is the predominant structure expressed in resting human lymphocytes. An inducible form, type II, is found in lymphocytes when they are stimulated by phytohemagglutinin (T cells) or transformed by Epstein-Barr virus (B cells). When stimulated, the type II gene is strongly expressed. The type II isoform of IMPDH is five times more sensitive to MPA than is the type I isoform (1). Thus, rapidly dividing lymphocytes are most susceptible to mycophenolic acid (i.e., the relative susceptibility of lymphocytes to mycophenolic acid is enhanced by their dependence on the type II isoform of IMPDH when activated).

## In Vitro Effects of Mycophenolic Acid

Mycophenolic acid, by strongly inhibiting IMPDH, depletes GTP, the precursor for RNA synthesis, and deoxy-GTP

(dGTP), the precursor for DNA synthesis in activated peripheral blood lymphocytes and human T- and B-lymphocytic cell lines, locking them in S phase (9). Guanosine monophosphate and adenosine monophosphate must be reduced to deoxydiphosphates and then converted to deoxytriphosphates to be substrates for DNA synthesis. In cells lacking the salvage pathway (those lacking hypoxanthine guanine phosphoribosyl transferase) the addition of deoxyguanosine results in restoration of deoxy-guanosine triphosphate, but not guanosine triphosphate. The restoration of the deoxy version allows DNA synthesis and cellular proliferation. This demonstrates that the depletion of deoxyguanosine triphosphate, the key substrate for DNA polymerase, and therefore for DNA synthesis, is the principal reason that proliferation is inhibited by MPA. In addition to its specific targeting of lymphocytes, MPA also decreases pools of deoxyguanosine triphosphate in human peripheral blood monocytes; however, it does not decrease deoxy-GTP in neutrophils (1). Physiologic concentrations of MPA inhibit the in vitro proliferative responses of human peripheral blood mononuclear cells to phytohemagglutinin, a T-cell mitogen; pokeweed mitogen, a T-cell–dependent B-cell mitogen; and *Staphylococcus* protein A sepharose, a B-cell mitogen (Fig. 5.2) (10). Mycophenolic acid also inhibits the mixed lymphocyte response. Importantly, the

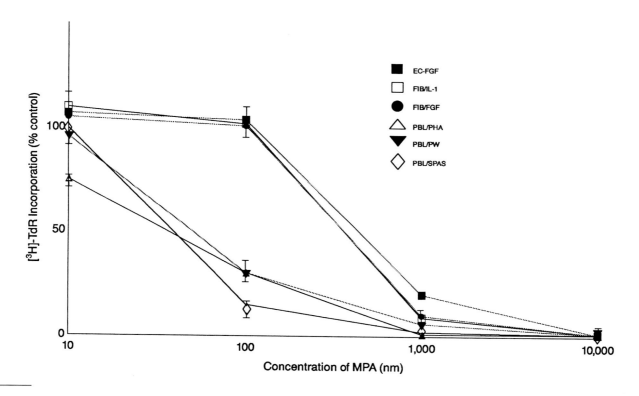

**FIGURE 5.2.** *Inhibition by MPA of human peripheral blood lymphocyte (PBL) proliferation in response to stimulation by PHA, PWM, and a B-cell mitogen (staphylococcal protein A sepharose). Higher concentrations of MPA are required to inhibit the proliferation of human dermal fibroblasts (FIB) responding to IL-1β and human umbilical vein endothelial cells (EC) responding to basic fibroblast growth factor.*

inhibiting concentration 50% (IC$_{50}$) is always less than 100 nmol/L, a concentration shown to have no antiproliferative effect on fibroblasts, endothelial cells, and most other cell types studied. Unlike the calcineurin inhibitors, MPA has no effect on IL-2 production by activated lymphocytes (10,11). However, when it is added to a mixed lymphocyte reaction 72 hours after initiation, it is still strongly inhibitory, implying that MPA works at a late stage in T-cell activation. Indeed, consistent with its inhibitory effect on DNA synthesis, cells treated with MPA are blocked at the G$_1$ to S transition stage (9).

An important secondary effect of purine nucleoside inhibition by MPA may be the disruption of the synthesis of adhesion molecules. Adhesion molecules such as the integrins and selectins are critical in the recruitment of leukocytes to sites of inflammation or rejection. They mediate the attachment of these cells to appropriate substrate cells. Both the recruitment of lymphocytes and their activation are decreased in the absence, or with reduced concentrations, of appropriate cell-adhesion molecules such as ICAM-1 and its complementary ligand, LFA-1 (12,13). Glycosylation of proteins and lipids, a required step in the creation of these molecules occurs through nucleotide intermediates. Thus, it follows that MPA, by depleting the purine nucleotide pools in the cells, could inhibit the transfer of the appropriate sugars to nascent membrane glycoproteins. This effect has been confirmed experimentally by measuring the transfer of labeled sugars to glycoproteins and assaying the density of glycoproteins via flow cytometric analysis (14). Thus, MPA may inhibit rejection by attenuating the recruitment of mononuclear cells to rejection sites and by reducing the ability of the lymphocytes to interact with endothelial cells once at the proper location.

In vitro antibody formation by polyclonally activated human B lymphocytes is almost completely inhibited by 100 μmol/L of MPA (10). In contrast to cyclosporine treatment, human spleen cells exposed to tetanus toxoid in the presence of MPA were found to produce no secondary response or subsequent antibody production (15). This may be important in the attenuation of chronic graft rejection.

A second possible mechanism through which MMF may reduce the potential for chronic rejection is through its ability to inhibit human arterial smooth muscle proliferation (Fig. 5.3) (1). Clinically attainable concentrations of MPA inhibit the proliferation of human arterial smooth muscle cells in culture. This has obvious implications for a possible therapeutic benefit with respect to the cellular intimal thickening found in chronic rejection.

The cellular effects of MPA are summarized in Table 5.1.

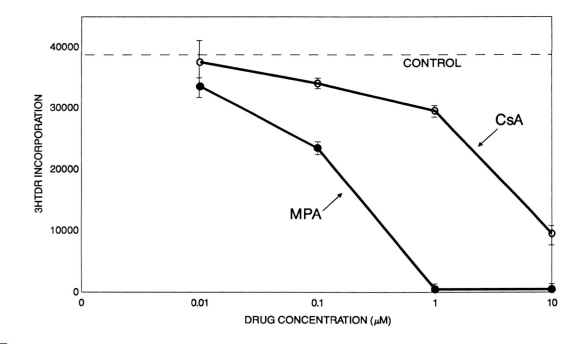

**FIGURE 5.3.**    *The effect of MPA and cyclosporine on the proliferation of human arterial smooth muscle cells in culture. MPA attenuated the proliferative response of human arterial smooth muscle cells grown in culture. This effect occurred at clinically attainable concentrations of MPA (1 to 10 μmol/L) and therefore, might be expected to contribute to a reduction in the arterial wall proliferative response in chronic rejection. Note that the inhibitory concentration for human smooth muscle cells, 10 times greater than that required for inhibition of lymphocytes in culture, was similar to that required for endothelial cells and fibroblasts (see Fig 5.2).*

**Table 5.1.** The Cellular Effects of Mycophenolic Acid

1. Blocks the proliferative response of both T and B cells.
2. Inhibits adhesion molecule production by inhibiting glycosylation.
3. Inhibits antibody production.
4. Inhibits medial smooth muscle proliferation.

## In Vivo Studies

That MPA is lymphocyte selective in vivo was first demonstrated by Eugui et al (16). Mice were given subcutaneous injections of the antigen ovalbumin, which is known to stimulate DNA synthesis in lymph nodes draining the site of injection by stimulating a secondary response. The mice were then given intraperitoneal [³H]-TdR to illuminate the sites of active DNA synthesis. Two groups were evaluated: a control group, which was given the vehicle only, and a treatment group, which was given 100 mg/kg/day of oral MPA. Incorporation of tritiated thymidine into DNA was measured in the appropriate lymph nodes, the spleen, and the testes. MPA strongly inhibited DNA synthesis in the lymph nodes, but had no detectable effect on DNA synthesis in the testes or small intestinal epithelial cells. The spleen was affected, as expected, but there was no effect noted on neutrophils or platelets. Next, mice were challenged with allogeneic tumor cells placed intraperitoneally. The mice treated with MPA had a dose-dependent reduction in the generation of cytotoxic T lymphocytes, and in contrast to untreated mice, they were unable to eliminate tumor cells from their peritoneum.

The effects of MPA on lymphocytes are rapidly and fully reversible (1). Peripheral blood mononuclear cells separated from the plasma of patients treated with MMF respond normally to mitogenic stimulation, whereas that response is strongly attenuated in the presence of the patient's plasma.

Modification of the in vivo antibody response by MMF has been evaluated in rats and mice. Mycophenolate mofetil given orally to mice inhibited the formation of antibodies in a dose-dependent manner (16). When given to rats, it nearly abolished the formation of xenoantibodies, and suppressed resynthesis after plasmapheresis (16,17). Antibody formation from human B cells cultured from the spleen was also inhibited by MMF (15,18).

The effect of MMF on cytokines has been studied by Nagy et al, who demonstrated that in contrast to cyclosporine, which inhibited all cytokines studied at all time points, MMF produced no early (6 to 24 hours) inhibition of cytokine production (19). It did, however, inhibit superantigen-induced cytokine production after 48 hours (only IL-3). This finding was seen in preparations induced with either superantigen or mitogen stimulation. That MPA does not affect IL-2 production was corroborated in a study of mitogen-activated human peripheral lymphocytes (10,11).

## STUDIES OF THE EFFECTS OF MYCOPHENOLATE MOFETIL ON ANIMAL ALLOGRAFTS

### Studies in Animal Models of Heart Transplantation

The first published reports on the use of MMF in a transplantation model were produced by Morris and co-workers, who studied the effect of MMF on the survival of rat cardiac allografts (20,21). Initially, they found that treatment with MMF prolonged median cardiac allograft survival from 8 to 60 days, and then with an increased dose in a subsequent study to 200 days. In addition, the authors showed that MMF could halt even rejection that was advanced at the onset of treatment (22). Indeed, there was no difference in rats who were treated with MMF from day 1 after transplant versus those begun on day 4 after transplant. When a lower dose of MMF was combined with cyclosporine, the drugs acted additively, further prolonging allograft survival. Rat cardiac allograft recipients surviving 200 days or more after the discontinuation of MMF were given two additional transplants: donor strain and third-party strain atrial allografts. The donor strain allografts were accepted and continued to beat for more than 100 days (suggesting that a state of tolerance may have been achieved). In stark contrast, the third-party atrial grafts were rejected within 14 days. An important additional observation was that graft coronary disease was diminished in the MMF-treated allograft recipients (23). MMF and sirolimus (rapamycin) were found to be synergistic in preventing heart, pancreas, and kidney allograft rejection and in reversing ongoing heart allograft rejection in a rat model (24).

To determine whether MMF might be useful in preventing hyperacute (antibody-mediated) or accelerated acute (T-cell–mediated) rejection, Knechtle et al studied its use in a rat model of sensitized cardiac allograft rejection (25). As shown in Table 5.2, untreated control Lewis recipients were found to have a median survival time of 6 days. Other Lewis rats sensitized with skin grafts from ACI rats were given ACI heart transplants. When untreated, allografts in sensitized rats survived for a median period of 2 days, whereas posttransplant MMF treatment prolonged median survival to 5 days. When given in combination with cyclosporine, MMF prolonged median survival to 14 days. Thus, hyperacute and accelerated acute rejection were prevented; however, acute cellular rejection could not be overcome with MMF alone or in combination with cyclosporine in these sensitized rats.

Investigators from Kobe University and from Syntex Research evaluated combination therapy consisting of MMF and brequinar in the heterotopic rat allograft model (26). Compared to controls, which survived an average of 7 days, animals treated with either MMF or brequinar had a median survival of 15 days. Combination therapy, however, increased median survival to 133 days with no toxic side effects noted. The effect of combination therapy with MMF and brequinar was also evaluated in the setting of rejection rescue

**Table 5.2.**     Allograft Survival in Previously Sensitized Recipients

| Group No. | Treatment | Graft Survival Time (Days) | Median Survival Time | P | Correlation Between Graft Survival Time and Cytotoxic Antibody Titer (P) |
|---|---|---|---|---|---|
| 1 | None | 1,1,1,1,1,1,2,2,3,4,4,4,4,4 | 2 | — | 0.99 |
| 2 | MMF (20 mg/kg/d) | 1,1,2,5,5,5,5,5,5[a],6,6[a],6 | 5 | 0.0002 vs. Group 1 | 0.15 |
| 3 | CsA (10 mg/kg/d) | 1,1,3,7,8,8,8,9,10,14,14,15[a] | 8 | 0.004 vs. Group 1<br>0.0016 vs. Group 2 | 0.61 |
| 4 | MMF + CsA | 1,3[a],5[a],11,12[a],13,17[a],18[a],20,24,35,37[b] | 15 | <0.01 vs. Groups 1, 2, 3 | 0.45 |
| 5 | 14 days MMF preoperatively, +MMP + CsA postoperatively | 1,3[a],3,5[a],9,13,14,14,15,16[a],22[a],33,35 | 14 | 0.05 vs. Group 3<br>0.39 vs. Group 4 | 0.92 |

Note: Last two columns represent long-rank tests comparing survival times and the correlation between graft survival and cytotoxic antibody titer.
[a]  Rat died.
[b]  Rat killed before rejection.
CsA = cyclosporine.

therapy (26). In this experiment, immunosuppressive therapy was withheld until the fifth postoperative day, after the establishment of acute rejection. At this point, treatment with MMF, brequinar, or both was begun. Recipients were evaluated on day 21, when it was noted that either drug by itself, and both in combination, significantly decreased the extent of rejection compared to control animals.

The effect of MMF in a combination therapy regimen was further evaluated in several subsequent studies, including one corroborating Morris' early results, demonstrating that combination therapy with cyclosporine and MMF prolongs rat cardiac allograft survival (27). Another study, in a strongly MHC-incompatible rat cardiac allograft model, evaluated the effect of MMF in combination with leflunomide or tacrolimus (28). It demonstrated that MMF alone or in combination with leflunomide significantly increased allograft survival. Morris et al subsequently demonstrated that MMF treatment significantly prolonged cardiac allograft survival in cynomolgus monkeys, futher supporting its clinical use (23).

### The Effect of Mycophenolate Mofetil on Renal Allografts in the Canine Model

The effect of MMF on kidney allograft survival in dogs was evaluated in several studies (29–31). Dogs that received either no treatment or treatment with subtherapeutic doses of cyclosporine and methylprednisolone had median allograft survivals of 8 days. In contrast, MMF prolonged mean survival to 36 days. The strongest effect was noted when MMF was combined with cyclosporine and methylprednisolone, which prolonged median allograft survival to 122 days. Gastrointestinal side effects, which had been seen in dogs receiving MMF alone, were significantly reduced with the lower doses employed in this combination therapy regimen.

A model of rescue therapy for acute renal allograft rejection in dogs was also evaluated (30). A subtherapeutic regimen of MMF, cyclosporine, and methylprednisolone, known from previous experiments to be inadequate for preventing acute allograft rejection, was given. As expected, severe allograft rejection occurred in all dogs within 5 to 10 days of transplantation. Methylprednisolone bolus therapy for 3 days only temporarily reversed this acute rejection, with no dog in this group surviving longer than 20 days after the diagnosis of acute rejection. In contrast, 14 of 16 dogs receiving high doses of MMF for 3 days and then returned to the scheduled combination therapy had complete reversal of rejection. The other two had partial reversal, and all had prolonged survival. Thus, high-dose MMF successfully reversed acute rejection in this canine renal allograft model.

### The Effect of MMF on Hepatic Allografts in the Canine Model

The effect of MMF on liver allograft rejection in dogs was also studied (32). As shown in Table 5.3, when used in combination with prednisone and cyclosporine, MMF significantly prolonged canine liver allograft survival. Specifically, this combination therapy, begun on day 1 and continued for up to two weeks, prolonged median survival from 7 days in untreated controls to 70 days in the treatment group. Again, the MMF was well tolerated.

### The Effect of MMF on Acute Rejection of Intestinal Allografts in the Animal Model

The effect of MMF on canine intestinal allograft survival was investigated by D'Alessandro et al (33). With no immunosuppressive therapy, median recipient survival was no longer than 10 days; however, triple therapy with MMF,

**Table 5.3.** Experimental Groups and Survival Following Allogeneic Liver Transplantation in Dogs

| Experimental Group | Survival Time (Days) | Mean ± SD | Median | P vs. Control |
|---|---|---|---|---|
| Control Group | 6,6,7,8,8 | 7 ± 1 | 7 | — |
| Prednisone 0.1 mg/kg | 6,8,9,11,11 | 9 ± 2 | 9 | NS |
| MMF 20 mg/kg | 9,9,10,11,24 | 13 ± 6 | 10 | <0.05 |
| CsA 5 mg/kg | 7,17,22,35,105,120 | 51 ± 49 | 29 | <0.05 |
| CsA 5 mg/kg, MMF 20 mg/kg | 27,36,68,90,110 | 66 ± 35 | 68 | <0.05 |
| CsA 10 mg/kg | 8,22,44,119,126 | 64 ± 55 | 44 | <0.05 |
| CsA 10 mg/kg, MMF 20 mg/kg (6 wks, then MMF 10 mg/kg) | 52,57,65,70,110,125,126 | 86 ± 33 | 70 | <0.01 |

NS = not significant; CsA = cyclosporine.

prednisone, and cyclosporine increased median survival to 136 days. In fact, no dog treated with this regimen died due to rejection of the intestinal allograft. This encouraging result was corroborated by a subsequent study of canine small bowel transplantation, which achieved excellent results using combination chemotherapy with prednisone, tacrolimus (FK506), and MMF (34). However, studies using rat models of intestinal transplantation failed to demonstrate increased survival with MMF (35,36).

## The Effect of Mycophenolate Mofetil on Animal Hind Limb Allograft Survival

Cyclosporine and MMF combination therapy also prolonged survival of rat hind limb allografts (37). Compared to controls, where the allografts were completely rejected within 10 to 12 days, five of six rats treated with cyclosporine had prolonged allograft survival; however, they demonstrated mild to moderate rejection on biopsy within six months. In contrast, five of six recipients receiving MMF had no rejection at 32 weeks' follow-up, while the remaining recipient demonstrated only slight rejection. Even better results were seen with combination immunosuppressive therapy using both MMF and cyclosporine, where no rejection was observed at all, and full sensation and partial function were observed in all animals. This work, suggesting that MMF was highly effective for immunosuppression in limb transplantation, was corroborated by a study of its efficacy in a rescue model of acute rat hind limb rejection. After being postponed for 7 to 9 days following transplantation, MMF treatment completely reversed rejection in all animals studied (38). A subsequent study using MHC-mismatched rat hind limb allografts—a highly antigenic model—corroborated this finding (39). MMF, along with cyclosporine and prednisone, has permitted successful transplantation of radial forelimb osteomyocutaneous flaps in a porcine model (40). Compared to untreated controls, where

all the grafts were completely rejected by day 7, 3 of 10 pigs treated with cyclosporine (CsA), MMF, and prednisone were free of rejection at 90 days, while 3 others developed stable mild-to-moderate rejection. Two pigs died and 2 flaps were lost (by day 29) from severe rejection.

## The Effect of MMF in Animal Models of Pancreatic Islet Cell Transplantation

The efficacy of MMF treatment on murine pancreatic islet cell allografts was studied by Howe and co-workers, who observed prolongation of islet survival with treatment (41–43). Allografted islets were transplanted under the kidney capsules of recipients that received either vehicle or 30 daily oral treatments with MMF. As documented by serial blood glucose levels, the authors noted that 9 of the 10 vehicle-treated controls rejected their grafts within 14 to 20 days, whereas 7 of the 11 MMF-treated mice had functioning grafts longer than 100 days after transplantation. No obvious toxic effects were observed. The recipients who maintained a functional allograft for at least 100 days were subsequently challenged with an intraperitoneal injection of donor spleen cells. Only one of the seven recipients then rejected the islet graft. Two weeks later, these recipients were simultaneously transplanted with donor strain and with third-party thyroid tissues. After 30 days, thyroid allograft function was assayed by measuring radioiodine uptake. The donor strain thyroid allografts continued to function, whereas third-party allografts did not, suggesting that not only had MMF reduced rejection of the original islet grafts, but that it had permitted the development of a state of donor-specific tolerance. MMF has also been shown to increase whole pancreas allograft survival in a rat model (44); in combination with IL-2 toxin, it was found to significantly prolong mouse thyroid allograft survival (45). The effects of MMF in animal models of allotransplantation are summarized in Table 5.4.

**Table 5.4.**    A Summary of the Effects of Mycophenolate Mofetil in Animal Models of Allotransplantation

| Transplanted Organ | Model | Findings |
|---|---|---|
| Heart | Rat and monkey | Prolongs graft survival<br>Reverses ongoing rejection (rescue therapy)<br>Inhibits hyperacute and accelerated acute rejection<br>Protection enhanced when used in combination with cyclosporine, tacrolimus, brequinar, and leflunomide<br>Reduces antibody production<br>Decreases graft coronary artery disease |
| Kidney | Dog | Prolongs graft survival<br>Reverses ongoing rejection (rescue therapy) |
| Liver | Dog | Prolongs graft survival |
| Intestinal | Dog | Prolongs graft survival |
| Hind limb | Rat | Prolongs graft survival<br>Reverses ongoing rejection (rescue therapy) |
| Islet cell | Mouse and rat | Prolongs graft survival |
| Thyroid | Mouse | Prolongs graft survival |
| Aorta | Rat | Decreases intimal proliferation |

**Table 5.5.**    A Summary of the Effects of Mycophenolate Mofetil in Animal Models of Xenotransplantation

| Organ | Combination | Effect |
|---|---|---|
| Heart | Hamster-to-rat | Prolongs graft survival |
|  | Monkey-to-baboon | Prolongs graft survival and decreases graft coronary artery disease |
| Islet | Rat-to-hamster | Prolongs graft survival |
|  | Pig-to-rat |  |

The effect of MMF on rejection of pancreatic islet cell xenografts has also been studied in a model where rat pancreatic islet cells were transplanted into hamsters (50). Treatment with MMF prevented rejection and maintained islet capillary perfusion, while the untreated islets suffered irreversible failure of capillary perfusion and died. Furthermore, in a pig islet-to-rat model, MMF in combination with cyclosporine and leflunomide prevented islet xenograft rejection (51). The effects of MMF in xenotransplantation are summarized in Table 5.5.

## THE EFFECT OF MYCOPHENOLATE ON ANTIBODY PRODUCTION IN ANIMAL ALLOGRAFTS

To study the effect of MMF on humoral rejection, Knechtle et al placed three successive skin grafts from ACI rats to Lewis recipients at 14-day intervals (25). Assaying antibody production by the chromium-51 release assay, the authors noted significantly higher titers of complement-fixing antibodies in the untreated group. Heterotopic rat cardiac allografts were then performed in the sensitized animals. Median survival of untreated cardiac allografts was 2 days. Treatment with MMF alone increased median survival to 5 days. However, the combination of cyclosporine and MMF increased median survival to 14 days.

## THE EFFECT OF MYCOPHENOLATE ON CHRONIC REJECTION IN TRANSPLANT VASCULOPATHY IN ANIMAL MODELS

There are three mechanisms through which MMF may decrease chronic rejection and the development of intimal disease in allografts. The first possible mechanism is through a reduction in acute rejection and the consequent reduction in endothelial injury. Endothelial injury results in a cascade of events triggered to effect repair of the defect—when exuberant, this results in ongoing cellular proliferation, fibrosis, and thus luminal compromise. A reduction in endothelial injury would attenuate this process. The second means through which MMF might decrease graft vascular disease is through its effect on antibody-mediated rejection. Antibodies attack endothelial antigens directly, resulting in endothelial damage, subsequent exuberant repair, fibrosis,

## The Effects of MMF on Animal Xenograft Models

Several studies have evaluated the efficacy of MMF in combination with cyclosporine in hamster-to-rat heart xenograft models (46,47). In untreated recipients and those treated with cyclosporine alone, rejection occurred on average at 4 days following transplantation. The combination of MMF and cyclosporine increased median survival to 6 days. When cyclosporine, MMF, and brequinar were used as a triple-therapy regimen, median survival was prolonged to 33 days.

MMF has been shown to be effective in increasing the survival of cynomolgus monkey cardiac xenografts transplanted into baboons (48,49). With no treatment, severe humoral and cellular rejection occurred, resulting in a mean graft survival of 9 days. In contrast, treatment with cyclosporine and prednisone increased graft survival to 77 days, while triple therapy with cyclosporine, prednisone, and azathioprine resulted in a mean graft survival of 94 days. However, baboons receiving daily cyclosporine, prednisone, and MMF (70mg/kg/day) fared best, with a mean graft survival of 296 days. Significantly diminished xenograft vascular disease was also observed in the baboons receiving MMF. Thus, rejection in the MMF-treated baboons occurred with less frequency, less severity, and with less development of vascular disease.

and narrowing of the lumen. The third mechanism through which MMF might decrease proliferative arteriopathy in transplant vessels is through its effect on smooth muscle cells. The endothelial lesions of chronic rejection tend to be concentric atherosclerotic lesions containing both cellular and fibrous elements. The cellular growth is attributed to proliferation of both smooth muscle cells and fibroblasts (1,52). Clinically attainable concentrations of MMF have been shown to inhibit the proliferation of human arterial smooth muscle cells in culture (1). The effect of MMF on chronic rejection was evaluated in the rat heterotopic allograft model; the incidence and severity of proliferative arteriopathy was found to be low in rats treated with mycophenolate compared to those treated with cyclosporine or FK506 (23). This evidence of an antiproliferative effect was corroborated in rats using an aortic allograft model (53). In this experiment, rats were given orthotopic aortic allografts and were treated with either MMF or no immunosuppression. After three months, the allografts were harvested and evaluated using morphometric analysis. Rats treated with MMF showed much less intimal thickening, with significantly decreased cellular proliferation compared to the control group. Syngeneic aortas, used to control for nonimmunologic effects, did not develop proliferative arteriopathy. These findings are supported by data from the cynomolgus monkey heart-to-baboon recipient model described previously (49); the extent of xenograft coronary artery disease was markedly decreased in animals treated with triple therapy including MMF compared to those treated with azathioprine. Furthermore, in a canine model of allogeneic saphenous vein vasculopathy, cyclosporine and MMF reduced the development of intimal disease. In these animals both humoral and cellular responses were inhibited (54). Thus, animal allograft models suggest that MMF may be effective in attenuating chronic rejection.

## CLINICAL STUDIES

The first clinical use of MPA was in the treatment of severe psoriasis. Two studies performed in the 1970s demonstrated attenuation of psoriatic lesions following MPA administration (55,56). It was also used at that time as an antiproliferative agent in the treatment of malignancy (57,58). However, absorption of MPA was poor, and the doses used were high and poorly tolerated. Thus, interest in its use waned until the current development of its prodrug, MMF, as an immunosuppressant for use in transplantation.

### Kidney Transplantation

Based on the strong evidence from animal and in vitro models suggesting that MMF both protects against rejection and has a mild side-effect profile, clinical trials were begun. The first trial was a phase I trial designed to test the safety of MMF and to determine proper dosing. Escalating doses of MMF (100–3500 mg/day orally) were administered in

combination with cyclosporine and prednisone to patients receiving renal allografts (59–61). The efficacy of MMF and its side effect profile were evaluated in eight groups of six patients at eight different dosages. Significant correlations were observed between the MMF dose, the incidence of rejection, and the number of rescue treatments required to treat acute rejection. The most important finding was that the drug was well tolerated, and especially that there was no nephrotoxicity or hepatotoxicity. The most common side effects were gastrointestinal problems, including mild ileus, gastritis, nausea, and vomiting. The only serious side effect observed was a case of hemorrhagic gastritis, which occurred in one patient receiving 1000 mg/day. The study suggested that doses of 2000 mg/day or higher were most efficacious. Dose reduction was required in five patients because of untoward effects, including nausea and vomiting (two patients), diarrhea, myelosuppression (persistent leukopenia), and prolonged elevation in liver function tests (in a patient with hepatitis C infection). Overall, MMF was tolerated at doses of up to 3500 mg/day for up to two years. Thus, this early clinical study demonstrated that MMF could safely replace azathioprine in a triple-drug regimen.

The next investigation was a multicenter study evaluating the effect of MMF as a rescue agent (60). Seventy-five patients who had previously undergone antirejection therapy with high-dose steroids, OKT-3, or both treatments were entered into the study. Treatment consisted of MMF in doses of either 1000 mg or 1500 mg twice daily, begun within 48 hours of a biopsy confirming acute rejection by Banff criteria. During treatment, maintenance doses of cyclosporine and prednisone were maintained. Successful rescue, defined as stabilization or improvement in renal function, was achieved in 52 of the 75 patients (69%). In patients having a serum creatinine of ≤4 mg/dl at initiation of MMF therapy, a success rate of 79% was noted. No significant nephrotoxicity, hepatotoxicity, or myelosuppression were observed. Thus, this study suggested that MMF was effective for treatment of refractory renal allograft rejection.

The effect of MMF on refractory renal allograft rejection was subsequently studied in a larger trial—an open-labeled, multicenter trial in which it was compared to treatment with high-dose intravenous steroids (62). The trial assigned 150 patients randomly to either MMF or intravenous steroid treatment. Six months after enrollment, graft loss or death was 45% lower in the MMF group compared to the high-dose steroid group. This significant reduction was maintained for the subsequent 12 months. Adverse events were gastrointestinal and hematologic, primarily leukopenia. The frequency of opportunistic infections for each group was similar, and at 35% was comparable to that of previous studies.

### Heart Transplantation

The first use of MMF to treat mild rejection in cardiac patients was in an eight-week-long phase I trial (64). Oral doses of 500–3000 mg/day of MMF were substituted for azathioprine in a triple therapy regimen. In 20 of the 30 patients with biopsy-proven rejection, rejection resolved within four weeks. The authors concluded that MMF was safe in cardiac patients, and that MMF-based triple therapy was at least as effective as azathioprine triple therapy. In addition, less myelosuppression was noted with MMF than with azathioprine.

Another group also studied the use of MMF to treat recurrent or persistent heart allograft rejection (65). Seventeen patients with biopsy-proven rejection at a mean of 5.4 months following transplantation were given 3000–3500 mg/day of MMF instead of azathioprine in a standard triple therapy regimen. Of the 17 patients, 14 were doing well 10 months from the start of the MMF triple therapy regimen, and the frequency of rejection episodes was decreased following institution of MMF therapy. Gastrointestinal intolerance was the only limiting factor to the use of MMF in this group of patients. These two studies demonstrated that MMF was safe and effective for heart transplant patients.

A randomized, multicontinental trial of the effect of MMF in heart transplant recipients demonstrated that MMF decreased both mortality and rejection within the first year after cardiac transplantation (66). In this study, 650 patients in 28 centers were randomized to receive, in addition to cyclosporine and corticosteroids, 3000 mg/day of MMF or 1.5–3.0 mg/kg/day of azathioprine. The use of MMF resulted in a significant reduction in both mortality at one year (from 11% to 6%, $P = 0.03$) and the requirement for treatment of rejection within the first 6 months after transplantation (from 74% to 66%, $P = 0.03$). More patients in the MMF group were rejection free at 6 months (34% versus 26%, $P = 0.04$). In addition, high-grade rejection (grade 3 or greater) was also reduced (from 53% to 45%, $P = 0.06$). Despite reduced requirements for OKT-3 or ATGAM (from 21% to 15%, $P = 0.06$), patients receiving MMF had a greater incidence of opportunistic infections—mostly herpes simplex (55% versus 44%, $P = 0.02$). No difference between groups in the rate of CMV infection was detected. Significantly more MMF-treated patients had diarrhea (45% versus 34%, $P = 0.008$). Leukopenia, in contrast, was more common in the azathioprine group (39% versus 30%, $P = 0.04$). There was no difference between groups in the risk of lymphoma.

## Liver Transplantation

The use of MMF as rescue therapy to treat liver rejection has also been evaluated (67). In this study, patients on a standard immunotherapy regimen of cyclosporine, prednisone, and azathioprine who had biopsy-proven persistent acute rejection after initial treatment with high-dose steroids and OKT-3 were begun on MMF therapy. In 21 of 23 patients there was a significant decrease in the extent of rejection, with complete resolution in 14 of the 23 patients. There was minimal toxicity of MMF noted.

A second study evaluated the treatment of rejection in liver transplant patients with a combination of MMF and prednisone (68). Four patients with established rejection were begun on the MMF and prednisone regimen, with resolution of the rejection in all four cases. Only one patient subsequently developed recurrent rejection, which was treated with OKT-3. It was felt that MMF could be used either to eliminate or to reduce the dose of cyclosporine in patients intolerant of that drug.

Recently, Eckhoff et al (69) published a retrospective analysis of their experience with the use of MMF in liver transplantation in which 130 consecutive liver transplant recipients were studied. The first 80 recipients received tacrolimus and prednisone, while the subsequent 50 recipients received tacrolimus, prednisone, and MMF (1 g orally twice a day, tapered monthly by 250 mg twice a day until discontinuation at 3 months after transplantation). Although there were no differences in 6-month patient and graft survival between groups, the incidence of acute rejection decreased· from 61% to 28% ($P = 0.007$). All patients with rejection in the MMF group responded to a steroid bolus, whereas 3 patients in the non-MMF group required the addition of monoclonal antibody therapy (and 2 others required supplemental MMF). In addition, renal function one month after transplantation was better in the MMF-treated group (creatinine = 1.1 versus 1.5, $P = 0.0001$). No difference was observed between groups in the rate of CMV infection. Glucose intolerance after transplantation, however, was greater in the combined therapy group (26% versus 12%, $P = 0.005$).

The use of MMF with tacrolimus in liver transplantation to allow for early steroid withdrawal has been evaluated by Stegall et al (70). Of the 71 patients studied, 35 were randomized to receive tacrolimus and MMF and 36 to receive cyclosporine and MMF. In all patients, prednisone was tapered off by day 15 after transplantation. No immunologic graft loss occurred in either group and biopsy-proven rejection within the first 6 months was similarly low in both groups (46% for the tacrolimus–MMF group, 42% for the cyclosporine–MMF group). Another study comparing tacrolimus to cyclosporine in liver transplant patients receiving MMF also demonstrated excellent results with both regimens. Indeed, rejection within 6 months of transplantation occurred in only 19% of patients for both groups (71).

The use of MMF in liver transplantation does not appear to increase the risk of infection in recipients (72). In a retrospective study from the University of Pittsburgh, 16 patients who received MMF to permit reduction in the doses of tacrolimus (required because of neurotoxicity or nephrotoxicity) were compared to 136 patients who received tacrolimus and prednisone, but no MMF. Despite a decrease in the incidence of rejection within the first 6 months from 30% to 6% with MMF, no significant increase in CMV infection or disease, PCP pneumonia, fungal infection, or recurrence in hepatitis C was observed. There was an increase in bacterial infections noted in the MMF group

(69% versus 36%, *P* = 0.02), but longer intensive care unit stays for patients in this group may have accounted for the difference.

## Pancreas Transplantation

MMF has been an extremely important addition to the arsenal of immunosuppression in pancreas transplantation. It has decreased rejection in pancreas transplantation so dramatically that it has allowed the switch from bladder drainage to enteric drainage and is responsible for the recent success with transplantation of the pancreas alone. Sollinger et al, summarizing their experience with simultaneous pancreas–kidney (SPK) transplantation, demonstrated marked improvements in allograft survival, with 2-year renal and pancreas graft survival rates increasing from 86% to 95% (*P* = 0.02) and 83% to 95% (*P* = 0.02), respectively, in the MMF era (versus azathioprine) (73,74). Patient survival rates at 2 years also improved, from 95% to 99% (*P* = NS). These increases in survival were largely due to markedly decreased rejection, with renal allograft rejection decreasing from 75% to 31% (*P* = 0.001) with MMF. Steroid refractory rejection was also reduced, from 24% to 7% (*P* = 0.01).

Similar improvements in patient and graft survival in pancreas transplantation were observed by Gruessner et al (75). Evaluating 61 SPK transplants, 44 pancreas-after-kidney (PAK) transplants, and 15 pancreas transplants alone (PTA), they observed that in the SPK population pancreas survival at one year increased from 79% to 86% versus azathioprine (*P* = NS) and kidney survival increased from 86% to 96% (*P* = NS). The incidence of rejection was significantly reduced with the use of MMF (in combination with tacrolimus), from 43% for azathioprine (AZA) to 15% with MMF (*P* = 0.0003). Notably, 50% of recipients in this series developed GI toxicity (toxicity responded to reduction of the dose of MMF or to switching to AZA, which occurred in 14% of patients within 1 year). A third, smaller analysis of the use of MMF in SPK transplantation also demonstrated similar reductions in rejection (76). In this study, patients who received tacrolimus and MMF (18 patients) or cyclosporine and MMF (18 patients) were compared to recipients who received cyclosporine and AZA. Biopsy-proven rejection within the first 6 months of transplantation was reduced from 77% in the AZA group (a historical group) to 11% for both MMF groups (*P* = 0.01).

## PHASE III CLINICAL TRIALS OF MMF IN THE PREVENTION OF ACUTE RENAL ALLOGRAFT REJECTION

The large body of experimental and clinical evidence summarized above indicated that MMF is a powerful immunosuppressant with a favorable side-effect profile and led to worldwide evaluation of the drug in renal transplantation. Three international, multicenter, randomized, phase III clinical trials of MMF as an immunosuppressant for renal allo-

graft rejection were initiated. These studies have now been completed, and the success of the drug demonstrated by these studies prompted rapid FDA approval of MMF for the prevention of renal allograft rejection.

The US multicenter study, a prospective, randomized, double-blind study that enrolled 499 patients in 14 states, used standard four-drug therapy (77). All patients received ATGAM for induction therapy, along with a triple-drug immunosuppression regimen consisting of cyclosporine and corticosteroid therapy, accompanied by either 2 mg/kg/day of azathioprine (166 patients), 2 g/day of MMF (167 patients), or 3 g/day of MMF (166 patients). As shown in Table 5.6, biopsy-proven acute rejection episodes or treatment failures were significantly decreased with MMF. MMF-treated patients had a 31% rate of treatment failure or acute rejection for both the 2-g/day and 3-g/day treatment groups. This was in contrast to a 48% failure rate in the azathioprine group. These were statistically significant differences. In addition, patients in the azathioprine group required a significantly greater number of full courses of antirejection therapy compared to both MMF groups. Most important, the rate of biopsy-proven rejection was essentially cut in half with MMF therapy, dropping from 38% in the azathioprine group, to 20% in the 2 g/day MMF group, and 18% in the 3 g/day MMF group. The incidence of leukopenia and tissue-invasive cytomegalovirus (CMV) disease was slightly higher in the MMF groups. Otherwise, the toxicities were similar. A study comparing the cost effectiveness of MMF 2 g/day and AZA in the patients enrolled in the US multicenter study revealed that, despite its greater cost, MMF, by decreasing rejection, dialysis, and graft failure (without changing the cost of treating opportunistic infections), yielded slightly lower first-year costs than AZA (US$29,158 versus US$27,807) (78).

The European Mycophenolate Mofetil Cooperative Study Group evaluated the effect of mycophenolate as a component of triple therapy in 491 patients receiving cadaveric renal allografts (79). This also was a randomized, double-blind, controlled trial. Patients were given standard

**Table 5.6.** Incidence of Treatment Failure, Early Termination, and Rejection in US MMF Versus Azathioprine Study of Renal Allograft Rejection[a]

| | AZA | MMF 2 g/day | MMF 3 g/day |
|---|---|---|---|
| Number of patients | 166 | 167 | 166 |
| All treatment failures | 48% | 31% | 31% |
| Biopsy-proven rejection | 38% | 20% | 18% |
| Biopsy-proven or presumptive rejection | 46% | 26% | 24% |
| Early termination[b] | 6% | 10% | 13% |

[a] Regimen included antithymocyte globulin induction therapy.
[b] Without prior acute rejection; does not include death and graft loss.
AZA = azathioprine; MMF = mycophenolate mofetil.

immunotherapy with corticosteroids, cyclosporine, and either placebo, MMF 2 g/day, or MMF 3 g/day. Biopsy-proven allograft rejection or treatment failure for any other reason were considered the primary efficacy variables. Acute rejection was treated with high-dose intravenous corticosteroids, and if necessary, with antilymphocyte agents. As shown in Table 5.7, MMF in the setting of triple therapy significantly reduced the incidence of rejection episodes or treatment failures. Indeed, the reduction was greater than 50%. The placebo group had a 56% incidence of treatment failure, in contrast to 30% for the 2 g/day MMF group and 39% for the 3 g/day MMF group. These were statistically significant differences. The need for treatment of rejection with corticosteroids or antilymphocyte agents dropped as well, from 59% in patients receiving placebo to 29% for those receiving 2 g/day of MMF and to 24% for those receiving 3 g/day of MMF. With the exception of usually mild gastrointestinal problems, leukopenia, and opportunistic infections, the frequency of adverse events was similar in all treatment groups. These findings corroborated the US study, demonstrating that MMF was effective in the prevention of renal allograft rejection and was well tolerated.

The largest study, a tricontinental study, took place at 21 sites in Australia, Canada, and Europe. The efficacy of MMF as a component of triple therapy was compared to that of azathioprine (80). A total of 503 patients were randomly assigned to one of three treatment groups, receiving corticosteroid and cyclosporine treatment, as well as either 100–150 mg/day of azathioprine (166 patients), 2 g/day of MMF (173 patients), or 3 g/day of MMF (164 patients). Again, biopsy-proven rejection or treatment failure for any reason occurring within the first 6 months of transplantation was the primary determinant of efficacy. As summarized in Table 5.8, patients receiving MMF had significantly fewer treatment failures than did the patients receiving azathioprine therapy; MMF patients also had significantly fewer episodes of rejection. Specifically, 36% of the azathioprine-treated patients had biopsy-proven rejection versus 20% of those in the 2 g/day MMF treatment group and 16% of

those in the 3 g/day MMF treatment group. Although the side-effect profiles of the drugs were similar, the MMF treatment groups did have higher rates of attrition for non-rejection-related events.

The 3-year follow-up to this study (which was not designed for the evaluation of long-term end points) demonstrated continued improved patient and graft survival for the recipients receiving MMF, but the differences were not statistically significant (81). With 50% of the patients remaining in the study at 3 years, by intent to treat, the total rate of graft loss was 20% for the AZA group, 18% for the MMF 2 g/day group, and 15% for the MMF 3 g/day group. Excluding death as a cause of graft loss, the rates for graft loss were 15% for the AZA group, 15% for the MMF 2 g/day group, and 8% for the MMF 3 g/day group. There was no difference in creatinine or the incidence of proteinuria between groups at 3 years, suggesting that there was no major difference in the effect on chronic rejection. As had been seen at one year, the MMF groups had slightly greater gastrointestinal toxicity, infection, and malignancy. There were no differences in lymphoproliferative disorders: PTLD occurred in 1 patient (0.6%) in the AZA group, 2 patients (1.2%) in the MMF 2 g/day group, and 3 patients (1.8%) in the MMF 3 g/day group. Perhaps the most important finding was that there was no change in the adverse event profile of MMF from that observed at 1 year; thus, long-term treatment with MMF appears to be safe.

The data from all three international phase III studies has been pooled and analyzed as a single study (82). This combined analysis revealed no real differences in results from the individual studies, but strengthened their findings. Specifically, 1-year graft survival for the 1493 patients from the three studies was 90% for the MMF 2 g/day group, 89% for the MMF 3 g/day group, and 88% for the placebo–AZA group ($P$ = NS). There was also no significant difference between groups in patient survival at one year: 95% for the placebo–AZA and MMF 3 g/day groups, and 96% for the MMF 2 g/day group. Graft loss due to rejection, however, was significantly greater in the placebo–AZA group (6%) than in the MMF groups (3% for MMF 2 g/day, 4% for MMF 3 g/day, $P$ = 0.004). This reflected significantly greater

**Table 5.7.**    Incidence of Rejection, Graft Loss/Death, and Other Treatment Failures at 6 Months for the European MMF Versus Placebo Study of Renal Allograft Rejection

|  | Placebo | MMF 2 g/day | MMF 3 g/day |
|---|---|---|---|
| Number of patients | 166 | 165 | 160 |
| All treatment failures (biopsy-proven rejection, graft loss/death, other) | 56% | 30% | 39% |
| Biopsy-proven rejection | 46% | 17% | 14% |
| Graft loss/death | 2% | 2% | 3% |
| Other (any reason) | 7% | 12% | 23% |

MMF = mycophenolate mofetil.

**Table 5.8.**    Incidence of Treatment Failure, Early Termination, and Biopsy-Proven Rejection in Tricontinental (Australia, Canada, and Europe) MMF Versus Azathioprine Study of Renal Allograft Rejection

|  | AZA | MMF 2 g/day | MMF 3 g/day |
|---|---|---|---|
| Number of patients | 166 | 173 | 164 |
| All treatment failures | 50% | 38% | 35% |
| Biopsy-proven rejection | 36% | 20% | 16% |
| Early termination* | 10% | 14% | 15% |

\* Without prior acute rejection; does not include death and graft loss.
AZA = azathioprine; MMF = mycophenolate mofetil.

rates of rejection at 6 months in the placebo–AZA group (41%) than in the MMF 2 g/day group (20%) and in the MMF 3 g/day group (16%) (*P* < 0.001). Consequently, the requirement for antilymphocyte therapy to treat steroid-resistant rejection was greatest in the placebo–AZA group at 20%, versus 9% in the MMF 2 g/day group and 5% in the MMF 3 g/day group. Thus, with no increase in mortality compared to AZA, MMF provided better protection from rejection and graft loss due to rejection.

Similar survival rates and rates of rejection were noted in another placebo-controlled, multicenter study performed in Europe (83). The rates of biopsy-proven rejection within the first year dropped from 46% in the placebo group to 18% in the 2 g/day and 14% in the 3 g/day MMF groups (*P* < 0.001). The requirement for antibody therapy for rejection dropped commensurately.

The use of MMF to treat established rejection has also been evaluated (84). In this double-blinded, controlled trial in 221 renal transplant recipients, MMF, in combination with a corticosteroid bolus and taper, was found to be more effective in treating established rejection than a cortico-steroid–AZA regimen. The addition of MMF to the regimen significantly reduced the requirement for antilymphocyte therapy compared to the addition of AZA. This suggests that if a patient is not on MMF at the time of rejection, then it should be started to enhance the response to the steroid bolus.

The efficacy of MMF in the African-American population was evaluated in a reexamination of the data from the US Renal Transplant Mycophenolate Mofetil Study Group (85). African-American recipients of renal transplants benefited from MMF, but required a higher dose (3 g/day) than the non-African Americans. Of the 495 patients studied, 117 (24%) were African American. Biopsy-proven rejection (Banff criteria) in African Americans was diminished from 48% for AZA to 32% for MMF 2 g/day and 12% for MMF 3 g/day (*P* = NS). Similar efficacy was observed in the non-African-American population, but an MMF dose of 2 g/day was adequate. Specifically, 36% of the non-African-American recipients on AZA rejected within the first 6 months, compared to 16% on MMF 2 g/day and 19% on MMF 3 g/day. When rejection and treatment failure (graft loss, death, or withdrawal from the study for any reason without prior rejection) were considered together, the requirement for greater doses of MMF in African Americans became more evident. Fifty-seven percent of African Americans in the AZA group and 32% in the MMF 2 g/day group experienced rejection or treatment failure. In contrast, only 24% in the MMF 3 g/day group experienced such an adverse event (*P* = 0.0008 versus AZA). For the non-African-American patients, 44% in the AZA group, 27% in the MMF 2 g/day group (*P* = 0.007 versus AZA), and 33% in the 3 g/day group (*P* = 0.08 versus AZA) had an adverse event.

The inadequacy of 2 g/day of MMF in African-American recipients of renal transplants was also observed in a single center study that compared MMF 2 g/day to

AZA (86). For Caucasians, biopsy-proven rejection at 6 months dropped from 42% to 17% (*P* < 0.001) with MMF. In contrast, for African Americans receiving 2 g/day of MMF, it only decreased from 37% to 31% (*P* = 0.4).

Thus, three large international, multicenter, randomized studies have demonstrated that MMF is significantly more efficacious than azathioprine or placebo in preventing acute kidney allograft rejection. Now the major concern is not the efficacy of the drug, but the gastrointestinal intolerance to MMF. There is also concern that the stronger immuno-suppression effected by MMF might result in greater rates of opportunistic infections, such as CMV and other viruses.

The use of MMF in combination with tacrolimus in renal transplant patients has also been studied. Roth et al (87) retrospectively compared 72 patients who received MMF, tacrolimus, and corticosteroids to 98 patients who received only tacrolimus and corticosteroids. They observed significantly reduced rejection in the MMF group (8% versus 21%, *P* = 0.003). This difference persisted when the recipient's race was considered, with rejection declining from 22% to 14% in Caucasians and from 28% to 10% in African Americans. One-year patient and graft survival did not differ between treatment groups. There also was no difference in post-transplant diabetes mellitus (18% in the MMF group versus 21% in the no MMF group). CMV viremia, however, was significantly more common in patients who received MMF (15% versus 2%, *P* = 0.0001).

## MMF IN THE TREATMENT OF CHRONIC REJECTION

With the demonstrated in vitro attenuation of B-cell, fibroblast, and smooth muscle cell activity, it has been hypothesized that MMF might also inhibit the development of chronic rejection. No large studies evaluating the effect of MMF on chronic rejection have been published, but early analyses of its long-term efficacy in the phase III studies have not identified a major impact on chronic rejection. Indeed, no significant difference in graft survival or serum creatinine at 3 years was detected in MMF and AZA groups in the Tricontinental Mycophenolate Mofetil Renal Transplantation Study Group (which was not designed for evaluation of the effects of MMF on chronic rejection) (68a). However, encouraging results have been obtained from several small, preliminary studies of the use of MMF as a replacement for, or to permit reduction of the dose of, cyclosporine in patients with chronic cyclosporine-associated nephrotoxicity (88–91).

## THE EFFECT OF MMF ON ANTIBODY PRODUCTION IN HUMANS

A study by Kimball et al evaluated the effect of MMF on anti-ATGAM (IgG) antibody formation in renal transplant recipients (63). Forty-seven patients receiving ATGAM and standard therapy with prednisone and cyclosporine were randomized to receive, in addition, either azathioprine or MMF. Anti-ATGAM antibody was detected in 67% of patients receiving azathioprine, in 17% of those receiving MMF at 25 mg/kg/day, and in only 10% of those receiving MMF at 30 mg/kg/day ($P < 0.02$).

Suppression of the humoral immune response by MMF has also been demonstrated by Smith et al (92), who observed a profound (and statistically significant) depression in the response to influenza vaccination in patients immunosuppressed with MMF. Fifty percent of the nonimmunosuppressed controls responded to the vaccination, 33% of the recipients who received AZA responded, but only 10% of the recipients who received MMF responded.

These studies provide further evidence that MMF attenuates the humoral arm of the human immune system.

## PHARMACOKINETICS

As noted earlier, mycophenolate mofetil, a prodrug, was developed by researchers at Syntex who were searching for a conjoiner of MPA with increased oral bioavailability. MMF, the morpholinoethyl ester of MPA (Fig. 5.4) was thus developed. It was initially found in primates to have twice the bioavailability of MPA (93,94). MMF is rapidly hydrolyzed by gastrointestinal tract esterases to MPA, its active metabolite. This metabolism is so rapid and complete that no measurable concentrations of MMF in the plasma have been obtained in healthy volunteers or transplant patients after oral administration (95,96). Mycophenolic acid is then converted in the liver (and likely elsewhere) to its glucuronide metabolite, mycophenolic acid glucuronide (MAPG), which is pharmacologically inactive (see Fig. 5.4). The glucuronide moiety is excreted in the urine; in fact, an average of 90% of radiolabeled drug was recovered in the

urine after oral administration to healthy volunteers (97). This confirms that MAPG is indeed the primary metabolite of MPA, and that urinary excretion is its primary route of clearance. MAPG undergoes significant enterohepatic circulation, which results in considerable deglucuronidation and reabsorption as MPA. Enterohepatic circulation produces secondary peaks occurring between 6 and 12 hours following ingestion, and again at approximately 24 hours (96,97). Thus, the mean elimination half-life is approximately 16 hours. The pharmacologic activity of MMF is a function of the concentration of free MPA in the plasma (96,97). MPA is extensively bound to serum albumin in humans. Cyclosporine, FK506, and prednisone do not alter this binding (98). As shown in healthy volunteers, MPA reaches its peak plasma concentration at approximately 1 hour following MMF dosing. However, absorption is delayed for approximately 1 hour in the presence of food (96). The area under the plasma concentration time curve (AUC) for MPA increases in a dose-dependent fashion (59). In the phase I trial, it was noted that blood concentrations of MPA were low in the initial post-transplant period; however, they significantly increased over time. In addition, considerable variation in peak and trough concentrations of MPA were seen between individual patients. The long elimination half-life and the extensive protein binding of MPA may be the cause of the variation in blood concentration between that seen early after renal transplantation and that seen later on. Differences in absorption of MMF do not seem to play a role early on, as there is no significant difference in the AUC between oral and intravenous administration immediately after transplantation (oral and IV MMF have equivalent bioavailabilities) (99). Renal impairment has no effect on the pharmacokinetics of MPA, but it does decrease the clearance of MPAG (as a function of glomeru-

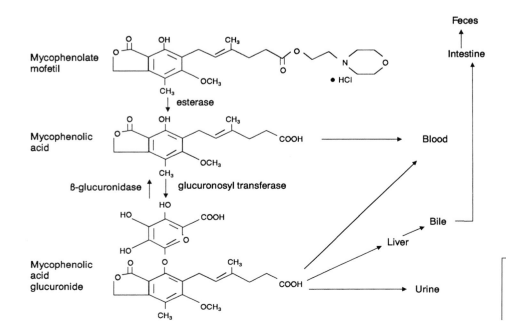

**FIGURE 5.4.**    *The chemical structures of mycophenolate mofetil, mycophenolic acid, and the glucuronide metabolite.*

lar filtration rate). Indeed, the AUCs for MPAG, which is inactive, can increase two to threefold with renal dysfunction after transplantation. Serum levels of the drug are not significantly affected by hemodialysis (96). In addition, the pharmacokinetics of MMF are not changed by coadministration of ganciclovir (100).

## THERAPEUTIC DRUG MONITORING

Plasma levels of MPA are measured using high-pressure liquid chromatography. Clinical pharmacokinetic studies suggest a strong correlation between the area under the MPA 24-hour curve and the prevention of rejection (60,97,101). Only free MPA is active (95,97,102). Although direct measurement of MPA is useful, new modes of evaluation to determine the most effective plasma levels for MPA are being developed. Specifically, IMPDH activity in whole blood can be monitored to determine the degree of inhibition of this enzyme by MPA (103,104). Langman et al (105) studied such monitoring in normal patients and in renal transplant recipients. They demonstrated that, in vitro, the maximum inhibition of IMPDH in intact cells in whole blood is 60% to 70%. Fifty percent inhibition occurred at 2–5 mg/L and complete inhibition of IMPDH activity was achieved in lysed cells with 20 mg/L. In vivo, the expected inverse relationship between MPA concentration and IMPDH activity was observed. The maximal inhibition detected, at peak concentrations (occurring 1 hour after dosing), produced 40% inhibition of IMPDH activity. Thus, perhaps only downregulation, not complete inhibition, is required to achieve immunosuppression. Inhibition of IMPDH activity persisted for 8 hours after dosing and little or no inhibition was detected at 12 hours after dosing, suggesting that an 8-hour dosing interval might maintain optimal inhibition of IMPDH. In the 23 normal subjects tested in this study, IMPDH activity followed a gaussian distribution and exhibited considerable variation between subjects (the standard deviation was relatively large with respect to the mean). Such variability might indicate that IMPDH activity in patients should be monitored. To justify widespread monitoring of IMPDH activity, however, the dose–activity relationship must be confirmed in large populations and the minimal activity level required for adequate immunosuppression must also be determined. In practice, drug concentrations or activity measurements may not be needed because interindividual variability in MPA concentrations has been relatively low and the therapeutic, yet tolerable dose range of MMF (2–3 g/day) remains narrow (99). Multicenter trials are required to determine whether MPA levels or IMPDH activity should be routinely monitored.

## ADVERSE EFFECTS

The effects of MMF have been studied in over 1500 patients. The major adverse effects of MMF are gastrointestinal and hematologic. Most of the adverse effects are mild, and discontinuation of MMF is seldom required. The most common gastrointestinal side effects are abdominal

**Table 5.9.**    Infections and Adverse Effects from the US Renal Transplant Mycophenolate Mofetil Study Group

| Group | AZA (1–2 mg/kg) | MMF (1 g/BID) | MMF (1.5 g/BID) |
|---|---|---|---|
| Patients enrolled | 166 | 167 | 166 |
| Patients with 1 or more opportunistic infection | 46% | 45% | 47% |
| CMV viremia syndrome | 15% | 15% | 13% |
| Tissue-invasive CMV | 6% | 9% | 11% |
| Herpes simplex | 14% | 13% | 15% |
| Herpes zoster | 4% | 5% | 7% |
| *Candida* | 23% | 19% | 22% |
| Diarrhea | 24% | 32% | 37% |
| Esophagitis | 3% | 6% | 7% |
| Gastritis | 0% | 6% | 4% |
| Gastrointestinal hemorrhage | 1% | 4% | 4% |
| Lymphoma/lymphoproliferative disorder | 0% | 1% | 1% |
| Neutropenia (absolute neutrophil count <500/μL) | 1% | 1% | 1% |
| Thrombocytopenia (<50/mL in the first 30 days) | 1% | 1% | 3% |
| Severe anemia (hemoglobin <6.5 mg/dL) | 4% | 4% | 8% |

Mild anemia and hypertension, like diarrhea, were relatively common, but their rates (37% for anemia and 31% for hypertension) did not differ between treatment groups. Leukopenia (1%) and sepsis (1%), which also occurred at similar rates between groups, were the most frequent adverse events leading to discontinuation of the drug.

pain, nausea, diarrhea, gastroenteritis, and gastritis. The most common hematologic disorders are leukopenia and thrombocytopenia, with occasional pancytopenia. As with other immunosuppressive modalities, opportunistic infections, especially with CMV, are somewhat common. Lymphomas have been reported infrequently, and there is reason to believe that the antiproliferative effect of MMF may decrease the rates of lymphoma. The adverse effects observed in the US multicenter study are listed in Table 5.9.

## DRUG INTERACTIONS

The serum concentrations of cyclosporine and tacrolimus are unaltered by MMF. However, tacrolimus appears to increase the immunosuppressive activity of MMF (106). Absorption of MMF is close to 100%, but antacids containing magnesium and aluminum can interfere with absorption, and should not be given concurrently with MMF (96). Cholestyramine decreases enterohepatic recycling, and therefore, decreases the 24-hour AUC for MPA. Thus, bile acid binders should be avoided (95,96).

## CONCLUSION

The introduction of MMF into clinical transplantation may be the most important advance since the introduction of the immunophilin binders cyclosporine and tacrolimus. The theoretical considerations of Allison, Nelson, and Eugui have been borne out in the clinical trials of MMF in transplantation. Other than infrequent myelosuppression and gastrointestinal toxicity, which is usually mild, there are minimal untoward effects from treatment with MMF. Because of its greater immunosuppressive activity, however, there does appear to be a higher incidence of tissue-invasive CMV disease.

With the major advances achieved in the treatment of acute allograft rejection, attention is now being focused on chronic rejection. There are several theoretical considerations suggesting that MMF may play a significant role in reducing the severity of chronic rejection. This remains to be seen as long-term data from treatment with MMF become available. Thus, MMF proven safe and efficacious for prevention of rejection in renal allografts, is now being evaluated in the prevention and treatment of rejection in other solid organs. In addition, MMF may have uses outside the realm of transplantation.

## COMMENTARY

*Carl G. Groth and Christina Brattström*

During the past two decades, immunosuppressive protocols have been based on cyclosporine. More recently, tacrolimus has emerged as an interesting alternative. Both of these drugs are characterized by high efficacy but also by dose-limiting, multiorgan toxicity. The goal for the future is to find more specific, less toxic immunosuppressive agents.

Mycophenolate mofetil (MMF) has been introduced as a novel immunosuppressive agent with significant efficacy, high specificity, and low toxicity. Over 3000 patients have by now been enrolled in studies of this drug. Its toxicity differs distinctly from that of cyclosporine and tacrolimus, as the toxic symptoms arise mainly in the gastrointestinal tract and the hematologic system (1). In this commentary, we have elected to focus on the safety of MMF. Also, we have some comments concerning ways of using the drug in clinical practice.

## CLINICAL TRIALS

Pioneer studies in animals and humans were performed by Morris (2), Sollinger (3), and their colleagues in the early 1990s. In 1992, three large, prospective, randomized, multicenter studies in renal transplant recipients were launched. One study was located in Europe (4), one covered three continents (5), and the third was done in the United States (6). Each of the studies recruited nearly 500 patients, making this the most ambitious scheme ever employed in evaluating an immunosuppressive agent. The three studies were similar in design, patient population, and timing. All patients received cadaveric renal transplants, and the baseline immunosuppression used was cyclosporine and prednisolone. In the US study the patients were also given antithymocyte globulin (ATG) for induction (6).

In each study the patients were randomized into three groups: 1) control patients, 2) patients given MMF, 2 g/day, and 3) patients given MMF, 3 g/day. In the European study, control patients were given placebo. In the two other studies they received azathioprine. The primary end point of the studies was treatment failure or the occurrence of acute rejection.

Findings in the three studies were remarkably similar, in that the frequency of acute rejection in patients given MMF was approximately half of that in the control groups, whether the latter patients had received azathioprine or placebo (4–6). However, the graft and patient survival figures at 6 and 12 months after transplantation were no better in patients given MMF.

## SAFETY OF MMF

The European study, comparing MMF with placebo, was particularly relevant in regards to assessing the toxicity of MMF (4).

In the placebo group, 4% of the patients suffered adverse events that led to discontinuation of the treatment. The corresponding figures were 8.5% in the MMF 2 g/day, and 18% in the MMF 3 g/day groups. Gastrointestinal problems were the most common adverse events. Some symptoms, such as diarrhea, abdominal pain, and dyspepsia, were equally prevalent in all three groups. Stomach and duodenal ulcers, which occurred in a few patients, were also equally distributed between the three groups. Nausea, gastroenteritis, and vomiting, however, were more common in the MMF-treated patients, and these symptoms were most frequently seen in the MMF 3 g/day patients. Life-threatening complications—gastrointestinal hemorrhage, large bowel perforation, and pancreatitis—occurred in a small number of patients treated with MMF, but not in any patient given placebo (Table 5C.1).

Hematologic problems comprised the second largest group of adverse events. Thus, leukopenia had an approximately threefold higher incidence in the MMF-treated patients than in the placebo-treated patients. Anemia was also observed more frequently in the two MMF groups. Thrombocytopenia was equally common in all three groups. Pancytopenia occurred in two MMF 2 g/day patients, and agranulocytosis occurred in two of the MMF 3 g/day patients. All four patients recovered after cessation of MMF (Table 5C.2).

**Table 5C.1.**   Gastrointestinal Adverse Events, European Study

| | Placebo (n = 166) | MMF 2 grams (n = 165) | MMF 3 grams (n = 160) |
|---|---|---|---|
| Diarrhea | 21 (12.7%) | 21 (12.7%) | 25 (15.6%) |
| Abdominal pain | 18 (10.8%) | 19 (11.5%) | 18 (11.3%) |
| Dyspepsia | 9 (5.4%) | 5 (3.0%) | 8 (5.0%) |
| Nausea | 4 (2.4%) | 7 (4.2%) | 10 (6.3%) |
| Gastroenteritis | 2 (1.2%) | 4 (2.4%) | 7 (4.4%) |
| Vomiting | 2 (1.2%) | 4 (2.4%) | 6 (3.8%) |
| Stomach ulcer | 3 (1.8%) | 2 (1.2%) | 2 (1.3%) |
| Duodenal ulcer | 1 (0.6%) | 2 (1.2%) | 1 (0.6%) |
| Gastrointestinal hemorrhage | 0 | 0 | 2 (1.3%) |
| Rectal hemorrhage | 0 | 1 (0.6%) | 1 (0.6%) |
| Duodenal ulcer hemorrhage | 0 | 1 (0.6%) | 0 |
| Hemorrhagic pancreatitis and gastritis | 0 | 0 | 1 (0.6%) |
| Large intestine perforation | 0 | 2 (1.2%) | 2 (1.3%) |

**Table 5C.2.**   Hematologic/Lymphatic Adverse Events, European Study

| | Placebo (n = 166) | MMF 2 grams (n = 165) | MMF 3 grams (n = 160) |
|---|---|---|---|
| Leukopenia | 7 (4.2%) | 18 (10.9%) | 22 (13.8%) |
| Anemia | 3 (1.8%) | 7 (4.2%) | 11 (6.8%) |
| Thrombocytopenia | 8 (4.8%) | 7 (4.2%) | 5 (3.1%) |
| Pancytopenia | 0 | 3 (1.8%) | 0 |
| Agranulocytosis | 0 | 0 | 2 (1.3%) |
| Other | 8 (4.8%) | 17 (10.3%) | 8 (5.0%) |

**Table 5C.3.**   Opportunistic Infections, European Study

| | Placebo (n = 166) | MMF 2 grams (n = 165) | MMF 3 grams (n = 160) |
|---|---|---|---|
| CMV viremia/ syndrome | 22 (13.3%) | 26 (15.8%) | 24 (15.0%) |
| CMV tissue-invasive disease | 4 (2.4%) | 5 (3.0%) | 11 (6.9%) |
| Herpes simplex | 10 (6.0%) | 24 (14.5%) | 18 (11.3%) |
| Herpes zoster | 3 (1.8%) | 11 (6.7%) | 8 (5.0%) |
| *Candida* | 13 (7.8%) | 16 (9.7%) | 9 (5.6%) |
| *Pneumocystis carinii* pneumonia | 4 (2.4%) | 0 | 0 |
| *Aspergillus/Mucor* | 1 (0.6%) | 0 | 0 |

**Table 5C.4.**   Adverse Events Excluding Infections, Tricontinental Study

| | AZA 100–150 mg (n = 162) | MMF 2 grams (n = 171) | MMF 3 grams (n = 164) |
|---|---|---|---|
| **Gastrointestinal** | | | |
| Diarrhea | 17% | 28% | 31% |
| Abdominal pain | 23% | 26% | 31% |
| Nausea | 20% | 14% | 20% |
| Vomiting | 6% | 12% | 16% |
| **Hematologic** | | | |
| Leukopenia | 30% | 19% | 35% |
| Anemia | 10% | 15% | 9% |
| Thrombocytopenia | 12% | 9% | 5% |

Since patients in the MMF arms were given an additional immunosuppressive drug, they ran an obvious risk of developing opportunistic infections. Indeed, herpes zoster and herpes simplex were more common in the MMF-treated patients, and CMV tissue-invasive disease was overrepresented in the MMF 3 g/day group (Table 5C.3). Cytomegalovirus (CMV) viremia/syndrome, however, was equally common in the three groups, as were candidal infections.

In the tricontinental study comparing MMF to azathioprine, gastrointestinal and hematologic symptoms were again the main adverse events (5). Interestingly, the overall incidence of these events was quite similar in all three treatment arms. Diarrhea seemed more common in the MMF-treated patients, whereas thrombocytopenia was perhaps less common (Table 5C.4).

The more severe GI complications in MMF 3 g/day patients included enteric infections (n = 9), colitis (n = 3), and hepatitis (n = 5). These conditions, along with nausea, were the main events leading to discontinuation or interruption of the MMF treatment. With regard to infectious events, CMV tissue-invasive disease occurred more frequently in patients who were given 3 g/day MMF than in those given 2 g/day MMF or azathioprine (Table 5C.5).

In the US study, which also made a comparison with azathioprine, the toxicity findings were very similar to those of the tricontinental study (6). However, the incidence of CMV tissue-invasive disease was no higher in the MMF 3 g/day group than in the MMF 2 g/day or azathioprine group.

Data from the placebo-controlled study (4) thus confirmed early findings (1) that MMF may cause significant GI and hematologic toxicity. In most instances these adverse events were mild or moderate, but in some instances life-threatening conditions occurred. As could be expected, adding MMF to cyclosporine and prednisolone caused an increased incidence of viral infections.

**Table 5C.5.**    Infections, Tricontinental Study

| | AZA 100–150 mg (n = 162) | MMF 2 grams (n = 171) | MMF 3 grams (n = 164) |
|---|---|---|---|
| Opportunistic infections | 44% | 46% | 46% |
| CMV viremia/ syndrome | 12% | 12% | 11% |
| CMV tissue-invasive disease | 6% | 7% | 11% |
| Herpes simplex | 25% | 21% | 25% |
| Herpes zoster | 7% | 7% | 8% |
| Candida | 12% | 12% | 12% |
| P. carinii pneumonia | 2 | 0 | 0 |
| Aspergillus/Mucor | <1% | <1% | <1% |

Taken together, the tricontinental and the US study included approximately 300 patients who were given azathioprine. The monitoring of these patients has provided an up-to-date database regarding the safety of this classic drug. It is noteworthy that the incidences of leukopenia and anemia were very similar with the azathioprine and MMF treatments. Surprisingly, the incidence of gastrointestinal adverse events was no less in azathioprine-treated patients than in those given MMF—azathioprine is apparently more toxic in this respect than hitherto reported. Regarding viral infections, the findings were very similar in patients given azathioprine and those given MMF.

## FUTURE CLINICAL APPLICATIONS OF MMF

Initially, MMF was tried in patients with renal allograft rejection during cyclosporine-based treatment. When these patients had MMF added, more than half of the grafts were rescued (7). More recently, similar results were obtained in a larger study where MMF or steroids were given for refractory rejection (8). Thus, MMF can be used for graft rescue, as has been done with tacrolimus.

The three large multicenter studies have proved that MMF effectively prevents renal graft rejection. A case can therefore be made for employing the drug routinely in all renal transplant recipients. However, some groups have chosen a more restricted use. One reason for this is that the 1-year patient and graft survival figures have not shown significant improvement by MMF treatment. The patients selected for MMF treatment may be immunologically high-risk patients or those who are particularly vulnerable for steroid treatment.

Thus, it may seem rational to limit MMF treatment to the first 6 or perhaps 12 months, as most acute rejection episodes occur within this time. Cost containment could favor such a policy. Such short-term treatment, however, would preclude or reduce the possible gains in regard to chronic rejection.

Because of its ability to suppress B-cell and antibody production, and to inhibit vascular smooth-muscle cell proliferation, MMF has been heralded as a drug that could be effective in chronic rejection. Long-term evaluation of patients in the prevention studies will, hopefully, elucidate this matter. Studies aimed at treatment of chronic rejection are also being contemplated. Patients developing chronic rejection could be randomized to receive MMF or placebo, with renal function and graft histology serving as study parameters. However, no such study has yet been implemented.

On the basis of the findings in the three multicenter studies, the preferred dose of MMF seems to be 2 g/day. This dose was just as effective as 3 g/day in preventing rejection and it has significantly less toxicity. However, MMF at 3 g/day may be used in selected patients. In case of toxicity, a temporary reduction in doses can be made, but prolonged treatment with doses below 2 g/day may not provide adequate immunosuppression. Doses above 3 g/day should not be used, for toxicity reasons.

With the advent of a new immunosuppressive drug, an important question is whether the drug will permit sparing of the old drugs. Indeed, studies in which MMF is given in conjunction with reduced doses of steroids or cyclosporine are in progress. The results are eagerly awaited.

A combination of MMF with other new immunosuppressive drugs offers another highly interesting possibility. Two ongoing studies in renal transplant recipients are exploring such combinations. In a European multicenter phase II study, the efficacy and safety of MMF given in combination with tacrolimus are being assessed. A similar study explores the use of MMF given in conjunction with rapamycin.

## CHAPTER REFERENCES

1. Allison AC, Eugui EM, Sollinger HW. Mycophenolate mofetil (RS-61443): mechanisms of action and effects in transplantation. Transplant Rev 1993;7:129–139.
2. Giblett ER, Anderson JE, Cohen F, et al. Adenosine deaminase deficiency in two patients with severely impaired cellular immunity. Lancet 1972;2:1067.
3. Allison AC, Hovi T, Watts RWE, et al. Immunological observations on patients with the Lesch-Nyhan syndrome, and on the role of de novo purine synthesis in lymphocyte transformation. Lancet 1975;2:1179.
4. Franklin TJ, Cook JM. The inhibition of nucleic acid synthesis by mycophenolic acid. Biochem J 1969;113:515.
5. Verham R, Meek TD, Hedstrom L, et al. Purification, characterization and kinetic analysis of inosine-5-monophosphate dehydrogenase of *Trichomonas foetus*. Mol Biochem Parasitol 1987;24:1.
6. Penn I. Tumors of the immunocompromised patient. Annu Rev Med 1988;39:63.
7. Natsumeda Y, Ohno S, Kawasaki H, et al. Two distinct cDNAs for human IMP dehydrogenase. J Biol Chem 1990;265:5292.
8. Konno Y, Natsumeda Y, Nagai M, et al. Expression of IMP dehydrogenase types I and II in *Escherichia coli* and distribution in normal lymphocytes and HL-60 leukemic cells. Cancer Res 1992;52:258.
9. Suthanthiran M, Morris RE, Strom TB. Immunosuppressants: cellular and molecular mechanisms of action. Am J Kidney Dis 1996;28:159–172.

10. Eugui EM, Almquist S, Muller CD, et al. Lymphocyte-selective cytostatic and immunosuppressive effects of mycophenolic acid in vitro: role of deoxyguanosine nucleotide depletion. Scan J Immunol 1991;33:175.

11. Dayton JS, Turka LA, Thompson CB, et al. Comparison of the effect of mizoribine with those of azathioprine 6-mercaptopurine and mycophenolic acid on T-lymphocyte proliferation and purine ribonucleotide metabolism. Mol Pharmacol 1992;41:671.

12. Altmann DM, Hoff N, Trowsdale J, et al. Cotransfection of ICAM-1 and HLA-DR reconstitutes human antigen-presenting mouse L cells. Nature 1989;338:512.

13. Isobe M, Yagita H, Okumura K, et al. Specific acceptance of cardiac allograft after treatment with antibodies to ICAM-1 and LFA-1. Science 1992;225:1125.

14. Allison AC, Kowalski WJ, Muller CJ, et al. Mycophenolic acid and brequinar, inhibitors of purine and pyrimidine synthesis, block the glycosylation of adhesion molecules. Transplant Proc 1993;25(suppl 2):67.

15. Grailer A, Nichols J, Hullet D, et al. Inhibition of human B-cell responses in vitro by RS-61443, cyclosporine A, and FK-506. Transplant Proc 1991;23:314.

16. Eugui EM, Mirkovich A, Allison AC. Lymphocyte-selective antiproliferative and immunosuppressive effects of mycophenolic acid in mice. Scand J Immunol 1991;33:175–183.

17. Kozlowski T, Tibell A, Morpurgo E, et al. Suppression of immunoglobulin resynthesis after plasmapheresis: efficacy of various immunosuppressive drugs—a study in rats. Transplant Proc 1995;27:3545–3546.

18. Burlingham WJ, Grailer AP, Hullett DA, Sollinger HW. Inhibition of both MLC and in vitro IgG memory response to tetanus toxoid by RS-61443. Transplantation 1991;51:545–547.

19. Nagy SE, Andersson JP, Andersson UG. Effect of mycophenolate mofetil (RS-61443) on cytokine production: inhibition of superantigen-induced cytokines. Immunopharmacology 1993;26:11–20.

20. Morris RE, Hoyt EG, Eugui EM, Allison AC. Prolongation of rat heart allograft survival by RS61443. Surg Forum 1989;40:337.

21. Morris RE, Hoyt EG, Murphy MP, Eugui EM. Mycophenolic acid morpholinoethylester (RS-61443) is a new immunosuppressant that prevents and halts cardiac rejection by selective inhibition of T- and B-cell purine synthesis. Transplant Proc 1990;22:1659–1662.

22. Morris RE, Hoyt EG, Eugui EM, Allison AC. Prolongation of rat heart allograft survival by RS-61443. Surg Forum 1989;40:337.

23. Morris RE, Wang J, Blum JR, et al. Immunosuppressive effects of the morpholinoethyl ester of mycophenolic acid (RS-61443) in rat and nonhuman primate recipients in heart allografts. Transplant Proc 1991;23(suppl 2):19–25.

24. Vu MD, Qi S, Xu D, et al. Synergistic effects of mycophenolate mofetil and sirolimus in prevention of acute heart, pancreas, and kidney allograft rejection and in reversal of ongoing heart allograft rejection in the rat. Transplantation 1998;66:1575–1580.

25. Knechtle SJ, Wang J, Burlingham WJ, et al. The influence of RS-61443 on antibody-mediated rejection. Transplantation 1992;53:699–701.

26. Kawamura T, Hullett DA, Suzuki Y, et al. Enhancement of allograft survival by combination RS-61443 and DUP-785 therapy. Transplantation 1993;55:691.

27. Ostraat O, Qi Z, Olausson M, et al. Additive immunosuppressive effect of combined mycophenolate mofetil and cyclosporin A in experimental rat cardiac transplantation. Transplant Proc 1995;27:3540.

28. D'Silva M, Antoniou E, DeRoover A, et al. Immunosuppressive effect of RS-61443 on rat cardiac allograft survival in combination with leflunomide or FK 506. Transplant Proc 1996;28:930–931.

29. Platz KP, Sollinger HW, Hullett DA, et al. RS-61443: a new, potent immunosuppressive agent. Transplantation 1991;51:27.

30. Platz KP, Bechstein WO, Eckhoff DE, et al. RS-61443 reverses acute allograft rejection in dogs. Surgery 1991;110:736.

31. Platz KP, Eckhoff DE, Hullett DA, Sollinger HW. RS-61443 studies: review and proposal. Transplant Proc 1991;23(suppl 2):33.

32. Bechstein WO, Schilling M, Steele DM, et al. RS-61443/cyclosporine combination therapy prolongs canine liver allograft survival. Transplant Proc 1993;25:702.

33. D'Alessandro AM, Rankin M, McVey J, et al. Prolongation of canine intestinal allograft survival with RS-61443, cyclosporine, and prednisone. Transplantation 1993;55:695.

34. Nakajima K, Ochiai T, Nagata M, et al. Effects of triple therapy of cyclosporine, FK 506, and RS-61443 on allogeneic small bowel transplantation in dogs. Transplant Proc 1993;25:595.

35. D'Alessandro AM, Rankin MA. Heterotopic rat intestinal transplantation: effect of cyclosporine and RS-61443 on graft-vs-host disease and rejection. Transplant Proc 1994;26:1611.

36. Shaffer D, Blakely ML, Gottschalk R, Monaco AP. Small bowel transplantation in rats using RS-61443: effect on GVHD and rejection. Transplant Proc 1992;24:1159.

37. Benhaim P, Anthony JP, Lin LY-T, et al. A long-term study of allogeneic rat hindlimb transplants immunosuppressed with RS-61443. Transplantation 1993;56:911.

38. van den Helder TBM, Benhaim P, Anthony JP, et al. Efficacy of RS-61443 in reversing acute rejection in a rat model of hindlimb allotransplantation. Transplantation 1994;57:427.

39. Benhaim P, Anthony JP, Ferreira L, et al. Use of combination of low-dose cyclosporine and RS-61443 in a rat hindlimb model of composite tissue allotransplantation. Transplantation 1996;61:527–532.

40. Ustuner ET, Zdichavsky M, Ren X, et al. Long-term composite tissue allograft survival in a porcine model with cyclosporin/mycophenolate mofetil therapy. Transplantation 1998;66:1581–1587.

41. Hao L, Lafferty KJ, Allison AC, Eugui EM. RS-61443 allows islet allografting and specific tolerance induction in adult mice. Transplant Proc 1990;22:876.

42. Lafferty KJ. Facilitation of specific tolerance induction in adult mice by RS-61443. Transplantation 1992;53:590.

43. Hao L, Wang Y, Chan S-M, Lafferty KJ. Effect of mycophenolate mofetil on islet allografting to chemically induced or spontaneously diabetic animals. Transplant Proc 1992;24:2843.

44. Qi S, Chen H, Xu D, Daloze P. Prolongation of pancreas allograft survival by mycophenolate mofetil in the rat. Transplant Proc 1996;28:932–933.

45. Hullett DA, Landry AS, Eckhoff DE, et al. DAB486-IL-2 (IL-2-toxin) in combination with low-dose RS-61443 (mycophenolate mofetil) prolongs mouse murine thyroid allograft survival. Transplant Proc 1993;25:756.

46. Hullett DA, Kawamura T, Fujino Y, et al. Prolongation of allograft and xenograft survival with mycophenolate mofetil (RS-61443) and brequinar sodium (DUP-785). Transplant Proc 1993;25:700.

47. Fujino Y, Kawamura T, Hullett DA, Sollinger HW. Evaluation of cyclosporine, mycophenolate mofetil, and brequinar sodium combination therapy on hamster-to-rat cardiac xenotransplantation. Transplantation 1994;57:41.

48. McManus RP, O'Hair DP, Komorowski R, Scott JP. Immunosuppressant combinations in primate cardiac xenografts. Ann NY Acad Sci 1993;696:281.

49. O'Hair DP, McManus RP, Komorowski R. Inhibition of chronic vascular rejection in primate cardiac xenografts using mycophenolate mofetil. Ann Thorac Surg 1994;58:1311.

50. Beger C, Vajkoczy P, Menger MD, Messmer K. Effects of RS-61443 on pancreatic islet xenografts. Transplant Proc 1994;26:759.

51. Wennberg L, Wallgren AC, Sundberg B, et al. Immunosuppression with cyclosporin A in combination with leflunomide and mycophenolate mofetil prevents rejection of pig-islets transplanted into rats. Transplant Proc 1996;28:819.

52. Foegh ML. Chronic rejection-graft arteriosclerosis. Transplant Proc 1990;22:119.

53. Steele DM, Hullett DA, Bechstein WO, et al. Effects of immunosuppressive therapy on the rat aortic allograft model. Transplant Proc 1993;25:754.

54. Wagner E, Roy R, Marois Y, et al. Fresh venous allografts in peripheral arterial reconstruction in dogs: effects of histocompatibility and of short-term immunosuppression with cyclosporine A and mycophenolate mofetil. J Thorac Cardiovasc Surg 1995;110:1732–1744.

55. Lynch WS, Roenigk HH Jr. Mycophenolic acid for psoriasis. Arch Dermatol 1977;113:1203–1208.

56. Epinette WW, Parker CM, Jones EL, Greist MC. Mycophenolic acid for psoriasis: a review of pharmacology, long-term efficacy, and safety. J Am Acad Dermatol 1987;17:962–971.

57. Carter SB, Franklin TJ, Jones DF, et al. Mycophenolic acid: an anti-cancer compound with unusual properties. Nature 1969;223:848–850.

58. Williams RH, Lively DH, DeLong DC, et al. Mycophenolic acid: antiviral and antitumor properties. J Antibiot 1968;21:463–464.

59. Sollinger HW, Eugui EM, Allison AC. RS-61443: mechanism of action, experimental and early clinical results. Clin Transplant 1991;5:523–526.

60. Sollinger HW, Deierhoi MH, Belzer FO, et al. RS-61443: phase I clinical trial and pilot rescue study. Transplantation 1992;53:428–432.

61. Deierhoi MH, Sollinger HW, Diethelm AG, et al. One-year follow-up results of phase I trial of mycophenolate mofetil (RS-61443) in cadaveric renal transplantation. Transplant Proc 1993;25:693–694.

62. The Mycophenolate Mofetil Renal Refractory Rejection Study Group. Mycophenolate mofetil for the treatment of refractory, acute cellular renal transplant rejection. Transplantation 1996;61:722–729.

63. Kimball JA, Pescovitz MD, Book BK, Norman DJ. Reduced human IgG anti-ATGAM antibody formation in renal transplant recipients receiving mycophenolate mofetil. Transplantation 1995;60:1379–1383.

64. Ensley RD, Bristow MR, Olsen SL, et al. The use of mycophenolate mofetil (RS-61443) in human heart transplant recipients. Transplantation 1993;56:75–82.

65. Kirklin JK, Bourge RC, Naftel DC, et al. Treatment of recurrent heart rejection with mycophenolate mofetil (RS-61443): initial clinical experience. J Heart Lung Transplant 1994;13:444–450.

66. Kobashigawa J, Miller L, Renlund D, et al. A randomized active-controlled trial of mycophenolate mofetil in heart transplant recipients. Transplantation 1998;66:507–515.

67. Klintmalm GB, Ascher NL, Busuttil RW, et al. RS-61443 for treatment-resistant human liver rejection. Transplant Proc 1993;25:697.

68. Freise CE, Hebert M. Osorio RW, et al. Maintenance immunosuppression with prednisone and RS-61443 alone following liver transplantation. Transplant Proc 1993;25:1758–1759.

69. Eckhoff DE, McGuire BM, Frenette LR, et al. Tacrolimus (FK506) and mycophenolate mofetil combination therapy versus tacrolimus in adult liver transplantation. Transplantation 1998;65:180–187.

70. Stegall MD, Wachs ME, Everson G, et al. Prednisone withdrawal 14 days after liver transplantation with mycophenolate. Transplantation 1997;64:1755–1760.

71. Fisher RA, Ham JM, Marcos A, et al. A prospective randomized trial of mycophenolate mofetil with Neoral or tacrolimus after orthotopic liver transplantation. Transplantation 1998;66:1616–1621.

72. Paterson DL, Singh N, Panebianco A, et al. Infectious complications occurring in liver transplant recipients receiving mycophenolate mofetil. Transplantation 1998;66:593–598.

73. Sollinger HW, Odorico JS, Knechtle SJ, et al. Experience with 500 simultaneous pancreas-kidney transplants. Ann Surg 1998;228:284–296.

74. Odorico JS, Prisch JD, Knechtle SJ, et al. A study comparing mycophenolate mofetil to azathioprine in simultaneous pancreas-kidney transplantation. Transplantation 1998;66:1751–1759.

75. Gruessner RWG, Sutherland DER, Drangstveit MB, et al. Mycophenolate mofetil in pancreas transplantation. Transplantation 1998;66:318–323.

76. Stegall MD, Simon M, Wachs ME, et al. Mycophenolate mofetil decreases rejection in simultaneous pancreas-kidney transplantation when combined with tacrolimus or cyclosporin. Transplantation 1997;64:1695–1700.

77. Sollinger HW, for the U.S. Renal Transplant Mycophenolate Study Group. Mycophenolate mofetil for the prevention of acute rejection in primary cadaveric renal allograft recipients. Transplantation 1995;60:225–232.

78. Sullivan SD, Garrison LP, Best JH, et al. The cost effectiveness of mycophenolate mofetil in the first year after primary cadaveric transplant. J Am Soc Nephrol 1997;8:1592–1598.

79. European Mycophenolate Mofetil Cooperative Study Group. Placebo-controlled study of mycophenolate mofetil combined with cyclosporin and corticosteroids for prevention of acute rejection. Lancet 1995;345:1321–1325.

80. The Tricontinental Mycophenolate Mofetil Renal Transplantation Study Group. A blinded, randomized clinical trial of mycophenolate mofetil for the prevention of acute rejection in cadaveric renal transplantation. Transplantation 1996;61:1029–1037.

81. Mathew TH, for the Tricontinental Mycophenolate Mofetil Renal Transplantation Study Group. A blinded, long-term, randomized multicenter study of mycophenolate mofetil in cadaveric renal transplantation. Transplantation 1998;65:1450–1454.

82. Halloran P, Mathew T, Tomlanovich S, et al. for the International Mycophenolate Mofetil Renal Transplant Study Groups. Mycophenolate mofetil in renal allograft recipients. Transplantation 1997;63:39–47.

83. Weisel M, Carl S, for the European Mycophenolate Mofetil Cooperative Study Group. A placebo controlled study of mycophenolate mofetil used in combination with cyclosporin and corticosteroids for the prevention of acute rejection in renal allograft recipients: 10 year results. J Urol 1998;159:28–33.

84. The Mycophenolate Mofetil Acute Rejection Study Group. Mycophenolate mofetil for the treatment of a first acute renal allograft rejection. Transplantation 1998;65:235–241.

85. Neylan JF, for the U.S. Renal Transplant Mycophenolate Mofetil Study Group. Immunosuppressive therapy in high risk transplant patients. Transplantation 1997;64:1277–1282.

86. Schweitzer EJ, Yoon S, Fink J, et al. Mycophenolate mofetil reduces the risk of acute rejection less in African-American than in Caucasian kidney recipients. Transplantation 1988;65:242–248.

87. Roth D, Colona J, Burke GW, et al. Primary immunosuppression with tacrolimus and mycophenolate for renal allograft recipients. Transplantation 1998;65:248–252.

88. Weir MR, Anderson L, Kink JC, et al. A novel approach to the treatment of chronic allograft nephropathy. Transplantation 1997;64:1706–1710.

89. Ducloux D, Fournier V, Bresson-Vautrin C, et al. Mycophenolate mofetil in renal transplant recipients with cyclosporin-associated nephrotoxicity. Transplantation 1998;65:1504–1506.

90. Zanker B, Schneeberger H, Rothenpieler U, et al. Mycophenolate mofetil-based, cyclosporin-free induction and maintenance immunosuppression. Transplantation 1998;66:44–49.

91. Hueso M, Bover J, Seron D, et al. Low-dose cyclosporin and mycophenolate mofetil in renal allograft recipients with suboptimal renal function. Transplantation 1998;66:1727–1731.

92. Smith KGC, Isbel NM, Catton MG, et al. Suppression of the humoral immune response by mycophenolate mofetil. Nephrol Dial Transplant 1998;13:160–164.

93. Pirsch JD, Sollinger HW. Mycophenolate mofetil—clinical and experimental experience. Ther Drug Monit 1996;18:357–361.

94. Lee WA, Gu L, Miksztal AR, et al. Bioavailability improvement of mycophenolic acid through amino ester derivitization. Pharm Res 1990;7:161–166.

95. Shaw LM, Nowak I. Mycophenolic acid: measurement and relationship to pharmacologic effects. Ther Drug Monit 1995;17:685–689.

96. Bullingham RES, Nicholls A, Hale M. Pharmacokinetics of mycophenolate mofetil (RS-61443): a short review. Transplant Proc 1996;28:925–929.

97. Shaw LM, Sollinger HW, Halloran P, et al. Mycophenolate mofetil: a report of the consensus panel. Ther Drug Monit 1995;17:690–699.

98. Nowak I, Shaw LM. Mycophenolic acid binding to human serum albumin: characterization and relation to pharmacodynamics. Clin Chem 1995;41:1011–1017.

99. Bullingham RES, Nichols AJ, Kamm BR. Clinical pharmacokinetics of mycophenolate mofetil. Clin Pharmacokinet 1998;34:429–455.

100. Wolfe EJ, Mahtur V, Tomlanovich S, et al. Pharmacokinetics of mycophenolate mofetil and intravenous ganciclovir alone and in combination in renal transplantation patients. Pharmacotherapy 1997;17:591–598.

101. Takahashi K, Ochiai T, Uchida K, et al. Pilot study of mycophenolate mofetil (RS-61443) in the prevention of acute rejection following renal transplantation in Japanese patients. Transplant Proc 1995;27:1421–1424.

102. Li S, Yatscoff RW. Improved high-performance liquid chromatographic assay for the measurement of mycophenolic acid in human plasma. Transplant Proc 1996;28:938–940.

103. Langman LJ, LeGatt DF, Yaatscoff RW. Pharmacodynamic assessment of mycophenolic acid-induced immunosuppression by measuring IMP dehydrogenase activity. Clin Chem 1995;41:295–299.

104. Langman LJ, Shapiro AMJ, Lakey JRT, et al. Pharmacodynamic assessment of mycophenolic acid-induced immunosuppression by measurement of inosine monophosphate dehydrogenase activity in a canine model. Transplantation 1996;61:87–92.

105. Langman LJ, LeGatt DF, Halloran PF, et al. Pharmacodynamic assessment of mycophenolic acid induced immunosuppression in renal transplant recipients. Transplantation 1996;62:666–672.

106. Zucker K, Esquenazi V, Rosen A, et al. Unexpected augmentation of MMF pharmacokinetics in renal transplant patients receiving Prograf and CellCept in combination therapy, and analogous in vitro findings. Proceedings of the American Society of Transplant Surgeons 22nd Annual Scientific Meeting 1996:79.

## COMMENTARY REFERENCES

1. Sollinger HW, Dierhof MH, Belzer FO, et al. RS-61443—a phase I clinical trial and pilot rescue study. Transplantation 1992;53:428–432.

2. Morris RE, Hoyt EG, Eugui EM, Allison AC. Prolongation of rat heart allograft survival by RS-61443. Surg Forum 1989;40:337.

3. Platz KP, Sollinger HW, Hullett DA, et al. RS-61443, a new, potent immunosuppressive agent. Transplantation 1990;51:27–31.

4. European Mycophenolate Mofetil Cooperative Study Group. Placebo-controlled study of mycophenolate mofetil combined with cyclosporin and corticosteroids for prevention of acute rejection. Lancet 1995;345:1321–1325.

5. The Tricontinental Mycophenolate Mofetil Renal Transplantation Study Group. A blinded, randomized clinical trial of mycophenolate mofetil for the prevention of acute rejection in cadaveric renal transplantation. Transplantation 1996;61:1029–1037.

6. Sollinger HW for the US Renal Transplant Mycophenolate Mofetil Study Group. Mycophenolate mofetil for the prevention of acute rejection in primary cadaveric renal allograft recipients. Transplantation 1995;60:225–232.

7. Sollinger HW, Belter FO, Deierhoi MH, et al. RS-61443 (mycophenolate mofetil). A multicenter study for refractory kidney transplant rejection. Ann Surg 1992;216:513–519.

8. The Mycophenolate Mofetil Renal Refractory Rejection Study Group. Mycophenolate mofetil for the treatment of refractory acute, cellular renal transplant rejection. Transplantation 1996;61:722–729.

# New Small Molecule Immunosuppressive Agents

Ferda Senel  Barry D. Kahan

The study of neoplastic agents led to the use of small molecule cytostatic antiproliferative agents, such as 6-mercaptopurine (6-MP), methotrexate (MTX), and cyclophosphamide, as the first immunosuppressive agents. These agents, however, displayed only modest activity when used in the clinical transplant setting, because their nonspecific modes of action caused serious bone marrow suppression with consequent impairment of host resistance and increased infection rates. More recently it was demonstrated that certain agents, namely cyclosporine (CsA), tacrolimus (TRL), and sirolimus (SRL), act selectively on the adaptive host response at different stages of the T- and B-cell cycles and spare nonspecific host resistance (Fig. 6.1). Unfortunately, owing to their significant toxic effects, it has been difficult to optimize the use of individual agents in monotherapy. Therefore, there has been interest in the use of combinations of these immunosuppressants as well as in the introduction of new small molecule agents that specifically alter T-cell function, such as 15-deoxyspergulain (DSG) and FTY720, which offer promising modes of immunosuppression.

## NEW NUCLEOSIDE SYNTHESIS INHIBITORS

### Mycophenolate Mofetil

Mycophenolate mofetil (MMF; RS-61443, Syntex, San Jose, CA) is the 2-morpholinoethyl ester of mycophenolic acid (MPA; Fig. 6.2), which is produced by several species of *Penicillium* (1). MMF, which is converted primarily in the liver to its active drug, MPA, by ester hydrolysis, was initially used in clinical trials for the treatment of psoriasis and rheumatoid arthritis (2–6) before being applied in experimental animal transplant models and in clinical transplantation by Sollinger et al (7,8). MMF has now been approved by many countries for use in the prophylaxis, but not rever-

sal, of rejection episodes. (See Chapter 5 for a more detailed discussion of mycophenolate mofetil.)

### *Molecular Mode of Action*

MPA noncompetitively and reversibly inhibits inosine monophosphate dehydrogenase (IMPDH) activity during the synthesis (S phase) of the cell cycle (Table 6.1). Because the salvage pathway of purine synthesis in lymphocytes is somewhat less active than the de novo pathway, lymphocytes depend on the conversion of 5-phosphoribosyl-1-phosphate (PRPP), which is synthesized from ribose-5P and adenosine triphosphate (ATP) by PRPP synthetase to inosine monophosphate (IMP). In turn, IMP is converted to guanosine monophosphate (GMP) by IMPDH. Some GMP, in contrast, is formed by the salvage pathway, in which guanine is converted to GMP by the action of hypoxanthine-guanine phosphoribosyltransferase (HGPRTase). MPA inhibits isozyme 2 (9,10), the primary isoform in human lymphocytes, and is upregulated in other cells upon stimulation. The mechanism of action of MMF is similar to that of mizorbine (MZB; Bredinin, C9H13N306, Tojo Pharma, Tokyo, Japan) (11,12) and is far more selective than that of azathioprine (Aza; Imuran, Burroughs-Wellcome, Research Triangle Park, NC), which exerts inhibitory effects on multiple enzymes in the de novo pathway. Eugi et al (13) found that MPA significantly reduced guanine triphosphate (GTP) levels, an effect that was reversed upon addition of deoxyguanosine ribonucleotides (13,14).

MPA inhibits the proliferation of T and B cells because their generation predominantly depends on de novo purine synthesis. After it was serendipitously discovered that MPA possessed immunosuppressive properties, Allison and Eugi (15) observed that MPA inhibited in vitro proliferative responses even when added 72 hours after stimulation with phytohemagglutinin (PHA) or pokeweed mitogen (PWM)

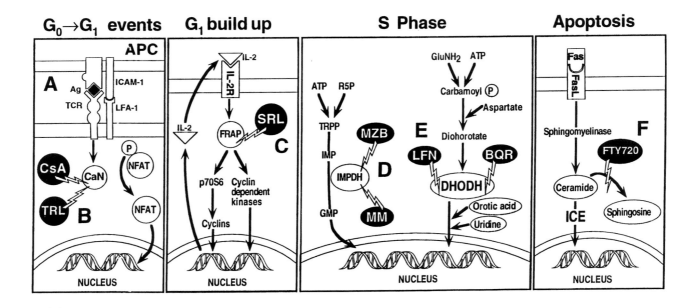

**FIGURE 6.1.** *Putative sites of T-cell–specific immunosuppressive agents. The sites of action can be classified in the $G_0$ to $G_1$ transition, wherein the intercellular adhesion molecule-1 (ICAM-1) antisense phosphorothioate oligonucleotide (PS-Oligo), denoted by A, inhibits the antigen presenting cell function of binding to lymphocyte function antigen-1 (LFA-1) (94). Also, engineered major histocompatibility complex (MHC) antigens act as altered peptide ligands (96). Cyclosporine (CsA) or tacrolimus (TRL) inhibits calcineurin (CaN), denoted by B, in the $G_0$ to $G_1$ pathway. During the $G_1$ buildup, sirolimus (SRL), denoted by C, inhibits the FK-RAPA associated protein (FRAP). In the S phase, mycophenolic acid or its analogue, mycophenolate mofetil (MM), as well as mizorbine (MZB), inhibits purine synthesis (denoted by D), and brequinar (BQR) or leflunomide (LFN) inhibits pyrimidine de novo biosynthesis (denoted by E). FTY720, denoted by F, favors the apoptotic pathway by possibly blocking ceramide degradation, thereby leading to ceramide accumulation and induction of apoptosis.*

**Table 6.1.** Site of Action of New Small Immunosuppressants During Cell Cycle Progression of Lymphocytes

| Phase of Cell Cycle | Inhibitory Drug(s) |
|---|---|
| $G_0$ | FTY720 |
| $G_0 \rightarrow G_1$ | CsA, TRL |
| $G_1$ | SRL |
| S | MMF, BQR, LFN |

(13). At concentrations of 100 nmol/L, MPA did not inhibit proliferation of nonstimulated fibroblasts or endothelial cells. Unlike CsA and TRL, MPA, at concentrations up to 100 nmol/L, did not affect interleukin (IL)-2 production (16). The depletion of intracellular guanosine-diphosphate intermediates not only affects DNA synthesis but may also inhibit the transfer of mannose and fucose to glycoproteins (17) such as the intercellular adhesion molecules (ICAMs) and very late antigen (VLA)-4 (18), and thereby may impair lymphocyte interactions with target cells (19).

### Pharmacokinetics

MMF appears to have a 1.5-fold greater bioavailability than the parent compound MPA (20,21). After single-dose oral administration (20 mg/kg) to cynomolgus monkeys, MMF had a shorter time to peak concentration ($t_{max}$; 1.3 ± 0.6 hours) and a higher peak concentration ($C_{max}$) value (34 ± 11 µg/mL) than MPA (13 ± 6.5 hours and 6.9 ± 2.5 µg/mL, respectively) (20). After rapid oral absorption, the prodrug MMF is hydrolyzed in the liver to the active metabolite MPA, which is metabolized principally by hepatic glucuronyl transferase to form an inactive phenolic glucuronide (MPAG), which is secreted into the bile (7). Intestinal glucuronidase converts the inactive compound back into active MPA, which may explain the gastrointestinal toxicity of the drug and enterohepatic recycling (7).

MPA is almost exclusively found in the plasma fraction. Of the MPA in plasma, 7.2% to 16.5% is unbound, less than 10% is bound to lipoproteins, and the rest is primarily bound to nonalbumin proteins (22). Analysis of the pharmacokinetic profiles of cadaveric kidney transplant recipients treated with escalating doses of MMF (1000–1750 mg twice a day) showed that the values for the $C_{max}$ and area under the concentration-time curve over a 24-hour period ($AUC_{0-24}$) increased in dose-proportionate fashion. For MMF, the $C_{max}$ and $AUC_{0-24}$ values ranged from 1.0 to 3.2 µg/mL and 6.4 to 37.6 µg/hr/mL, respectively. The presence of food lowered the $C_{max}$ by 40% but had no effect on the AUC values. The terminal half-life ranged from 2.3 to 9.6 hours. The $AUC_{0-24}$ values on day 1 after transplant were

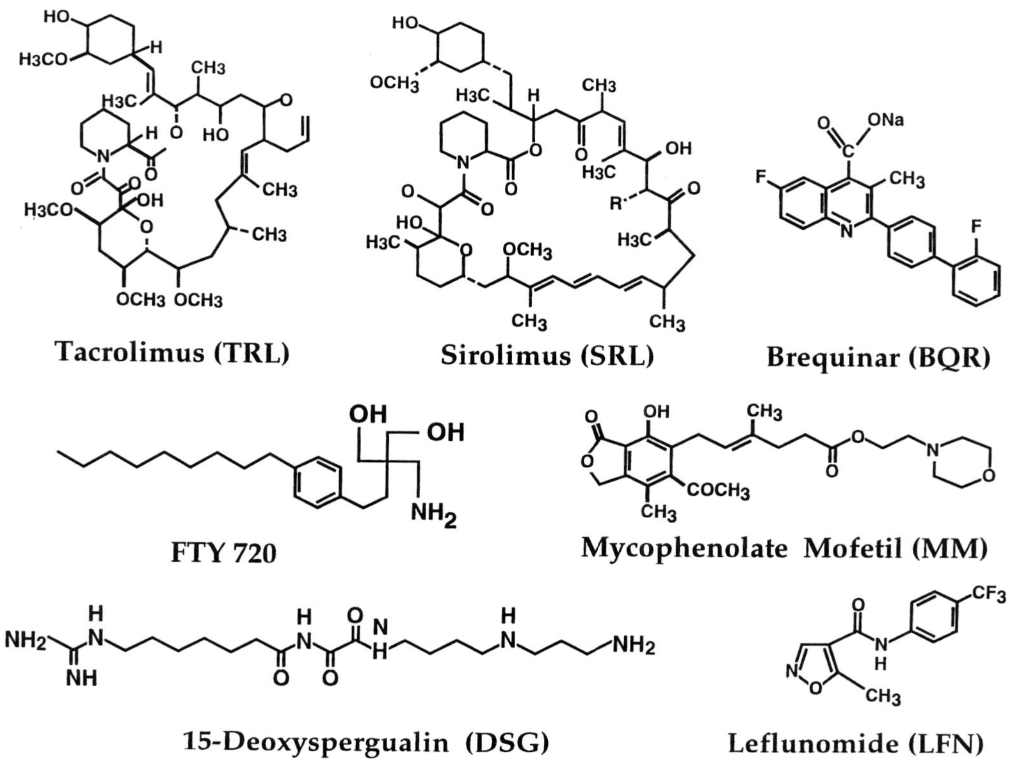

**Tacrolimus (TRL)**     **Sirolimus (SRL)**     **Brequinar (BQR)**

**FTY 720**     **Mycophenolate Mofetil (MM)**

**15-Deoxyspergualin (DSG)**     **Leflunomide (LFN)**

**FIGURE 6.2.**     *Molecular structures of the small molecule immunosuppressants tacrolimus, sirolimus, brequinar, FTY720, mycophenolate mofetil, 15-deoxyspergualin, and leflunomide.*

significantly lower compared to those at day 20, suggesting improved absorption upon resolution of gastrointestinal ileus. In addition, there was also substantial interindividual variation in AUC values (23).

### Clinical Applications

**Clinical Toxicity in Transplantation and Psoriasis: Phase I Trials**
Jones et al (4) found that 14 of 29 psoriasis patients showed a clearing of their skin lesions; however, there was a high incidence of gastrointestinal side effects, including nausea, diarrhea, and anorexia. Other studies in psoriasis patients reported an increased incidence of neoplasms (0.08%) (5,6) as well as herpes zoster infections (11.6%) (6,24). Long-term studies in which 1600–7368 mg/day MPA was administered to psoriatic patients revealed that 72.4% of the patients experienced gastric toxicity (6,25), a side effect that was also observed among patients with refractory severe rheumatoid arthritis who were treated with MPA (1.0–1.5 g) twice daily (3,26).

A phase I study that enrolled 48 cadaveric kidney recipients showed that MMF used at doses of 100–3500 mg/day caused a dose-dependent gastrointestinal toxicity (gastritis, mild ileus) with no evidence of bone marrow suppression (23). An open-label single-center trial in which MMF was administered to 21 cadaveric renal transplant recipients at doses ranging from 250–3500 mg/day together with a

CsA-prednisone maintenance immunosuppression regimen demonstrated that the limiting side effects of MMF include diarrhea, nausea, elevated liver enzymes, and an increased rate of infections, the most common of which was cytomegalovirus (CMV) (27). In liver transplant recipients, no significant differences were observed in infectious complications between MMF-treated and untreated patients (28).

**Prophylaxis of Acute Rejection: Phase II Trials**   MMF was administered to primary cadaver kidney recipients at doses ranging from 100–3500 mg/day in conjunction with Minnesota Anti-Lymphocyte Globulin (MALG), CsA, and prednisone. A dose-dependent reduction in the incidence of rejection episodes occurred at doses of 2 g/day or more. Moreover, at these doses, there was a less frequent need to use OKT-3 to treat refractory rejection episodes (23). In small cohorts of patients, MMF reduced the incidence of acute rejection episodes among pediatric recipients of cadaveric donor renal allografts and reduced the rate of persistent or recurrent acute rejection episodes among 17 heart transplant patients (29). More recent studies in high-risk renal allograft recipients revealed that acute rejection is best prevented in African Americans (AAs) by an MMF dosage of 3000 mg/day, whereas 2000 mg/day provided a superior benefit/risk ratio for non-AAs (30).

**Pilot Studies of Rescue Treatment**   An open-label study in 20 kidney transplant recipients, who were defined by the investigators as experiencing "refractory allograft rejection," suggested that the episodes were "reversed" in 4 of 5 (80%) living-related donor (LRD) grafts and in 7 of 15 (47%) cadaveric donor grafts (23). A multicenter study (31) of 75 kidney transplant recipients with biopsy-proven rejection episodes that were refractory to at least one course of anti-lymphocyte globulin (ALG)–OKT-3 revealed that MMF (2000–3500 mg/day) "rescued" the grafts in 52 of 75 (69%) patients, particularly among patients with an entry serum creatinine value below 4 mg/dL (Table 6.2). Another study randomly assigned 150 renal allograft recipients suffering refractory acute cellular rejection to treatment with MMF or steroids. Graft loss or death occurred in 14.3% of the MMF-treated group as compared with 26% of the steroid-treated patients ($P = 0.08$) (32). Prominent side effects included nausea, diarrhea, and a 40% overall infection rate with drug discontinuation required for patients who experienced pancreatitis, CMV colitis, and severe gastrointestinal complications. Upon review of these and other studies, the United States FDA did not consider the evidence for rejection reversal with MMF compelling.

**Prophylaxis of Acute Rejection: Phase III Trials** The European, double-blind, placebo-controlled multicenter study (33) enrolled 491 kidney transplant recipients who were randomized to receive placebo (n = 166), 2 g/day MMF (n = 165), or 3 g/day MMF (n = 160) in combination with CsA–prednisone therapy. Biopsy-proven rejection episodes occurred in 17.0% and 13.8% of patients treated with 2 g/day and 3 g/day MMF, respectively, versus a 46.4% rejection episode rate in the placebo group. For all groups, however, no improvement was observed in the six-month graft loss rate, which was 6.7% for 2 g/day MMF, 8.8% for 3 g/day MMF, and 10.2% for placebo. The US double-blind multicenter study (34) included 495 renal transplant recipients who were randomized to receive 2 g/day MMF (n = 167), 3 g/day MMF (n = 166), or 1–2 mg/kg/day Aza (n = 166) together with a CsA–prednisone regimen and antithymocyte globulin (ATG) induction therapy. Compared with a 38.0% rate of rejection episodes among patients in the Aza

group, the rates for the 2 g and 3 g MMF groups were 19.8% and 17.5%, respectively, with similar six-month patient and graft survival rates. The time to first biopsy-proven rejection episode or to treatment failure was significantly greater for patients treated with 2 g MMF ($P = 0.0036$) or 3 g MMF ($P = 0.0006$) than for those treated with Aza. MMF also appeared to reduce the severity of the rejection episodes. The side effects associated with MMF treatment included diarrhea, leukopenia, tissue-invasive CMV disease, gastrointestinal toxicity, anemia, hypertension, and sepsis.

**Potential Effects on Chronic Allograft Vasculopathy** MMF has been reported to reduce intimal thickening and graft coronary disease in rats. To four Lewis (LEW; RT1$^l$) recipients of Brown Norway (BN; RT1$^n$) heart allografts, MMF was administered in doses of 30 mg/kg/day from day 1 through day 50, and 20 mg/kg/day from day 51 through day 100. At day 100 one graft had no coronary disease, two grafts had mild intimal proliferation, and one had moderate intimal thickening (35). A subsequent experiment found significantly ($P = 0.011$) reduced intimal proliferation in ACI aortic allografts transplanted into LEW recipients that received MMF at 40 mg/kg/day for 14 days followed by 30 mg/kg/day thereafter (36). Some researchers, however, failed to document a benefit of MMF in preventing graft vessel disease in a F344-to-LEW heterotopic heart transplant model; similar degrees of arterial intimal thickening in treated versus untreated animals were found (37). Among F344 renal allografts in LEW hosts, administration of MMF (15 mg/kg/day) starting at either day 1 (n = 5) or week 8 after transplant (n = 5) reduced the chronic histologic changes of interstitial fibrosis, tubular atrophy, glomerulosclerosis, and arterial obliteration, and the incidence of proteinuria (38). MMF (40 mg/kg PO for 13 days) also appeared to reduce the degree of arterial intimal thickening in four Sprague-Dawley rats exposed to mechanical injury by balloon dilatation, particularly when combined with sirolimus (1.5 mg/kg). However, there is no evidence that MMF affects the progression of graft vessel disease or chronic rejection in clinical studies.

**Table 6.2.** Potential Clinical Indications for the Use of Small Molecular Immunosuppressants

| Indications | Agent | | | | | |
|---|---|---|---|---|---|---|
| | MMF | BQR | TRL | SRL | 15DS | FTY720 |
| Presensitized response | 0 | ? | 0 | 0 | ? | 0 |
| Rejection prophylaxis | ++[a,b] | ++[b] | ++[a,c] | +++[b] | 0 | ++[b] |
| Rejection reversal | 0 | 0 | 0 | + | ++[c] | 0 |
| Rejection rescue | + | + | + | ++ | 0 | 0 |
| Chronic rejection | ? | ? | 0 | ? | 0 | 0 |

[a] FDA-approved indication for drug use.
[b] Use in combination with CsA.
[c] Use in combination with corticosteroids.

In summary, three randomized clinical studies have shown that MMF decreases the incidence and severity of acute rejection episodes, but fails to improve overall graft or patient survival rates. A recent update failed to show improvement in the three-year graft survival or histopathology among patients treated with CsA–MMF–steroid versus CsA–Aza–steroid or CsA–steroid (39). Nevertheless, MMF is being incorporated into immunosuppressive regimens with increasing frequency for allograft recipients (40). Despite its putatively selective role for T-cell action, clinical experience has documented that MMF inhibits multiple types of rapidly dividing cells, which results in the major side effects of bone marrow suppression and gastrointestinal toxicity, particularly diarrhea. These adverse reactions together with its high cost may limit the long-term application of MMF in future immunosuppressive regimens, unless it can be documented that it reduces the incidence of chronic rejection or permits substantial CsA dose reduction.

## Brequinar

Brequinar (BQR; DUP785) was originally developed as an antitumor agent (41), because it inhibits pyrimidine biosynthetic pathways (42). Its high bioavailability and long serum half-life are major advantages, but the drug displays considerable dose-related toxicity.

### *Molecular Mode of Action*

BQR is a synthetic difluoroquinolone carboxylic acid derivative [6-fluoro-2-(2′-fluoro-1,1′biphenyl-4-yl)-3-methyl-4-quinolinecarboxylic acid sodium salt; DuPont-Merck, Wilmington, DE] that inhibits the growth of a wide range of human solid tumors implanted in nude mice (41). BQR displays antitumor effects over a wide range of concentrations, but only displays antilymphocyte effects over a relatively narrow range (22 to 185 nmol/L) (43). In vitro BQR (25 to 75 μM) kills 50% of clone A human colon tumor cells when incubated within 24 hours and 99% after 48 to 72 hours of incubation. Intracellular uridine triphosphate (UTP) and cytidine triphosphate (CTP) pools were depleted to 50% at 3 hours and to undetectable levels (<0.3 pmol) after 24 hours. The addition of exogenous uridine or cytidine to cell cultures reversed the cytotoxic effect.

At concentrations ranging from 15 to 105 nmol/L (44), BQR noncompetitively inhibits dihydro-orotate dehydrogenase (DHO-DH), the enzyme that converts dihydro-orotate into orotic acid. This conversion is a critical step, leading to the formation of uridine- and cytidine-MP. DHO-DH, which blocks the synthesis of DNA and RNA, is the fourth enzyme in the de novo pyrimidine synthesis pathway, located on the outer side of the inner mitochondrial membrane (45). Because lymphocyte pyrimidine pool is limited, activated lymphocytes depend primarily on de novo synthesis, producing a high degree of sensitivity to BQR during the S phase of the immune response (46). In C57Bl/6 mice bearing colon cancer transplants (Colon 38), BQR (50 mg/

kg) inhibited plasma and tissue uridine levels to 10% and depleted DHO-DH activity, which persisted for several days, by more than 90% (47).

### *In Vitro and In Vivo Immunosuppressive Effects*

BQR inhibits mixed lymphocyte reaction (MLR) in various species, but most sensitively in human (48). MLR cultures admixing lymphocytes from ACI and LEW rats display a BQR $IC_{50}$ of 0.15 μg/mL (49), and cultures using allogenic human peripheral blood lymphocytes (PBLs), 0.01 μg/mL. Although the $IC_{50}$ concentration is identical to that of CsA, BQR produces 90% inhibition ($IC_{90}$) at 0.07 μg/mL, a concentration that is considerably lower than that required for CsA (1.2 μg/mL) (50). Just as it inhibited the growth of tumor cells, BQR (10 mg/kg) significantly inhibited the DHO-DH activity in the lymph node cells of antigen-sensitized mice. The delayed-type hypersensitivity response induced by 2,4-dinitrofluorobenzene (DNFB) was 90% inhibited by a BQR dosage of 10 mg/kg, a 10-fold lower dose than that required for CsA. BQR produced dose-dependent inhibition of cytotoxic T-cell proliferation and antibody responses to antigens in C57BL/6 mice. A 50% inhibition of specific lysis was produced by 1.6 mg/kg BQR. There was a strong correlation between drug blood levels and the inhibition of the mitogen-induced lymphocyte proliferation (50). BQR produces synergistic inhibition with CsA toward in vitro human MLR with combination index values ranging from 0.06 to 0.003 at the 95% inhibition level. BQR also displays strong synergism with sirolimus, with $CI_{95}$ values ranging from 0.08 to 0.02. The maximum inhibition degree of lymphocyte proliferation in response to mitogen or MLR–driven stimulation was observed with the triple combination CsA–sirolimus–BQR, with CI values less than 0.0001 over the inhibition range 60% to 95% (51).

BQR inhibits the IgM antibody-mediated xenograft rejection responses in hamster-to-rat heart xenograft models. While the IgM level increased from 218.3 ± 88.4 mg/L to 1631 ± 359.8 mg/L (n = 6, $P < 0.01$) in untreated animals, it did not increase in BQR-treated animals (52). At high doses (12 mg/kg, three times a week), BQR prevented both IgM and IgG production in ACI heart allotransplants into skin graft–sensitized LEW rat hosts (53).

The high sensitivity of lymphocytes to the action of BQR compared to comparable purine inhibitors has been attributed to the 100-fold smaller pyrimidine pool than purine pool in these cells (54).

### *Pharmacokinetics*

BQR, a water-soluble compound, is rapidly absorbed from the gastrointestinal tract. The bioavailability is 90%, reaching peak plasma levels between 2 and 4 hours (55). The drug is bound to serum proteins and has a $t_{1/2}$ of 15 hours, a volume of distribution of 15.5 ± 6.0 L/m², and a mean plasma clearance of 9.2 ± 7.7 mL/min/m². Serum levels of BQR are measured with a reverse phase high-performance liquid chromatography assay (56). After a series of five single daily IV injections of doses ranging from 135 to 300 mg/m$^2$, the AUC increased linearly as a function of dose (r: 0.85). At higher doses (300 to 2250 mg/kg$^2$), BQR displayed non-linear pharmacokinetics. BQR is believed to be metabolized in the liver by the P450 cytochrome oxidase system, and excreted primarily in feces (66%) and to a lesser extent in urine (23%) (41). The oral administration of BQR to rats for 1 month did not affect CsA pharmacokinetics (57). Its high bioavailability and long half-life allow BQR to be administered orally on an alternate-day dosing schedule.

### Experimental Transplantation

**Prevention of Acute and Accelerated Allograft Rejection**
BQR monotherapy prolongs heart, liver, and kidney allograft survival in rat transplant models. BQR (12 mg/kg, three times a week for 30 days) prolonged cardiac allografts in the ACI-to-LEW rat strain combination from 7.0 ± 0.69 to 45.5 ± 12.26 days. Grafts were rejected approximately 2 weeks after discontinuation of treatment. The same dose of BQR produced graft survivals of more than 230 days for 12 of 26 orthotopic liver transplants and more than 87 days for all kidney transplants. Challenge of long-term liver graft survivors with repeat donor-type (but not with third-party BN cardiac) transplants resulted in permanent survival, demonstrating donor-specific tolerance (49). BQR monotherapy (4 mg/kg orally three times each week) prolonged the survival of heterotopic cardiac allografts in cynomolgus monkeys from 8 ± 0.5 to 20.0 ± 21.5 days (52). BQR (3 mg/kg/day for 90 days) also prolonged mean survival time of hamster heart xenotransplants in LEW recipients from 4.0 ± 0.48 to 24.5 ± 42.2 days. Four animals survived over 90 days (52). BQR administered at a dose of 12.5 mg/kg three times a week from day −10 to day +30 also prevented accelerated rejection of ACI cardiac allograft in LEW recipients that had been presensitized by ACI skin graft placement 7 days prior to transplantation. This regimen prolonged survival from 2.5 ± 0.9 days to 40.0 ± 14.0 days, while CsA (5–15 mg/kg/day for 30 days) was not effective (53).

**Combinations with Other Immunosuppressive Drugs**    In various animal transplant models, the immunosuppressive effect of BQR is potentiated by combination with other agents. The combination of BQR (6 mg/kg) with CsA (1 mg/kg) prolonged liver allograft survival to 220.6 ± 110.3 days, compared with 13.5 ± 83.5 days for BQR alone and 10.0 ± 77.8 days for CsA alone (49). Median effect analysis documented the interaction of CsA and BQR to be synergistic. Administration of BQR (0.25–2.0 mg/kg/day for 14 days) with CsA (0.5 mg/kg) and SRL (0.01 mg/kg) improved the survival of BUF heterotopic heart allografts in Wistar-Furth (WF; RT1$^u$) recipients from 20.8 ± 2.7 days to 56.6 ± 5.2 days, with a CI value of 0.06 (51). In mice, the addition of BQR (0.125 mg/kg) to the combination of CsA (90.25 mg/kg/day) and sirolimus (SRL) (0.01 mg/kg) prolonged the graft survival from 8.2 ± 1.5 days to 56.6 ± 22.1 days, with a CI of 0.01 (58). In other experiments using a limited array of dose combinations, the addition of MMP

to BQR treatment was claimed to prolong significantly the survival of ACI heterotopic heart allografts in LEW recipients (59). In primates, the combination of BQR and CsA also prolonged graft survival. BQR (2 mg/kg three times weekly) and CsA (2 mg/kg) increased graft survival from 8.0 ± 0.5 days in the untreated group and from 22 and 20 ± 21.5 days in both single-drug groups, respectively, to 43 days in the combination group.

Dogs are more sensitive than monkeys or humans to drug-induced myelosuppressive and gastrointestinal (GI) toxic effects, presumably because these tissues undergo rapid cell turnover (47,49). BQR (5 mg/kg) treatment of Sprague-Dawley rats for 1 month caused anemia, leukopenia, bone marrow hypocellularity, GI epithelial growth inhibition, and intestinal mucosal atrophy. The combination of BQR with CsA (10 mg/kg) increased the mortality rate in rats to 69% (22/32) (57), caused hypoplastic changes in the white pulp area of the spleen, and produced mucosal erosive changes in the small intestine and colon in monkeys (60).

### Clinical Applications

**Phase I Studies**    Administration of BQR to 45 cancer patients by single daily IV infusion for 5 days over a dose range of 36–300 mg/m$^2$/day produced dermatitis, mucositis, phlebitis, reversible transaminase elevations, and thrombocytopenia (61). Short-term (10- to 60-minute) IV infusion of BQR repeated every three weeks at doses above 1200 mg/m$^2$ caused a wide range of dose-dependent side effects, including severe thrombocytopenia, leukopenia, mucositis, nausea, vomiting, and skin rash (56). Phase II studies in cancer using BQR doses of 1800 mg/m$^2$ failed to reduce the tumor growth (62). There was a strong correlation between the AUC and thrombocytopenia. In a study of 67 cancer patients, 10-minute daily IV infusion of BQR for five consecutive days produced dose-limiting myelosuppression with severe thrombocytopenia; the maximum tolerable doses ranged from 210–350 mg/m$^2$ (56). BQR was administered at doses ranging from 0.5–4.0 mg/kg to 36 renal (Kahan BD, unpublished data) and 18 orthotopic liver (63) stable adult allograft recipients. The drug was generally tolerated, except for stomatitis, occasional mild diarrhea, and rare viral infections. Concentration-dependent changes occurred in platelet but not in white blood cell counts.

**Phase II Studies**    An initial phase II study in cadaveric kidney recipients failed to document that addition of BQR to a CsA–prednisone regimen reduces the incidence of acute allograft rejection episodes (DuPont-Merck, unpublished data). The study design was flawed, however, and the phase II assessment will need to be repeated in order to draw a firm conclusion about the activity of BQR.

Like other nucleotide synthesis inhibitors, BQR is a potent blocker of the lymphocyte proliferation in vivo and in vitro; however, it also reduces the activity of other dividing cells, such as GI epithelium and bone marrow cells. In animal transplant models, BQR improves graft survival and overcomes accelerated rejection when used alone and acts synergistically with CsA and/or SRL. BQR's unique abilities to suppress antibody responses and to improve the survival of xenotransplants make it likely that the agent will become an important adjunct in clinical immunosuppression. However, the phase I toxicity studies, initially conducted in cancer patients (56,61,62) and then in transplant patients, documented that BQR must play this role only at reduced doses that are subtherapeutic as monotherapy.

## Leflunomide

Leflunomide (HWA 486; Hoechst, Basel, SZ), an isoxazol derivative [*N*-(4-trifluoro-methylphenyl)-5-methylisoxazol-4-carboxamide], was initially synthesized to be an agricultural herbicide (see Fig. 6.2). Leflunomide displays immunosuppressive activity in animal models of arthritis, autoimmune diseases, and graft rejection. The parent compound is metabolized quickly to an active metabolite, A771726, which is minimally water soluble. In rodents, A771726 displays a half-life of 10 to 30 hours, which is 10-fold longer in humans. Because the pharmacokinetic characteristics of leflunomide show significant interindividual variability, and because of the agent's severe adverse reaction profile, considerable effort is now underway to produce a less toxic analogue.

### Molecular Mode of Action

In vitro A771726 inhibits the proliferation of human PBL upon stimulation with allogeneic PBL in one-way MLR with anti-CD3 MAb plus phorbol myristate acetate (PMA), and with anti-CD28 MAb plus PMA (64,65). Although leflunomide partially inhibits IL-2 production, it does not affect IL-2R expression, and administration of exogenous IL-2 fails to restore T-cell proliferative responses. It has been hypothesized that leflunomide inhibits T-cell activation by inhibiting the lck and fyn families of tyrosine kinases, enzymes that are associated with transduction of many growth factor receptor signals, including IL-2, IL-3, and tumor necrosis factor (TNF)-$\alpha$, but not IL-1 (66,67). However, leflunomide does not affect the formation of the IL-2/IL-2R complex or initial signal transduction events, such as phosphotyrosine formation and Ca mobilization. These findings were initially interpreted to suggest that the agent principally inhibits the transformation from the $G_1$ to the S phase of the cell cycle (64–66). However, recent data show that A771726 does not inhibit T-cell receptor (TCR)-mediated signal transduction in Jurkat T cells stimulated by PHA or anti-CD3. Tyrosine kinase–dependent early signal transduction was not affected by A771726. There was no increase in the level of intracellular ionized $Ca^{2+}$.

Based on the observation that the addition of uridine and cytidine to T cells treated with A771726 restores proliferative responses, an alternate hypothesis has been proposed: A771726 inhibits pyrimidine synthesis (68), in a similar fashion as BQR, by inhibiting dihydro-orotate dehydrogenase (see Table 6.1).

### Experimental Animal Models

Leflunomide displays potent immunosuppressive activity against experimental autoimmune disorders, including arthritis (69), systemic lupus erythematosus (70), antibasement membrane antibody–induced glomerulonephritis (71), and tubulointerstitial nephritis (72). It prolongs rat (70) and dog (73) kidney and rat skin graft survival. Kuchle et al (74) demonstrated that treatment with leflunomide (5 and 10 mg/kg/day PO) prolonged BN kidney allograft survival in LEW rats from 8.2 ± 0.3 days to over 60 days. Treatment with 20 mg/kg/day leflunomide significantly prolonged DA skin graft survival in LEW recipients to 29.1 ± 1.8 days from 10.5 ± 1.1 days in untreated controls, and LEW skin graft survival in Fisher rat recipients to 33.8 ± 2.8 days from 16.2 ± 1.0 days in untreated controls. Spleen cells from long-surviving LEW recipients of DA grafts that were treated with leflunomide when transferred prolonged survival of donor-type skin grafts to naive nonirradiated LEW rats (75). Leflunomide monotherapy at daily doses of 0.63–10.0 mg/kg for 7 days significantly prolonged the survival of BN hearts in LEW rats (76). When treatment was extended to 21 days at a leflunomide dose of 5 mg/kg/day, 3 of 6 animals displayed indefinite graft survival. In the hamster-to-LEW rat cardiac xenotransplant model, leflunomide (2.5–20.0 mg/kg/day PO) initiated on day 0 prolonged survival from 3.9 ± 0.3 days to 71.3 ± 17.9 days (10 mg/kg group) (77). The high leflunomide doses (20 mg/kg/day) prolonged survival (MST = 50.9 ± 16.2 days), but caused significant anemia; 4 of 8 animals were lost due to toxicity.

In canine renal transplant models, McChesney et al (73) found that escalating doses of 2–16 mg/kg/day of leflunomide produced dose-dependent effects: 4 mg/kg/day extended survival from 9.0 ± 1.0 days to 15.5 ± 5.0 days with all dogs dying of rejection, and 16 mg/kg/day prolonged survival to 20.7 ± 2.0 days with all dogs dying due to inanition and anemia. The side effects included mild interstitial nephritis and superficial ulcerations of the stomach and jejunal mucosa, as well as anemia and anorexia that were attributed to the generation of an aniline metabolite by hepatic oxidation of the parent compound.

The severe adverse reaction profile of the present compound obviates clinical application of leflunomide. Research is underway to develop less toxic analogues of the A771726 metabolite of leflunomide.

## NEW AGENTS THAT SPECIFICALLY ALTER T-CELL FUNCTION

### Tacrolimus

During an intensive search to find antibiotics that inhibit IL-2 production in a similar fashion as CsA, the macrolide product of *Streptomyces tsukubaensis* No. 9993 was unearthed from soil samples from Tsukuba, Japan (78). The active compound, tacrolimus (TRL; FK506, Prograf, Fujisawa, Osaka, Japan; molecular weight = 804 daltons molecular weight), is a macrolide lactone with a hemiketal-masked $\alpha,\beta$-

diketoamide that is functionally incorporated in a 23-member ring (79) (see Fig. 6.2; see Chapter 4 for a more detailed discussion of tacrolimus).

### Molecular Mode of Action

TRL forms complexes with FK-binding proteins (FKBPs), which are abundant cytosolic enzymes with intrinsic rotamase activity (80,81), to inhibit the phosphatase activity of calcineurin (82–84), thereby preventing the emigration of the phosphorylated cytoplasmic nuclear factor of activated T cells (NFAT) from the cytoplasm to the nucleus (see Table 6.1). Because NFAT is critical for the upregulation of IL-2 gene transcription, the synthesis of this cytokine is disrupted (85,86) (see Fig. 6.2). Of the four FKBPs characterized to date, it seems most likely that TRL forms a complex with FKBP12, a 12-kd cytosolic protein, which then mediates the immunosuppressive effects of TRL (87).

### Pharmacokinetics

Although high-performance liquid chromatography (HPLC) methods unequivocally detect TRL and its metabolites (88), the drug is generally measured in human whole blood samples with an enzyme-linked immunosorbent assay (ELISA) (89). After intravenous administration of TRL, the median half-life is 11.3 hours, with a range of 3.5 to 40.5 hours (90,91). The plasma clearance rate ranges from 5.8 to 103 mL/min/kg. After oral administration, TRL is rapidly absorbed independent of the presence of bile, with a $t_{max}$ of 0.5 to 4.0 hours and a mean oral bioavailability of 25%. The agent is primarily metabolized by the hepatic cytochrome P450-IIIA4 enzyme system (66). Unfortunately, the intraindividual and interindividual variations in TRL pharmacokinetics are as great as those observed with CsA.

### Clinical Applications

**Prophylaxis of Acute Rejection: Phase III Trials**   In the phase III open-label, randomized European multicenter trial (92), which enrolled 545 liver transplant recipients, patients in the TRL treatment group displayed an approximately equal incidence of acute rejection episodes compared with those in the CsA treatment group (43.4% versus 53.6%; $P$ = NS). The modest delay in the time to diagnosis ($P$ = 0.04) does not seem important, because the trial was unblinded and time to rejection is a subjective measure. The patient and graft survival rates were similar: 82.9% and 77.5%, respectively, for the TRL-treated group, and 77.5% and 72.6%, respectively, for the CsA-treated group. Renal toxicity, altered glucose metabolism, and neurologic complications were more commonly experienced by patients in the TRL group.

The phase III US multicenter trial (93) included 478 adult and 51 pediatric recipients of orthotopic liver transplants. After one year, patients treated with immunosuppressive regimens based on TRL (n = 263) and CsA (n = 266) showed comparable patient and graft survival rates. It was claimed that TRL produced a delay in the onset of all rejection episodes and fewer episodes that were steroid-resistant, but TRL was also associated with substantially more adverse events that required discontinuation of therapy. In renal transplant recipients, acute rejection episodes were significantly reduced in the TRL-treated group and the side effects observed were similar to those in the CsA group (94). As with liver recipients, graft survival rates were not significantly different in the two groups. These findings led to FDA approval of TRL as an alternative to CsA for baseline immunosuppression for transplantation (see Table 6.2).

**Rescue Treatment for Acute Refractory Allograft Rejection**
TRL (0.3–0.15 mg/kg/day) was used by Starzl et al (95) to reverse refractory rejection in 7 of 10 liver allograft patients. The common side effects were nausea and vomiting. A pilot study by Jordan et al (96) found that 20 of 35 renal transplant patients who had been converted to TRL (0.3 mg/kg/day) because of either "uncontrolled" rejection or complications attributed to CsA or steroid therapy showed a return to baseline serum creatinine levels, improvement in histologic features of the allograft on renal biopsy, and/or freedom from chronic dialysis. The observed side effects included CMV or bacterial pneumonia, diabetes, hypertension, cecal perforation, and epistaxis. Another report claimed that with TRL treatment, 57 of 77 patients (74%) experienced "rescue" after refractory rejection episodes of liver, cardiac, and combined pancreas and kidney transplants (97). In a US multicenter trial (98), TRL (0.05–0.075 mg/kg/12 hr IV or 0.15 mg/kg/12 hr PO) was administered to 125 liver transplant recipients with rejection episodes that were refractory to OKT-3. It was reported that 54% of patients experienced beneficial effects after 28 days of treatment. Actuarial graft and patient survival rates were 50% and 72%, respectively, at 12 months after conversion. In 54 of 125 patients, the drug was prematurely discontinued because of treatment failure, severe adverse effects, death, or intercurrent illness.

Armitage et al (99) reported that 5 of 8 rejection episodes in cardiac transplant patients were reversed with TRL (0.2–0.4 mg/kg/day). Although they suggested that TRL therapy permits steroid withdrawal, particularly in pediatric cardiac transplant patients, CsA-based regimens also permit successful withdrawal (100). Based on these equivocal findings the FDA declined to approve TRL for the indication of reversal of refractory rejection.

TRL represents an alternative to CsA that displays greater potency in part due initially to the willingness of physicians to tolerate a greater degree of toxicity than what had been observed with CsA therapy, including hyperglycemia (31.4%), nephrotoxicity (27.1%), cardiac toxicity (18.6%; includes chest pain, chest discomfort, palpitations, abnormal EKG), abdominal distension (18.6%), and tremors (10%) in some reports (101). As further progress helped to clarify optimal dosing regimens for TRL therapy, the drug has become more widely used for recipients of all types of allografs including pancreas (102), kidney (103), and thoracic organs (104).

## Sirolimus

Sirolimus (Rapamycin, SRL; Rapamune, Wyeth-Ayerst, Princeton, NJ), a macrocyclic triene antibiotic produced by

*Streptomyces hygroscopicus* isolated from soil samples collected on Easter Island in 1975 (105,106), was originally developed as an anticandidal and antitumor agent (107,108). SRL is a 31-member macrocyclic lactone (molecular weight = 914.2 kd, C51H79N013) akin in structure to TRL by virtue of an unusual tricarbonyl array (carbons [C] 14–16) consisting of an amide, a ketone, a hemiketal, and a chemically sensitive retroaldol site (C31–C33). Importantly, unlike TRL, SRL also contains a triene segment (C1–C6) (109). The backbone of the macrolide ring is mainly derived from acetates and propionates (110) (see Fig. 6.2).

### Molecular Mode of Action

Although SRL binds to FKBP 25, the molecular mechanism of its effect is distinct from the calcineurin-based activity of TRL or even CsA. Sirolimus inhibits a variety of cytokine-mediated, protein kinase C–triggered, and lymphokine-mediated signal transduction pathways, particularly triggered by IL-2 or IL-6 (111). It is thought that SRL inhibits a 282-kd phosphatidylinositol (PI) 3-kinase (FK–Rapamycin Associated Protein, FRAP) (112) that appears necessary for the activation and subsequent protein synthesis of 70-kd S6 kinase ($p70^{S6k}$), a critical enzyme for the activation of the ribosomal protein S6 (113–115). In addition, SRL blocks the phosphorylation (presumably mediated by FRAP) of downstream factors, including: 1) $p34^{cdc2}$ kinase, which forms a heterodimeric complex with cyclin E to produce the maturation-promoting factor, 2) an ill-defined protein that prevents the elimination of $p27^{kip}$, which is a negative regulatory factor for cyclin-dependent kinases, and 3) the eukaryotic initiation factor (eIF-4E)-binding protein necessary for protein translation. The overall effect of these actions is interference with the progression of T cells from the $G_1$ to the S phase of the cell cycle (116–117).

### Pharmacokinetics

The HPLC techniques used to estimate whole blood concentrations of SRL in clinical practice display a detection limit of 2 ng/mL (118). Although liquid chromatography/mass spectrometry (LC/MS) methods are more sensitive, with a detection limit of 80 pg (119), clinical samples generally display concentrations of 5 to 30 ng/mL, and thus LC/MS methods are impractical for use in routine concentration monitoring of SRL. Most of the SRL is found in human red blood and tissue cells, with less than 3% in plasma (120). In contrast to CsA and TRL, the value of the SRL AUC correlates well with the terminal drug concentration ($C_{24}$; $r^2 = 0.9$). Because CsA, TRL, and SRL are all metabolized by cytochrome P450-IIIA4 3A/4, drug interactions have been observed in experimental animals (121) and in humans. High SRL trough levels correlate with high CsA average concentration ($C_{av}$) values (Meier-Kriesche, unpublished observations).

### Experimental Animal Models

**Prophylaxis of Acute Rejection**   SRL doses of 3 and 6 mg/kg for 13 days prolong the survival of heart allografts in rats

and mice, respectively (122). Single 12-mg/kg doses administered intraperitonealy produced indefinite survival of BN and (LxBN) heart allografts in LEW rats (123). Continuous intravenous infusion of SRL (0.08–0.80 mg/kg/day for 14 days) markedly prolonged transplant survival in rats: kidney graft survival was prolonged from 10 ± 0 to 90.2 ± 62.4 days, and small bowel graft survival from 11.6 ± 1.5 to 26.8 ± 3.7 days (124). In contrast, the pig is more sensitive to SRL: doses of 2 mg/kg SRL extended renal allograft survival from 15.1 to 76 days, although interstitial pneumonitis occurred in 5 of 9 pigs. In dogs, even subtherapeutic doses of 2 mg/kg SRL produced the toxic effects of thrombocytopenia and necrotizing fibrinoid vasculitis in the GI tract (125), a finding that was also observed in baboons (126,127). Interestingly, in all these animal models there was no pathohistologic change in kidney grafts associated with SRL therapy in situations where an equally immunosuppressive dose of CsA was nephrotoxic (128,129).

Passive transfer experiments from hosts demonstrating long-term graft survival to isogeneic virgin hosts demonstrated a unique mechanism of drug-induced unresponsiveness. In both rats and mice, SRL treatment induces the production of IgG-blocking antibodies (130). Serum passively transferred from SRL-treated WF recipients significantly prolonged Buffalo (BUF; $RT1^b$) heart allograft survival from 9.8 ± 1.2 days in controls to 74.4 ± 31.1 days ($P = 0.002$). The sera were directed toward donor foreign histocompatibility antigens rather than specific T-cell receptors.

**Rescue Treatment**   When SRL treatment (0.8 mg/kg/day) for 14 days was initiated on day 3 or 4, but not day 5, the rejection process of BUF heart allografts in WF recipients that had been treated with a subtherapeutic dose of CsA was reversed and the transplants enjoyed prolonged survival (131). The same SRL dose prevented accelerated cardiac allograft rejection in presensitized WF recipients, an effect that was also associated with significantly lower levels of donor-specific IgG compared with sensitized, untreated hosts (132).

**Prevention of Chronic Allograft Vasculopathy**   Treatment with SRL reduced intimal thickening and prevented development of experimental chronic allograft vasculopathy in two cardiac transplant models—LEW-to-F344 and BN-to-LEW rats (133,134). In untreated mice, at 30 and 50 days after cardiac transplantation, the incidences of intimal thickening were 55% and 60%, respectively. These rates improved with SRL treatment (135). In addition, the intimal thickening and endothelial proliferation observed in the carotid artery after mechanical balloon injury in rats were reduced by 85% after SRL therapy (136). Presumably these results are related to the immunosuppressive actions of SRL, as well as to its blockade of the proliferative effects of epidermal- and fibroblast-derived growth factors and/or of other cytokines that induce endothelial proliferation.

**Combination Therapy with Other Immunosuppressive Agents**
SRL acts synergistically with CsA in vivo and in vitro. The SRL–CsA combination displays a strong synergistic effect on the order of a 10- to 1000-fold augmentation of the potency of the individual agents to inhibit proliferative

responses (137) and reduce the generation of cytotoxic cells (138). The beneficial synergistic interactions noted by Meiser et al (139) and by Ochiai et al (140) in dogs were also documented in the rat by application of the rigorous median effect analysis (138). In contrast to the strong synergistic interaction of the combination of SRL (0.01 mg/kg/day) and CsA (0.05 mg/kg/day) to prolong rat cardiac allograft survival (157), the combination of SRL and TRL showed antagonism, perhaps due to mutual competition for FKBPs (82,141). SRL has been found to act synergistically with MMF in preventing heart, kidney, and pancreas allograft rejection in rat models (142).

### Clinical Applications

**Clinical Toxicity in Transplantation: Phase I Trial**   In a double-blinded randomized phase I study, Murgia et al (143) administered SRL or placebo for 14 days as twice daily doses to renal transplant recipients who had remained stable for at least 6 months on a CsA–steroid regimen. Thirty patients were divided into three groups: low-dose (1–3 mg/m$^2$/day), medium-dose (5–6 mg/m$^2$/day), and high-dose (7–13 mg/ m$^2$/day); 10 patients received placebo. The major toxic effect of SRL was hypertriglyceridemia. In addition, SRL produced a dose-dependent decrease in platelet counts and to a lesser extent in white blood cell counts. These effects were more pronounced in patients with initially low cell counts. However, SRL treatment did not affect the CsA AUC, blood pressure values, or kidney or liver function tests.

A phase I trial of ascending doses of SRL (0.5– 7.0 mg/m$^2$) administered de novo together with CsA and prednisone showed a reduction in the incidence of acute rejection within the first 6 months to 6.7% (2 of 30) in SRL-treated patients from 36.9% for a historical cohort of 65 patients who were treated with CsA–prednisone alone ($P = 0.02$) (144).

**Prophylaxis of Acute Rejection: Phase II Trial**   A multicenter trial of SRL (1, 3, or 5 mg/m$^2$/day) in combination with

CsA and prednisone confirmed that SRL treatment reduced the incidence of acute rejection episodes among 149 renal transplant recipients. Within 6 months the CsA–prednisone–placebo group showed a 40% incidence of rejection episodes, whereas the groups of patients treated adjunctively with 1 and 3 mg/m$^2$/day SRL experienced a 10% and 7% rejection incidence, respectively. The one-year graft survival was 96% and 87% in patients given placebo and SRL, respectively. A significant racial difference was observed in the incidence of rejection episodes when CsA doses were halved. Nonblack patients treated with a reduced-dose CsA regimen and 1, 3, or 5 mg/m$^2$ SRL experienced approximately a 10% incidence of rejection episodes, whereas black patients treated with a reduced-dose CsA regimen and the same doses of SRL experienced rejection rates comparable to patients treated with a full-dose CsA regimen without SRL (145).

In a subsequent phase II multicenter study, SRL with azathioprine and steroids was compared to CsA with azathioprine and steroids in cadaver donor renal transplant recipients (145). The incidence of rejection and graft survival rates at one year were similar in both patient groups. SRL had a favorable safety profile compared to CsA with regard to tremor, hirsutism, and renal function but produced more significant abnormalities in triglyceride and cholesterol levels.

More recently, SRL has been combined with CsA in phase II/III global multicenter dose-escalation trial for mismatched cadaveric or living-donor renal allograft recipients (146). The investigators noted a reduction in the incidence of acute rejection episodes to 11% from 29% in patients previously treated with CsA and prednisone (Fig. 6.3). The SRL-treated patients had more severe hyperlipidemia, thrombocytopenia, and leukopenia but could be withdrawn more successfully from adjunctive corticosteroid treatment. Additional clinical trials with this agent are underway.

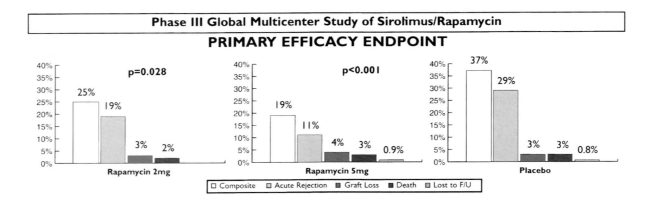

**FIGURE 6.3.**    *Data from 576 recipients of cadaveric or mismatched living-donor renal allografts randomized to receive Rapamycin (2 mg/day or 5 mg/day), or placebo together with CsA and steroids. (Adapted from Highlights of the Transplantation Society XVII World Congress. Montreal, 1998;1:1–2.)*

## 15-Deoxyspergualin

Spergualin (1-amino-19-guanitido-11,15-dihydroxy-4,9,12-triazanonadecane-10,13-dione), a water soluble peptide (molecular weight = 496 d) (147) fermentation product of *Bacillus laterosporus*, was synthetically dehydroxylated to produce 15-deoxyspergualin (DSG; Behringwerke, Marburg, Germany) (148), an agent with antibacterial, antitumor (148–150), and immunosuppressive properties (151–155). The DSG derivative, a racemic mixture of positive and negative enantiomers, has a broader range of activity and greater potency than DSG, but a similar toxicity profile to spergualin.

### Molecular Mode of Action

DSG only moderately inhibits Con-A-, LPS- or MLR-stimulated blastogenesis, as well as cytotoxic T-cell activity (154,156–158), without affecting IL-2 production. DSG is active even when added to cell cultures 3 or 4 days after stimulation (156), suggesting that DSG acts at a later stage during the cell cycle than CsA, perhaps during generation and/or differentiation of antigen-specific cytotoxic T lymphocytes. These immunosuppressive effects are antagonized by supplementation of the lymphocyte medium with IFN-γ, but not IL-2 (156,157,159–161). DSG (5 mg/kg) also dampens antibody production in immunotoxin-treated mice (162) and surface IgM expression after lipopolysaccharide or IFN-γ induction by a murine pre-B-cell line (163). Although the molecular mode of action of DSG is unknown, the compound specifically binds to Hsp70, a member of the heat shock protein family, which may represent a class of immunophilins distinct from the cis-trans proline isomerase immunophilins, cyclophilins, and FKBPs (164). In addition, DSG inhibits the monocyte/macrophage functions of liposomal enzyme release, superoxide production, class II antigen upregulation, and IL-1 production (165,166).

### Pharmacokinetics

DSG must be delivered parenterally because it is a highly polar molecule with poor (3% to 6%) oral bioavailability (167). After intravenous infusion (80–2160 mg/m²/day), DSG and its major (among 6) metabolite, desaminopropyl-DSG, reach steady-state concentration within 2 hours and show no accumulation over 5 days (168–171). The AUC of DSG correlates well with the administered dose ($r^2 = 0.97$). The drug is cleared in a biexponential manner. The α-phase half-life ranges from 5 to 30 minutes, the β-phase half-life ranges from 44 to 160 minutes, and the total body clearance rate ranges from 258 to 451 mL/min/m² (mean 364 ± 78 mL/min/m²) (168). The drug is primarily eliminated by the kidney, with 4% to 14% of the administered dose excreted unchanged in the urine (168,172).

### Experimental Animal Models

**Prophylaxis of Acute Rejection**   DSG modestly prolongs the survival of rat skin (154) or islet (151) allografts and mouse heart pinnal implants (173), as well as liver, pancreas, thyroid, and pancreaticoduodenal transplants in rats and mice (153,174). In canine models, DSG caused significant gastrointestinal toxicity, and in baboons 4 mg/kg/day DSG improved cardiac, but not renal, allograft survival (175). Furthermore, DSG modestly inhibited accelerated rejection responses in skin graft–sensitized rats, prolonging survival from 4.2 ± 0.5 days to 7.2 ± 0.5 days ($P < 0.01$).

**Rescue Treatment for Acute Allograft Rejection**   Because it was observed in rats that DSG was more effective if administered 10 days after skin transplantation rather than perioperatively (155,176), canine experiments were conducted and showed that DSG treatment (2.4 mg/kg/day for 12 days) reversed acute rejection episodes, although the dogs experienced severe gastrointestinal toxicity (177).

**Combination Therapy with Other Immunosuppressive Agents**   Although DSG adds little benefit to CsA immunoprophylaxis, there was no additive interaction between CsA and DSG (3–4 mg/kg/day) to improve the survival of monkey heart xenotransplants into chacme baboons (178). DSG showed a stronger interaction with the antirat T-cell receptor MAb R73 than with CsA. In a multimodality protocol, the combination of low doses of DSG (0.5 mg/kg/day), CsA (20 mg/kg/day), Aza (2.5 mg/kg/day), and ALG (2.5 mg/kg/day) treatment during a 14-day induction period showed an additive interaction to prolong canine islet graft survival in chacme baboons, which unfortunately suffered gastrointestinal toxicity.

### Clinical Applications

**Toxicity in Cancer Patients: Phase I Trials**   Administration of DSG (20–600 mg/m²) as a 3-hour infusion for 5 consecutive days to 28 cancer patients produced dose-dependent gastrointestinal toxicity (nausea/vomiting, anorexia), alopecia, tongue and perioral numbness, hypotension, and bone marrow suppression (granulocytopenia, leukopenia, and anemia) (169). There was extensive formation of the drug metabolite desaminopropyl-DSG, with less than 10% of the administered dose excreted unchanged in the urine (168).

**Prophylaxis of Rejection: Phase II Trials**   In a de novo treatment protocol in 10 patients, Koyama et al (179) administered the combination of DSG (2–5 mg/kg/day for 5 to 14 days), prednisone, CsA (4–6 mg/kg/day), and mizorbine (2–3 mg/kg/day) or Aza (1–2 mg/kg/day). They observed that facial numbness was the most common side effect, and bone marrow suppression was the most serious, albeit reversible, side effect. The most striking clinical result in phase II studies was that two patients with type I diabetes mellitus were insulin-independent at 9 months after simultaneous single donor islet and kidney transplants when treated with DSG, prednisone, MALG, and CsA (180).

**Rescue Treatment for Acute Allograft Rejection: Phase II Trials**   An initial study reported that DSG (40–220 mg/m²) produced remissions in 27 of 34 acute rejection episodes after renal transplantation (181), particularly when combined with methylprednisone (MP) (182). DSG (3–5 mg/kg) administered as seven daily 3-hour infusions produced a 76% rate of reversal of 260 acute rejection episodes within the first six months after transplantation. Among 30 rejection episodes graded by Banff criteria, DSG was more effective in reversing grade I (20 of 22; 88%) compared with grade IIa (3 of 8; 38%) episodes (183). In addition, DSG reversed 70% of steroid-resistant rejection episodes. However, the combination of DSG and MP produced the highest rate of rejection reversal (87.5%). The adverse effects observed in patients treated for allograft rejection included numbness of the face, lips, and limbs (14%), gastrointestinal toxicity (9%), bone marrow suppression (26 to 54% ), and the occurrence of infection (9%). These results led to approval of DSG in Japan in 1994 for the treatment of acute rejection episodes in kidney transplant recipients (184).

**Inhibition of Preformed Antibody Synthesis: Phase II Trials**
The combination of DSG (5 mg/kg/day for 5 days) with other agents (CsA, MP, and ALG) appears to inhibit secondary synthesis of preformed antibodies in ABO-incompatible or HLA-presensitized kidney transplant recipients. Combination therapy beginning de novo on postoperative day 1 was used with pretransplant plasmapheresis in 14 renal transplant patients. Five subjects did not experience rejection episodes, one lost his graft, and two died (one from a B-cell lymphoma and the other from cerebral hemorrhage) (185). Administration of DSG (4 mg/kg for 5 days) in three xenografted patients appeared to facilitate pig islet cell survival for several weeks to months, as manifested by urinary excretion of small amounts of porcine C-peptide (186).

Thus, although DSG seems to reverse allograft rejection episodes effectively, it displays a lower efficacy for prophylaxis of allograft rejection episodes than CsA. However, the clinical trials to date do not document the agent's therapeutic efficacy, but rather show its limitations, such as low oral bioavailability and severe gastrointestinal toxicity. Because of these characteristics, DSG must be administered systemically and for only limited periods of time.

# FTY720

Myriocin (ISP-1) is an immunosuppressive compound that was isolated from the culture broth of *Isaria sinclairii* (ATCC 24400) (187). Its semisynthetic derivative FTY720 (188), a phenyl ring inserted into the side chain (2-octadecyl-2-amino-1,3-propanediol) is less toxic than ISP-1 (189).

## *Molecular Mode of Action*
The parent compound ISP-1 inhibits the proliferation of lymphocytes in allogenic mouse MLR 5- to 10-fold more potently than CsA, but fails to dampen human leukemia cell proliferation. In vivo, ISP-1 inhibits T-cell–dependent antibody formation 10-fold and alloreactive CTL production 100-fold more effectively than CsA (187). In contrast, even at high (1000 nmol/L) concentrations, FTY720 does not inhibit the production of IL-2 or IL-3 (190), and therefore must act on a distinctive activation pathway. ISP-1, but not FTY720, inhibits serine palmitoyl transferase activity in IL-2–dependent CTLL-2 cells (191). One hypothesis advocated by Suzuki et al (192) suggests that antigen–induced apoptosis, as evidenced

by the formation of apoptotic bodies and the presence of DNA ladders on agarose gel analysis of rat spleen cells, is produced by a three-hour in vitro incubation with drug. A second hypothesis is based on the observation that administration of FTY720 (10 mg/kg) to rats causes peripheral lymphocytopenia within three hours, seemingly due to a reduced expression of $\alpha_4$-integrin. In contrast, FTY720 does not reduce the numbers of circulating polymorphonuclear leukocytes, peripheral B cells, bone marrow cells, or thymocytes, or the splenic content of B cells. Conversely, the numbers of T and B cells in mesenteric and peripheral lymph nodes increase, suggesting acceleration of lymphocyte homing, producing sequestration from the allograft. The effect may be mediated by upregulated expression $\alpha 4/\beta 7$-integrin on lymphocytes that bind Gly CAM-1 and Mad CAM-1, both of which are expressed on the cell surface of high endothelial venules (HEV) in lymph nodes and Peyer's patches (193).

## *Experimental Animal Models*
**Prophylaxis of Acute Rejection** Administration of ISP-1 at doses of 0.03–0.30 mg/kg intraperitoneally prolonged the survival of rat skin allografts in dose-dependent fashion, but with severe toxicity. FTY720 (0.1–10.0 mg/kg IV) prolonged LEW skin allograft survival in F344 rats (188). Administration of low doses (0.5 mg/kg) of FTY720 for 14 days prolonged ACI liver allograft survival in LEW rats from 11.5 to 27.5 days. A two-day course of FTY720 (5 mg/kg/day) initiated either one day before and on the day of transplant, or on days 3 and 4 after transplant, prolonged graft survival from 11.5 to 28.5 or 23 days, respectively. The former two-dose regimen of FTY720 administration prolonged the median survival time of canine kidney grafts from 9 to 21 days, a result that was not inferior to that obtained by administering a daily regimen of FTY720 (192).

**Combination Therapy with Cyclosporine** FTY720 (0.1 mg/kg) potentiated the immunosuppressive effects of CsA to prolong the survival of rat skin allografts (194). Subtherapeutic daily CsA doses (10 mg/kg PO) starting on day 1 in combination with 1 or 5 mg/kg/day doses of FTY720 starting on day 1 produced 36.5- or 74-day mean allograft survivals, respectively (192). Further studies showed that even lower FTY720 doses of 0.1 to 1.0 mg/kg/day in combination with CsA significantly prolonged canine renal graft survival compared with CsA alone (195). Median effect analysis of rat heart allograft survivals documented that combinations of FTY720 with CsA displayed a greater degree of synergism than did FTY720 with SRL (Kahan et al, unpublished observations). Phase I clinical trials studying an FTY720–CsA combination were begun in December of 1998.

# SUMMARY

During the past two decades, since the cyclosporine revolution, there has been an explosion of interest in the discovery and development of small molecule immunosuppressants that reduce the rate of acute allograft rejection episodes and increase graft and patient survival rates. The nonspecific cytostatic immunosuppressive chemicals are now being superseded by agents that act specifically on T-cell function. As a result, there has been a trend to eliminate azathioprine and corticosteroids, the primary components of the immunosuppressive regimens used from 1962 to 1982, from the regimens because of their adverse effects on elements of nonspecific host resistance. Although some physicians contend that the more selective purine synthesis inhibitor mycophenolate mofetil significantly reduces the incidence of acute allograft rejection episodes, others are concerned about the agent's well-documented side-effect profile. Although leflunomide and brequinar specifically inhibit de novo pyrimidine synthesis, their adverse effect of marked myelodepression results in a narrow therapeutic window and consequently little advantage over the purine synthesis inhibitors mycophenolate mofetil and mizorbine. In contrast, two new agents introduced since the advent of the cyclosporine era, tacrolimus and sirolimus, specifically disrupt cytokine generation by acting on T lymphocytes, and therefore may serve to improve graft survival in clinical transplantation. Although tacrolimus seems to be little more than an alternative to cyclosporine, sirolimus, particularly when combined with CsA, produces a synergistic interaction that reduces the incidence of acute rejection episodes, permits early steroid withdrawal, and/or allows marked CsA dose reduction. Among the other new agents, 15-deoxyspergualin, which has been used primarily by Japanese physicians to treat refractory renal allograft rejection, is not presently under clinical development, although it might play a future role in the treatment of allo-presensitized recipients or in xenotransplantation. In contrast, there is considerable excitement about the new agent FTY720, which may cause antigen-induced apoptosis and certainly interacts synergistically with CsA both in rodents and in dogs. The drug is currently being prepared to begin clinical trials.

As the enormous number of new small molecule compounds that display in vitro antilymphocyte activity are evaluated as immunosuppressants in rodent, canine, and primate models, we are likely to witness an evolution in immunosuppressive therapy. Soon, highly selective drug therapy may be based on our knowledge of the molecular events that lead to acute or chronic allograft rejection.

---

## COMMENTARY

*Karl Wagner*

The evolution of immunosuppressive therapy has reached the point where basic questions must be addressed. The development of cyclosporine (CsA) and its subsequent widespread use in highly differentiated protocols in combination with steroids resulted in a marked increase in short-term survival among transplant patients. Following renal transplantation, one-year patient and graft survival figures in excess of 95% and 85%, respectively, became achievable. Such an accomplishment is even more impres-

sive when we consider the relative expansion of indications for transplantation, the waiving of various contraindications for transplantation (including coronary heart disease), and the adoption of a more liberal use of organs from elderly donors during the past two decades. The questions raised now, therefore, include: What one-year survival rates can be achieved by using conventional immunosuppressive therapy in multimorbid patients? Can we further improve upon these results without inducing donor-specific tolerance? As we approach the magical limit of 100% one-year survival rates, the size of study groups that would be required to demonstrate the statistical superiority of a new immunosuppressive compound has become extraordinarily large. Since these numbers are seldom achievable, the efficacy of any new agent must compete at least with the results achieved using the "gold standard" CsA. Secondary end points including the occurrence of "immunologic catastrophes" (e.g., steroid-resistant rejection, life-threatening septicemias), changes in vascular risk (hypertension, lipid metabolism) profiles, the severity and clinical relevance of other complications, and economic analyses must, therefore, also be taken into consideration.

Despite the improvement of one-year survival rates with CsA, the subsequent rate of graft loss has not changed considerably over the past decade. This may be the consequence of chronic rejection that might have additional causes other than immunologic imbalance between donor and recipient. As there may be numerous mechanisms involved in the development of chronic rejection, further questions are: What potential role can new immunosuppressive agents play in preventing chronic rejection? Do immunosuppressive agents currently under evaluation exert their effects by any supplementary mechanisms that might be relevant for chronic rejection? Although clinical observations that can answer these questions will only be available from long-term investigations, we should certainly consider these points when evaluating new immunosuppressive agents.

The molecules discussed in this chapter can be divided into three groups: those with proven clinical relevance [mycophenolate mofetil (MMF) and tacrolimus (TRL, FK506)], a second group consisting of agents entering clinical investigation [sirolimus (SRL) and 15-desoxyspergualin (DSG)], and a final group where data are only available from animal experiments (leflunomide and the myriocin derivative, FTY720). With respect to the latter group and specifically leflunomide, the adverse reaction profile of the active compound A771726 obviates clinical application. Whether less toxic analogues can be developed remains to be evaluated. Clinical use of DSG may be limited because of the associated gastrointestinal toxicity; but perhaps more importantly, based on its very low oral bioavailability, it will need to be administered systemically. Although DSG has a proven efficacy in the reversal of ongoing rejection episodes (including steroid-resistant rejection), the assessment of Senel and Kahan that DSG is less efficacious than CsA in the prophylaxis of allograft rejection is supported by the fact that DSG has received formal approval only for the treatment of acute renal allograft rejection.

Thus, of the six compounds discussed in this chapter, only MMF, TRL, and SRL seem to be of current clinical relevance. Besides the different mechanisms of action, there is an additional major distinguishing point that must be recognized: Only TRL has, to date, been considered a primary immunosuppressant capable of replacing CsA, whereas MMF and SRL have been investigated mostly for use in conjunction with CsA.

Conclusions concerning SRL must reflect the fact that patient and graft survival from prospective randomized renal transplant trials are just becoming available. Survival and toxicity observations from the multi-institutional European trial will be of particular interest since this trial will evaluate SRL as primary therapy in place of CsA. Available data from the Sirolimus Multi-Center Study Group phase I/II trials indicate a dramatic reduction in the occurrence of rejection from 40% for the control group (CsA and steroids) to 10% and 7%, respectively, in patients treated with the addition of 1 and 3 mg/m$^2$/day of SRL. Combination therapy with SRL and CsA appears to exert, at least experimentally, a synergistic immunosuppressive effect. This implies, as shown by the Sirolimus Multi-Center Study Group, the possibility, at least in Caucasians, of reducing the CsA dose in conjunction with SRL with no detrimental effect on rejection rates. The experimental observation that SRL prevents chronic allograft vasculopathy by blockade of the proliferative effects of growth factors might have implications for its effect on chronic rejection. SRL, in conclusion, appears to be a promising substance. However, the data currently available do not yet enable us to answer whether patient and graft survival are comparable to those achieved with conventional CsA-based therapy.

MMF has undergone extensive investigations for the prophylaxis of rejection in prospectively randomized renal transplant recipients (see also Chapter 5). Over 1400 recipients were included in three different trials. One observation from these trials was the finding that conventional triple therapy (CsA, steroids, and azathioprine) offers only a 2% reduction in the incidence of rejection compared with dual therapy (CsA and steroids). The addition of MMF in doses of 2 or 3 g/day to dual therapy resulted in similar patient and graft survival but a significant reduction in rejection episodes (to below 20%). This was accompanied by a reduction in the severity of the rejection as assessed according to the Banff classification. This was paralleled by a reduction in the rate of steroid-resistant rejection and a lower use of OKT-3. The incidence of leukopenia was significantly reduced in patients receiving MMF compared with those treated with azathioprine. These positive effects were somewhat counter-balanced by the frequent occurrence of abdominal discomfort and a slightly higher incidence of viral infections. Since MMF has been shown

experimentally to reduce the formation of adhesion molecules, the MMF-treated patients in the above trials have been enrolled in continuing studies investigating the possible role of MMF in limiting the development of biopsy-proven chronic rejection.

It may be concluded that whenever the indication for an augmentation of immunosuppression with the addition of azathioprine is present, it is reasonable to consider incorporating MMF in its place. Whether this may have any impact on the development of chronic rejection can only be determined in further trials. Unfortunately, a misguiding pricing policy, which established the daily cost of MMF to be comparable to that of CsA and therefore far above that of azathioprine, may in the long run prevent the long-term use of MMF.

TRL differs markedly from the molecules discussed above (see also Chapter 4). First, it is the only new molecule thus far established to be effective as baseline immunosuppression in place of CsA. Second, initial clinical experience was gained in liver transplantation. Its mechanism of action, at least in part, seems to be similar to that of CsA. However, TRL complexes with a different intracellular binding protein and its immunosuppressive potency seems to be far higher than that of CsA. In phase III liver transplant studies comparing CsA-based triple therapy and TRL-based dual therapy, patient and graft survival were numerically higher in the TRL treatment groups, although these differences failed to reach statistical significance. In addition, TRL was associated with significant reductions in the incidence of acute and steroid-resistant rejection episodes and a consequent lower usage of OKT-3. In some trials, a reduced incidence of hypertension and smaller disturbances in lipoprotein metabolism were also noted. Subsequent renal transplant studies have now yielded similar results: comparable patient and graft survival in the TRL and CsA treatment groups, but significant reductions in the incidence of rejection and less frequent OKT-3 usage in TRL-treated patients. However, changes in the vascular risk profile (hypertension and lipoprotein metabolism) appeared to be somewhat less prominent. Adverse reactions associated with TRL are similar to those seen with CsA, although some differences are apparent. Nephrotoxicity is comparable, but both gingival hyperplasia and hirsutism are far less prevalent with TRL. A major difference in some trials is the higher diabetogenic effect of TRL, which may be controlled by steroid reduction.

TRL possesses a unique property not as evident with CsA. In numerous trials in both liver and renal transplant recipients, TRL has shown the capacity to reverse refractory allograft rejection. This effect appears to be independent of the preceding administration of antilymphocyte antibodies, and the use of TRL is therefore warranted even in the presence of steroid-resistant graft rejection or when treatment with antilymphocyte antibodies is ineffective or contraindicated. Based on experience with TRL in previous studies of primary immunosuppressive treatment and on the compelling evidence that the drug is effective in rescue therapy, its use in a primary immunosuppressive regimen for immunologic high responders should be considered.

In conclusion, with respect to the emerging clinical role of small molecule immunosuppressive agents, the short-term results appear similar to those achieved with CsA immunosuppression. However, as a result of their distinct properties, they may offer a more flexible individualization of immunosuppression and hopefully, in the long run, for improvement in long-term graft survival.

## REFERENCES

1. Gosio B. Ricerche bacteriologiche e chimiche sulle alterazioni del mais. Riv Igiene e Sanita Publica Ann 1896;7:825.
2. Platz KP, Sollinger HW, Hullett DA, et al. RS-61443—a new potent immunosuppressive agent. Transplantation 1991;51:27–31.
3. Schiff MH, Goldblum R, Rees MMC. 2-Morpholino-ethyl mycophenolic acid in the treatment of refractory rheumatoid arthritis. Arthritis Rheum 1990;33s:155.
4. Jones EL, Epinette WW, Hackney VC, et al. Treatment of psoriasis with oral mycophenolic acid. J Invest Dermatol 1975;65:537–542.
5. Lynch WS, Roesnigk HH Jr. Mycophenolic acid for psoriasis. Arch Dermatol 1977;113:1203–1208.
6. Epinette WW, Parker CM, Jones EL, Greist MC. Mycophenolic acid for psoriasis. J Am Acad Dermatol 1987;17:962–971.
7. Sollinger HW, Eugi EM, Allison AC. RS-61443: mechanism of action, experimental and early clinical results. Clin Transplant 1991;5s:523–526.
8. Giblett ER, Anderson JE, Cohen F, Meuwissen HJ. Adenosine deaminase deficiency of two patients with severely impaired cellular immunity. Lancet 1972;2:1067–1069.
9. Natsumeda Y, Carr SF. Human type I and II IMPDH as drug targets. Ann NY Acad Sci 1993;696:88.
10. Franklin TJ, Cook JM. The inhibition of nucleic acid synthesis by mycophenolic acid. Biochem J 1969;113:515–524.
11. Mizuno K, Miyazaki T. Synthesis and cytotoxicity of bredinine 5-monophosphate. Chem Pharm Bull 1976;24:2248–2250.
12. Mita A, Akiyama N, Nagao T, et al. Advantages of mizoribine over azathioprine in combination therapy with cyclosporine for renal transplantation. Transplant Proc 1990;22:1679–1681.
13. Eugi EM, Almquist S, Muller CD, Allison AC. Lymphocyte selective cytostatic and immunosuppressive effects of mycophenolic acid in vitro: role of deoxyguanosine nucleotide depletion. Scan J Immunol 1991;33:161–173.
14. Allison AC, Kowalski WJ, Muller CD, Eugi EM. Mechanisms of action of mycophenolic acid. Ann NY Acad Sci 1993;696:63.
15. Allison AC, Eugi EM. Inhibitors of de novo purine and pyrimidine synthesis as immunosuppressive drugs. Transplant Proc 1993; 25(Suppl 2):8–18.
16. Dayton JS, Turka LA, Thompson CB, et al. Comparison of the effects of mizoribine with those of azathioprine, 6-mercaptopurine or mycophenolic acid on T lymphocyte proliferation and purine metabolism. Molec Pharmacol 1992;141:671.
17. Laurent AF, Dumont S, Poindron P, Muller CD. Mycophenolic acid suppresses protein N-linked glycosylation in human monocytes and their adhesion to endothelial cells and to some substratcs. Exp Hematol 1996;24:59–67.
18. Alices M, Osborne L, Takada Y, Carause C. VCAM-1 on activated endothelium interacts with the lymphocytes integrin VLA-4 at a site distinct from the fiber nectin binding site. Cell 1990;60:577–584.
19. Allison AC, Kowalski WJ, Muller CJ, et al. Mycophenolic acid and brequinar, inhibitors of purine and pyrimidine synthesis, block the glycosylation of adhesion molecules. Transplant Proc 1993;25(3;Suppl 2):67–70.
20. Lee WA, Gu L, Miksztal AR, et al. Bioavailability improvement of mycophenolic acid through amino ester derivatization. Pharmaceut Res 1990;7:161–166.
21. Allison AC, Eugi EM. Immunosuppressive and long-acting anti-inflammatory effect of mycophenolic acid and derivatives, RS-61433. Br J Rheum 1991;30(Suppl 2):57–61.
22. Propper DJ, Woo J, Macleod AM, et al. The effects of rapamycin on humoral immunity in vivo: suppression of primary responses but not of ongoing alloantibody synthesis or memory responses. Transplantation 1992;54:1058.
23. Sollinger HW, Deierhoi MH, Belzer FO, et al. RS-61443: a phase I clinical trial and pilot rescue study. Transplantation 1992;53:428–432.
24. Marinairi R, Fleischmajer R, Schragger AH, Rosenthal AL. Mycophenolic acid in treatment of psoriasis: long term administration. Arch Dermatol 1977;113:930–932.
25. Jones EL, Frost P, Epinette WW, Gomez E. Mycophenolic acid: an evaluation of long-term safety. In: Faber M, ed. Psoriasis: Proceedings of the Second International Symposium. New York: Yorke, 1977:442–443.
26. Goldblum R, McHugh D, Schiff M, et al. 2-morpholino-ethyl mycophenolic acid (ME-MPA) inhibits lymphocyte mitogen responses in rheumatoid arthritis. J Clin Pharm Ther 1990;47:193.
27. Deierhoi MH, Kauffman RS, Hudson SL, et al. Experience with mycophenolate mofetil (RS61443) in renal transplantation at a single center. Ann Surg 1993;217:476–484.
28. Paterson DL, Singh W, Panebianco A, et al. Infectious complications occurring in liver transplant recipients receiving mycophenolate mofetil. Transplantation 1998;66:593–598.
29. Kirklin JK, Bouge RC, Naftel DC, et al. Treatment of recurrent heart rejection with mycophenolate mofetil: initial clinical experience. J Heart Lung Transplantation 1994;13:444–450.
30. Neylan JF for the U.S. Renal Transplant Mycophenolate Mofetil Study Group. Immunosuppressive therapy in high-risk transplant patients. Transplantation 1997;64:1277–1282.
31. Sollinger HW, Belzer FO, Deierhoi MH, et al. RS-61443: a multicenter study for refractory kidney transplant rejection. Ann Surg 1992;216:513–519.
32. The Mycophenolate Mofetil Renal Refractory Rejection Study Group. Mycophenolate mofetil for the treatment of refractory acute cellular renal transplant rejection. Transplantation 1996;61:722–729.
33. European Mycophenolate Mofetil Cooperative Study Group. Placebo-controlled study of mycophenolate mofetil combined with cyclosporin and corticosteroids for prevention of acute rejection. Lancet 1995;345:1321–1325.
34. Sollinger HW, for the US Renal Transplant Mycophenolate Mofetil Study Group. Mycophenolate mofetil for the prevention of acute rejection in primary cadaveric renal allograft recipients. Transplantation 1995;60:225–232.
35. Morris RE, Wang J, Blum JR, et al. Immunosuppressive effects of the morpholinoethyl ester of mycophenolic acid (RS-61443) in rat and nonhuman primate recipients of heart allografts. Transplant Proc 1991;23(Suppl 2):19–25.
36. Steele DM, Hullett DA, Bechtein WO, et al. The effects of immunosuppressive therapy on rat aortic allograft model. Transplant Proc 1993;25:754.
37. Schmid C, Heemann U, Azuma H, Tilney NL. Comparison of rapamycin, RS-61443, cyclosporine, and low-dose heparin as treatment for transplant vasculopathy in rat model of chronic allograft rejection. Transplant Proc 1995;27:438–439.
38. Azuma H, Binder J, Heeman U, et al. Effects of RS61443 on functional and morphological changes in chronically rejecting rat kidney allografts. Transplant Proc 1995;27(1):436–437.
39. Mathew TH for the Tricontinental Mycophenolate Mofetil Renal Transplantation Study Group. A blinded, long-term, randomized multicenter study of mycophenolate mofetil in cadaveric renal transplantation. Transplantation 1998;65:1450–1454.
40. Gruessner RWG, Sutherland DER, Drangsveit MB, et al. Mycophenolate mofetil in pancreas transplantation. Transplantation 1998;66:318–323.
41. Dexter DL, Hesson DP, Ardecky RJ, et al. Activity of a novel 4-quinolinecarboxylic acid, NSC368390 [6-fluoro-2-(2′fluoro-1,1′biphenyl-4-yl)-3-methyl-4-quinolinecarboxylic acid sodium salt], against experimental tumors. Cancer Res 1985;45:5563–5568.
42. Chen SF, Ruben R, Dexter D. Mechanism of action of the novel anti-cancer agent 6-fluoro-2-(2′-fluoro-1,1 byphenyl 4-yl)-3 methyl-4 quinolone carboxylic acid sodium salt. Inhibition of de novo pyrimidine nucleotide biosynthesis. Cancer Res 1986;46:5014.
43. Simon P, Townsend RM, Harris RR, et al. Brequinar sodium: inhibition of dihydro-orotic acid dehydrogenase, depletion of pyrimidine pools and consequent inhibition of immune function in vitro. Transplant Proc 1993;25(Suppl 2):77–80.
44. Chen SF, Papp LM, Ardecky RJ, et al. Structure-activity relationship of quinoline carboxylic acids: a new class of inhibitors of dihydro-orotate dehydrogenase. Biochem Pharmacol 1990;40:709–714.
45. Chen JJ, Jones ME. The ceullar location of dihydro-orotate dehydrogenase: relation to de novo biosynthesis of pyrimidines. Arch Biochem Biophys 1976;176:82–90.

46. Makowka L, Chapman F, Cramer DV. Historical development of brequinar sodium as a new immunosuppressive drug for transplantation. Transplant Proc 1993;25(Suppl 2):2–7.

47. Peters GJ, Nadal JC, Laurensse EJ, et al. Retention of in vitro antipyrimidine effects of brequinar sodium (DUP-785; NSC 368390) in murine liver, bone marrow, and colon cancer. Biochem Pharmacol 1990;39:134–144.

48. Makowka L, Sher LS, Cramer DV. The development of brequinar as an immunosuppressive drug for transplantation. Immunol Rev 1993;136:51.

49. Cramer DV, Chapman FA, Jaffee BD, et al. The effects of a new immunosuppressive drug: brequinar sodium on heart, liver and kidney allograft rejection in the rat. Transplantation 1992;53:303–308.

50. Jaffee BD, Jones EA, Loveless SE, Chen SF. The unique immunosuppressive activity of brequinar sodium. Transplant Proc 1993;25(Suppl 2):19.

51. Kahan BD, Tejpal N, Gibbons S, et al. The synergistic interactions in vivo and in vitro of brequinar sodium with cyclosporine or rapamycin alone and in triple combination. Transplantation 1993;55:894.

52. Cramer DV, Chapman FA, Jaffee BD, et al. The prolongation of concordant cardiac hamster-to-rat xenograft by brequinar sodium. Transplantation 1993;54:403–408.

53. Yasunaga C, Cramer DV, Chapman FA, et al. The prevention of accelerated cardiac allograft rejection in sensitized recipients following treatment with brequinar sodium. Transplantation 1993;56:898.

54. Eiras-Hreha G, Cramer DV, Cosenza C, et al. Brequinar sodium: monitoring immunosuppressive activity. Transplant Proc 1993;25(3;Suppl 2):32–36.

55. Shen HS, Chen SF, Behrens C, et al. Distribution of the novel anticancer drug candidate brequinar sodium (Du 785, NSC 36890) into normal and tumor tissues of nude mice bearing human colon carcinoma xenografts. Cancer Chemother Pharmacol 1988;22:183–186.

56. Schwartzmann G, Dodion P, Vermorken JB, et al. Phase I study with brequinar sodium (NSC 368390) in patients with solid malignancies. Cancer Chemother Pharmacol 1990;25:345–351.

57. Barnes TB, Campbell P, Zajac I, Gayda D. Toxicological and pharmacokinetic effects following coadministration of brequinar sodium and cyclosporine to Sprague-Dawley rats. Transplant Proc 1993;25(Suppl 2):71–74.

58. Stepkowski SM, Tu Y, Chou TC, Kahan BD. Synergistic interactions of cyclosporine, rapamycin, and brequinar on heart allograft survival in mice. Transplant Proc 1994;26:3025–3027.

59. Kawamura T, Hullet DA, Suzuki Y, et al. Enhancement of allograft survival by combination RS-61443 and DUP-785 therapy. Transplantation 1993;55:691–695.

60. Makowka L, Tixier D, Chaux A, et al. The use of brequinar sodium for preventing cardiac allograft rejection in primates. Transplant Proc 1993;25(Suppl 2):48–53.

61. Artega CL, Brown TD, Khun JG, et al. Phase I clinical and pharmacokinetic trial of brequinar sodium. Cancer Res 1989;49:4648.

62. Maorun J, Ruckdeschel J, Natale R, et al. Multicenter phase II study of brequinar sodium in patients with advanced lung cancer. Cancer Chemother Pharmacol 1993;32:64.

63. Sher LS, Eiras-Hreha G, Kornhauser DM, et al. Safety and pharmacokinetics of brequinar sodium in liver allograft recipients on cyclosporine and steroids. Hepatology 1993;18:746.

64. Chong AS-F, Gebel H, Finnegan A, et al. Leflunomide, a novel immunomodulatory agent: in vitro analyses of the mechanism of immunosuppression. Transplant Proc 1993;25(1):747–749.

65. Chong AS-F, Finnegan A, Jiang XL, et al. Leflunomide, a novel immunosuppressive agent: the mechanism of inhibition of T cell proliferation. Transplantation 1993;55:1361–1366.

66. Chong AS, Xiao F, Xu XL, Williams JW. In vivo and in vitro immunosuppression with leflunomide. New immunosuppressive drugs. Glenview, IL: Physicians and Scientists, 1995:163–176.

67. Bartlett RR, Dimitrijevic M, Mattar T, et al. Leflunomide (HWA 486), a novel immunomodulating compound for the treatment of autoimmune disorders and reactions leading to transplantation rejection. Agents Actions 1991;32:10–21.

68. Cao WW, Kao PN, Choa AC, et al. Mechanism of antiproliferative action of leflunomide. A77 1726, the active metabolite of leflunomide, does not block T-cell receptor-mediated signal transduction but its antiproliferative effects are antagonized by pyrimidine nucleosides. J Heart Lung Transplant 1995;14:1016–1030.

69. Bartlett RR, Schleyerbach R. Immunopharmacological profile of novel isoxazol derivative HWA 486, with potential antirheumatic activity-I. Disease modifying action on arthritis of the rat. Int J Immunopharmacol 1985;7:7–18.

70. Popovic S, Bartlett RR. The use of the murine chronic graft vs. host disease, a model for systemic lupus erythematosis, for drug discovery. Agents Actions 1987;21:284.

71. Ogawa T, Inazu M, Gotoh K, Hayashi S. Effects of leflunomide on glomerulonephritis induced by antibasement membrane antibody in rats. Agents and Actions 1990;31:321–328.

72. Thoenes GH, Sitter T, Langer KH, et al. Leflunomide (HWA 486) inhibits experimental autoimmune tubulointerstitial nephritis in rats. Int J Immunopharmac 1989;11:921–929.

73. McChesney L, Xiao F, Sankary H, et al. Evaluation of leflunomide in the canine renal transplantation model. Transplantation 1994;57:1717–1722.

74. Kuchle CCA, Thoenes GH, Langer KH, et al. Prevention of kidney and skin graft rejection in rats by leflunomide, a new immunomodulating agent. Transplant Proc 1991;23:1083–1086.

75. Schorlemmer HU, Seiler FR, Bartlett RR. Prolongation of allogeneic transplanted skin grafts and induction of tolerance by leflunomide, a new immunosuppressive isoxazol derivative. Transplant Proc 1993;25:763–767.

76. Williams JW, Xiao F, Foster P, et al. Leflunomide in experimental transplantation. Transplantation 1994;57:1223–1231.

77. Xiao F, Chong A, Foster P, et al. Effect of leflunomide in control of acute rejection in hamster-to-rat cardiac xenografts. Transplant Proc 1993;26:1263–1265.

78. Kino T, Hatanaka H, Hoshimata M, et al. FK 506, a novel immunosuppressant isolated from a streptomyces. I. Fermentation, isolation, and physicochemical and biological characteristics. J Antibiotics 1987;40:1249–1255.

79. Tanaka H, Kurado A, Marusawa H, et al. Structure of FK 506: a novel immunosuppressant isolated from a streptomyces. J Am Chem Soc 1987;109:5031–5033.

80. Harding MW, Galat A, Uehling DE, Schreiber SL. A receptor for immunosuppressant FK506 is a peptidyl prolyl cis-trans isomerase. Nature 1989;341:758–760.

81. Siekierka JJ, Hung SHY, Poe M, et al. A cytosolic binding protein for the immunosuppressive FK506 has peptidyl prolyl isomerase activity but is distinct from cyclophilin. Nature 1989;341:755–757.

82. Liu J. FK506 and cyclosporine, molecular probes for studying intracellular signal transduction. Immunol Today 1993;14(6):290–295.

83. Klee CB, Draetta GF, Hubbard MJ. Advances in enzymology and related areas of molecular biology. Vol. 61. New York: Wiley, 1988:49–209.

84. Fruman DA, Klee CB, Bierer BE, Burakoff SJ. Calcineurin phosphatase activity in T lymphocytes is inhibited by FK506 and cyclosporin A. Proc Natl Acad Sci 1992;89:3686–3690.

85. O'Keefe SJ, Tamura J, Kincaid RL, et al. FK-506 and CsA-sensitive activation of the interleukin-2 promoter by calcineurin. Nature 1992;357:692–694.

86. Tocci MJ, Matkovich DA, Collier KA, et al. The immunosuppressant FK506 selectively inhibits expression of early T cell activation genes. J Immunol 1989;143:718–726.

87. Bram RJ, Hung DT, Martin PK, et al. Identification of the immunophilins capable of mediating inhibition of signal transduction by cyclosporin A and FK506. Roles of calcineurin binding and cellular localization. Mol Cell Biol 1993;13:4760–4769.

88. Takada K, Oh-hashi M, Yoshikawa H, et al. Determination of a novel potent immunosuppressant (FK506) in rat serum and lymph by high-performance liquid chromatography with chemiluminescence detection. J Chromatography 1990;530:212–228.

89. Warty V, Zuckerman S, Venkataramanan R, et al. FK506 measurement: comparison of different analytical methods. Ther Drug Monit 1993;15:204–208.

90. Venkataramanan R, Jain A, Warty VW, et al. Pharmacokinetics of FK506 following oral administration: a comparison of FK506 and cyclosporine. Transplant Proc 1991;23:931–933.

91. Venkataramanan R, Jain A, Cadoff E, et al. Pharmacokinetics of FK506: preclinical and clinical studies. Transplant Proc 1990;22(Suppl 1):52.

92. European FK 506 Multicenter Liver Study Group. Randomised trial comparing tacrolimus (FK506) and cyclosporin in prevention of liver allograft rejection. Lancet 1994;344:423–428.

93. The U.S. Multicenter FK506 Liver Study Group. A comparison of tacrolimus (FK506) and cyclosporine for immunosuppression in liver transplantation. N Eng J Med 1994;331(17):1110–1115.

94. FK506 Kidney Transplant Study Group. A comparison of tacrolimus (FK506) and cyclosporine for immunosuppression after cadaveric kidney transplantation. Transplantation 1997;63:977–983.

95. Starzl TE, Todo S, Fung J, et al. FK 506 for liver, kidney and pancreas transplantation. Lancet 1989;2:1000–1004.

96. Jordan ML, Shapiro R, Jensen CWB, et al. FK 506 conversion of renal allografts failing cyclosporine immunosuppression. Transplant Proc 1991;23:3078–3081.

97. Jordan ML, Shapiro R, Vivas CA, et al. FK 506 "rescue" for resistant rejection of renal allografts under primary cyclosporine immunosuppression. Transplantation 1994;57:860–865.

98. The U.S. Multicenter FK506 Liver Study Group. Use of prograf (FK506) as rescue therapy for refractory rejection after liver transplantation. Transplant Proc 1993;25:679–688.

99. Armitage JM, Kormos RL, Griffith BP. A clinical trial of FK 506 as primary and rescue immunosuppression in cardiac transplantation. Transplant Proc 1991;23:1149.

100. McMaster P, Dousset B. The improved results of liver transplantation. Transplant Int 1992;5:125.

101. Japanese FK 506 Study Group. Japanese study of FK 506 on kidney transplantation: results of phase II study. Transplant Proc 1993;25:649–654.

102. Tacrolimus Pancreas Transplant Study Group. Tacrolimus in pancreas transplantation: a multicenter analysis. Clin Transplant 1997;11:299–312.

103. Laskow DA, Neylan JF, Shapiro RS, et al. The role of tacrolimus in adult kidney transplantation: a review. Clin Transplant 1998;12:489–503.

104. Keck BM, Bennett LE, Fiol BS, et al. Worldwide thoracic organ transplantation: a report from the UNOS/ISHLT International Registry for Thoracic Organ Transplantation. In: Terasaki PI, Cecka JM, eds. Clinical transplants 1997. Los Angeles: UCLA Tissue Typing Laboratory, 1998:29–43.

105. Vezina C, Kudelski A, Sehgal SN. Rapamycin (AY-22,989), a new antifungal antibiotic: I. Taxonomy of the producing streptomycete and isolation of the active principle. J Antibiot (Tokyo) 1975;28:721–732.

106. Sehgal SN, Baker H, Vezina C. Rapamycin (AY-22,989), a new antifungal antibiotic: II. Fermentation, isolation and characterization. J Antibiot (Tokyo) 1975;28:727–732.

107. Douros J, Suffness M. New antitumor substances of natural origin. Cancer Treatment Rev 1981;8:63.

108. Eng CP, Sehgal SN, Vezina C. Activity of rapamycin (AY-22,989) against transplanted tumors. J Antibiot 1984;37:2131.

109. Findlay JA, Radics L. On the chemistry and high field nuclear magnetic resonance spectroscopy of rapamycin. Can J Chem 1980;58:579–584.

110. Paiva NL, Demain AL, Roberts MF. Incorporation of acetate, proprionate, and methionine into rapamycin by *Streptomyces hygroscopicus*. J Nat Prod 1991;54:167.

111. Kahan BD. Immunosuppressive agents acting upon lymphokine synthesis and signal transduction. Clin Transplantation 1993;7:113–125.

112. Kunz J, Henriquez R, Schneider U, et al. Target of rapamycin in yeast, TOR2, is essential phosphatidylinositol kinase homolog required for G1 progression. Cell 1993;73:585–596.

113. Kahan BD, Ghobrial R. Immunosuppressive agents. In: Kahan BD, ed. Surgical clinics of North America: transplantation. Philadelphia: WB Saunders, 1994:1029–1054.

114. Sehgal SN, Molnar-Kimber, Ocain TD, Weichman BM. Rapamycin: a novel immunosuppressive macrolide. Medicinal Res Rev 1994;14(1):1–22.

115. Kuo CJ, Chung J, Fiorentino DF, et al. Rapamycin selectively inhibits interleukin-2 activation of p70S6 kinase. Nature 1992;358(6381):70–73.

116. Morris RE. Rapamycin: antifungal, antitumor, antiproliferative, and immunosuppressive macrolides. Transplantation Rev 1992;6(1):39–87.

117. Morice WG, Brunn GJ, Wiederrecht G, et al. Rapamycin induced inhibition of p34cdc2 kinase activation is associated with G1/S-phase growth arrest in T lymphocytes. J Biochem 1993;268:3734–3738.

118. Streit F, Christians U, Schiebel HM, et al. Sensitive and specific quantification of sirolimus (rapamycin) and its metabolites in blood and urine of kidney graft recipients using HPLC/electrospray-mass spectrometry. Clin Chem 1996;42:1417–1425.

119. Napoli KL, Kahan BD. Routine clinical monitoring of sirolimus whole-blood concentrations by HPLC with ultraviolet detection. Clin Chem 1996;42:1943–1948.

120. Zimmerman J, Kahan BD. The pharmacokinetics of sirolimus in stable renal transplant patients after multiple oral dose administration. J Clin Pharmacol 1997;37:405–415.

121. Stepkowski SM, Napoli KL, Wang ME, et al. The effects of the pharmacokinetic interaction between orally administered sirolimus and cyclosporine on the synergistic prolongation of heart allograft survival in rats. Transplantation 1996;62:986–994.

122. Morris RE, Meiser BM. Identification of a new pharmacologic action for an old compound. Med Sci Res 1989;17:877.

123. Morris RE, Meiser BM, Wu J, et al. Use of rapamycin for the suppression of the alloimmune reactions in vivo: schedule-dependence, tolerance induction, synergy with cyclosporine and FK 506 and effect on host-versus-graft and graft-versus-host reactions. Transplant Proc 1991;23:521–524.

124. Stepkowski SM, Chen H, Dalazo P, Kahan BD. Rapamycin, a potent immunosuppressive drug for vascularized heart, kidney, small bowel transplantation in rat. Transplantation 1991;51:22–26.

125. Calne RY, Collier DS, Lim S, et al. Rapamycin for immunosuppression in organ allografting. Lancet 1989;2:227.

126. Collier DS, Calne R, Thiru S, et al. Rapamycin in experimental renal allografts in dogs and pigs. Transplant Proc 1990;22:1674.

127. Collier DS, Calne RY, Pollard SG, et al. Rapamycin in experimental renal allografts in primates. Transplant Proc 1991;23:2246.

128. Whiting PH, Adam J, Woo J, et al. The effect of rapamycin on renal function in the rat: a comparative study with cyclosporine. Toxicol Lett 1991;58:169–179.

129. Di Joseph JF, Sehgal SN. Functional and histopathologic effects of rapamycin on mouse kidney. Immunopharmacol Immunotoxicol 1993;15:45–99.

130. Ferraresso M, Ghobrial R, Stepkowski S, Kahan BD. Mechanism of unresponsiveness to allografts induced by rapamycin and rapamycin/cyclosporine treatment in rats. Transplantation 1993;55:888–894.

131. Wang M, Stepkowski SM, Ferraresso M, et al. Rapamycin rescue therapy delays rejection of heart allografts in rats. Transplantation 1993;54:704.

132. Chen H, Wu J, Xu D, et al. Reversal of ongoing heart, kidney and pancreas allograft rejection and suppression of accelerated heart allograft rejection in the rat by rapamycin. Transplantation 1993;56:661–666.

133. Adams DH, Wyner LR, Karnovsky MJ. Cardiac graft arteriosclerosis in the rat. Transplant Proc 1993;25(2):2071–2073.

134. Meiser B, Reichart B. Graft vessel disease: the impact of immunosuppression and possible treatment strategies. Immunol Rev 1993;134:99–116.

135. Ardehali A, Billingsley A, Laks H, et al. Experimental cardiac allograft vasculopathy in mice. J Heart Lung Transplant 1993;12:730–735.

136. Gregory CR, Huang X, Pratt RE, et al. Treatment with rapamycin and mycophenolic acid reduces arterial intimal thickening produced by mechanical injury and allows endothelial replacement. Transplantation 1995;59:655–661.

137. Kimball PM, Kerman RH, Kahan BD. Rapamycin and cyclosporine produce synergistic but nonidentical mechanism of immunosuppression. Transplant Proc 1991;23(1):1027–1028.

138. Kahan BD, Gibbons S, Tejpal N, et al. Synergistic interactions of cyclosporine and rapamycin to inhibit immune performances of normal human peripheral blood lymphocytes in vitro. Transplantation 1991;51:232–239.

139. Meiser BM, Wang J, Morris RE. Rapamycin: a new highly active immunosuppressive macrolide with an efficacy superior to cyclosporine. Prog Immunol 1989;7:1195–1198.

140. Ochiai T, Gunji Y, Nagata M, et al. Effects of rapamycin in experimental organ allografting. Transplant 1993;56:15–19.

141. Bierer BE, Somers PK, Wandless TJ, et al. Probing immunosuppressant action with a nonnatural immunophilin ligand. Science 1990;250:556–559.

142. Vu MD, Qi S, Xu D, et al. Synergistic effects of mycophenolate mofetil and sirolimus in prevention of acute heart, pancreas, and kidney allograft rejection in the rat. Transplantation 1998;66:1575–1580.

143. Murgia MG, Jordan S, Kahan BD. The side effect profile of sirolimus: a phase I study in quiescent cyclosporine-prednisone-treated renal transplant patients. Kidney Int 1996;49:209–216.

144. Kahan BD. Sirolimus: a new agent for clinical renal transplantation. Transplant Proc 1997;29:48–50.

145. Groth CG, Brattström C, Claesson K, et al. New trials in transplantation: how to exploit the potential of sirolimus in clinical transplantation. Transplant Proc 1998;30:4064–4065.

146. Kahan BD, Podbielski J, Napoli KL, et al. Immunosuppressive effects and safety of a sirolimus/cyclosporine combination regimen for renal transplantation. Transplantation 1998;66:1040–1046.

147. Falf W, Ulrichs K, Muller-Ruchholtz W. 15-deoxyspergualin (a new guanidine-like drug) blocks T lymphocyte proliferation. Transplant Proc 1991;23:864–865.

148. Takeuchi T, Iinuma H, Kunimoto S, et al. A new antitumor antibiotic, spergualin: isolation and antitumor activity. Antibiotics 1981;34:1619–1621.

149. Hibashami H, Tsukada T, Suzuki R, et al. Deoxyspergualin, an antiproliferative agent, shows inhibitory effects on synthetic pathway of polyamines. Anticancer Res 1991;11:325–330.

150. Umeda Y, Moriguchi M, Kurond H, et al. Synthesis and antitumor activity of spergualin analogues: I. Chemical modification of 7-guanidine-3-hydroxyacyl moiety. J Antibiot 1985;38:886–898.

151. Walter P, Feifel G, Shorlemmer H, et al. A new immunosuppressive active antitumoral drug 15-deoxyspergualin prevents rejection of allogeneic transplanted islets. Transplant Proc 1986;18:1860–1861.

152. Ochiai T, Hori S, Nakajima K, et al. Prolongation of rat heart allograft survival by 15-deoxyspergualin. J Antibiot 1987;40:249–250.

153. Thies JC, Walter PK, Zimmermann FA, et al. Prolongation of graft survival in allogeneic pancreas and liver transplantation by 15-deoxyspergualin. Eur Surg Res 1987;19:129–134.

154. Umezawa H, Ishizuka M, Takeuchi K, et al. Suppression of tissue graft rejection by spergualin. J Antibiot 1985;38:283–284.

155. Masuda T, Mizutani S, Iijima M, et al. Immunosuppressive activity of 15-deoxyspergualin and its effect on skin allografts in rats. J Antibiot 1987;40:1612–1618.

156. Takahara S, Jiang H, Takano Y, et al. The in vitro immunosuppressive effects of deoxyspergualin in man compared with FK 506 and cyclosporine. Transplantation 1992;53:914–918.

157. Tepper MA, Nadler S, Mazzucco C, et al. 15-deoxyspergualin: a novel immunosuppressive drug: studies of the mechanism of action. Ann New York Acad Sci 1993;685:136–147.

158. Kerr PG, Atkins RC. The effects of deoxyspergualin on human cytotoxic T lymphocytes, NK cells, and LAK cells. Kidney Int 1990;38:557–558.

159. Nishimura K, Tokunaga T. Mechanism of action of 15-deoxyspergualin: suppressive effects on the induction of alloreactive secondary cytotoxic T lymphocytes in vivo and in vitro. Immunology 1989;68:66–71.

160. Nishimura K, Tokunaga T. Mode of action of 15-deoxyspergualin: effects on induction and effector function of cytotoxic T lymphocytes (CTL). Int J Immunopharmacol 1988;10:75.

161. Kerr PG, Atkins RC. The effects of deoxyspergualin on lymphocytes and monocytes in vivo and in vitro. Transplantation 1989;48:1048–1052.

162. Pai LH, FitzGerald DJ, Tepper MA, et al. Inhibition of antibody response to *Pseudomonas exotoxin* and an immunotoxin containing *Pseudomonas exotoxin* by 15-deoxyspergualin in mice. Cancer Res 1990;50:7750–7753.

163. Sterbenz KG, Tepper MA. Effects of 15-deoxyspergualin on the expression of surface immunoglobulin in 70Z/3.12 murine pre-B cell line. Ann New York Acad Sci 1993;685:205–207.

164. Nadler SG, Tepper M, Schacter B, Mazzucco CE. Interaction of the immunosuppressant deoxyspergualin with a member of the Hsp 70 family of heat shock proteins. Science 1992;258:484–486.

165. Waaga AM, Ulrichs K, Krzymanski M, et al. The immunosuppressive agent 15-deoxyspergualin induces tolerance and modulates MHC-antigen expression and interleukin-1 production in the early phase of rat allograft responses. Transplant Proc 1990;22:1613–1614.

166. Dickneite G, Shorlemmer HU, Sedlacek HH. Decrease of mononuclear phagocyte cell functions and prolongation of graft survival in experimental transplantation by 15-deoxyspergualin. Int J Immunopharmacol 1987;9:559–565.

167. Thomas FT, Tepper MA, Thomas JM, Haisch CE. 15-deoxyspergualin: a novel immunosuppressive drug with clinical potential. Ann New York Acad Sci 1993;685:175–192.

168. Muindi J, Lee S, Baltzer L, et al. Clinical pharmacology of deoxyspergualin in patients with advanced cancer. Cancer Res 1991;51:3096–3101.

169. Tamura K, Niitaji H, Ogawa M, Kimura K. Phase I and pharmacokinetic study of deoxyspergualin given by 3-hour infusion for 5 days. Proceedings of ASCO 1989;8:74.

170. Sprancmanis LA, Riley CM, Stobaugh JF. Determination of the anticancer drug, 15-deoxyspergualin, in plasma ultrafiltrate by liquid chromatography and precolumn derivatization with naphthalene-2,3-dicarboxyaldehyde/cyanide. J Pharmacol Biomed Anal 1990;8:165–175.

171. Hibasami H, Tsukada T, Suzuki R, et al. Deoxyspergualin, an antiproliferative agents, shows inhibitory effects on the synthetic pathway on polyamines. Anticancer Res 1991;11:325–330.

172. Morris RE. 15-deoxyspergualin: a mystery wrapped within an enigma. Clin Transplant 1991;5:530–533.

173. Yuh DY, Morris RE. The immunopharmacology of immunosuppression by 15-deoxyspergualin. Transplantation 1993;55:578–591.

174. Kamata K, Okubo M, Masaki Y, et al. Effect of 15-deoxyspergualin on the survival of thyroid allografts in mice. Transplant Proc 1989;21:1099–1103.

175. Reichenspeurner H, Hidebrandt A, Human P. 15-deoxyspergualin after cardiac and kidney allotransplantation in primates. Transplant Proc 1990;22:1618–1619.

176. Shorlemmer H, Dickneite G, Seiler F. Treatment of acute rejection episodes and induction tolerance in rat skin allotransplantation by 15-deoxyspergualin. Transplant Proc 1990;22:1626–1630.

177. Amemiya H, Suzuki S, Niya S, et al. A new immunosuppressive agent, 15-deoxyspergualin in dog renal allografting. Transplant Proc 1989;21:3468–3470.

178. Reichenspeurner H, Human P, Boehm DH, et al. Optimisation of immunosuppression after xenogeneic heart transplantation in primates. J Heart Transplant 1989;8:200–208.

179. Koyama I, Amamiya H, Taguchi Y, et al. Prophylactic use of deoxyspergualin in a quadruple immunosuppressive protocol in renal transplantation. Transplant Proc 1991;23:1096–1098.

180. Gores PF, Najarian JS, Stephanian E, et al. Insulin independence in type I diabetes after transplantation of unpurified islet from single donor with 15-deoxyspergualin. Lancet 1993;341:19.

181. Amemiya H, Suzuki S, Ota K, et al. A novel rescue drug, 15-deoxyspergualin. Transplantation 1990;49:337–343.

182. Amemiya H. Deoxyspergualin: clinical trials in renal graft rejection. Ann NY Acad Sci 1993;685:196–201.

183. Kyo M, Ichikawa Y, Fukunishi Y, et al. Histopathologic classification and clinical effects of kidney transplant rejection treated with 15-deoxyspergualin. Transplant Proc 1995;27:1012.

184. Amemiya and Japanese Collaborative Transplant Study Group of NKT-01. Immunosuppressive mechanism and action of deoxyspergualin in experimental and clinical studies. Transplant Proc 1995;27:31.

185. Takahashi K, Tanabe K, Ooba S, et al. Prophylactic use of a new immunosuppressive agent, deoxyspergualin, in patients with kidney transplantation from ABO incompatible or preformed antibody-positive donors. Transplant Proc 1991;23:1078–1082.

186. Groth CG. Deoxyspergualin in allogeneic kidney and xenogeneic islet transplantation: early clinical trial. Ann New York Acad Sci 1993;685: 193–195.

187. Fujita T, Inoue K, Yamamoto S, et al. Fungal metabolites. Part 11. A potent immunosuppressive activity found in *Isaria sinclairii* metabolite. J Antibiot 1994;47:208.

188. Adachi K, Kohara T, Nakao N, et al. Design, synthesis, and structure-activity relationship of 2-substituted-2-amino-1,3-propanediols: discovery of a novel immunosuppressant, FTY720. Bioorganic & Medicinal Chemistry Letters 1995;5:853–856.

189. Fujita T, Yoneta M, Hirose R, et al. Simple compounds, 2-alkyl-2-amino-1,3-propanediols have potent immunosuppressive activity. Bioorg Med Chem 1995;5:847.

190. Chiba K, Teshima A, Fujii A, et al. FTY720, a novel immunosuppressant, possessing unique mechanism. I. Relationship between immunosuppressive effects and selective decrease of peripheral mature T cells. San Francisco: 9th International Congress of Immunology, 1995:864.

191. Miyake Y, Kozutsumi Y, Nakamura S, et al. Abstracts of the 16th Symposium on the interaction between biological membranes and drugs. Kyoto, 1994:21.

192. Suzuki S, Enosawa S, Kakefuda T, et al. A novel immunosuppressant, FTY720, with a unique mechanism of action, induces long-term graft acceptance in rat and dog allotransplantation. Transplantation 1996;61:200–205.

193. Chiba K, Adachi K. FTY720. Drugs of the Future 1997;22:18.

194. Hoshino Y, Chiba F, Rahman F, et al. FTY720, a novel immunosuppressant, possessing unique mechanism. II. Synergistic prolongation of allograft survival in combination with cyclosporin in rat and dog. San Francisco: 9th International Congress of Immunology, 1995:864.

195. Suzuki S, Kakefuda T, Amemiya H, et al. An immunosuppressive regimen using FTY720 combined with cyclosporine in canine kidney transplantation. Transplant Int 1998;11:95–101.

196. Stepkowski SM, Tu Y, Condon TP, Bennett CF. Blocking of heart allograft rejection by intracellular adhesion molecule 1 antisense oligonucleotides alone or in combination with other immunosuppressive modalities. J Immunol 1994;153:5336.

# Principles of Action of Biologic Immunosuppressants

Lucienne Chatenoud

Polyclonal antilymphocyte sera (ALS) were the first biologic immunosuppressants to be introduced in clinical transplantation for both the prevention and the treatment of acute allograft rejection. This represented, in the late 1960s, a major advance. Prior to that time, prolonged survival of functioning allografts was difficult to achieve using corticosteroids and azathioprine exclusively (1). The introduction of ALS was, in addition, the first step toward the use of drugs having, as opposed to conventional chemical immunosuppressants, a selective activity on immunocompetent cells.

The advent of hybridoma technology in 1975 led to the development of potentially therapeutic monoclonal antibodies directed against T-lymphocyte receptors. This major technologic breakthrough made feasible the characterization of biologic agents that could selectively target functionally distinct cell subsets of immunocompetent cells (Fig. 7.1) (2). Monoclonal antibodies represent, in addition, an excellent alternative to polyclonal antisera, which are laborious to produce, screen, and standardize (see also Chapter 8, Table 8.8). They allow the use of small doses of an homogeneous antibody preparation with predefined specificity for a single cell surface or soluble molecule. More recently, by means of molecular engineering, a new generation of promising biologic agents has emerged in the form of "humanized" monoclonal antibodies and recombinant proteins—immunoadhesins targeting distinct immune cell receptors or products (i.e., cytokines) (Fig. 7.2) (3).

Experimental and clinical experience with biologic agents both in transplantation and in autoimmune disorders has clearly demonstrated that they may exhibit unique therapeutic properties not shared by conventional chemical immunosuppressants (e.g., corticosteroids, azathioprine, cyclosporine). They can, under some circumstances, promote immune tolerance defined operationally as an acquired state of antigen-specific immunologic unresponsiveness that is

durable in the absence of generalized chronic immunosuppression (4). The work of Monaco and his group in the early 1970s was seminal in pointing to the ability of ALS to induce tolerance to allografts in rodent skin transplant models (5). Since then, in several models it has been shown that anti-T-cell monoclonal antibodies can induce tolerance to foreign soluble antigens and to tissue alloantigens and autoantigens (6–16).

Understanding the cellular and molecular basis by which biologic agents control deleterious immune responses to allografts requires a discussion of the principal targets.

## MAIN TARGETS OF THERAPEUTIC BIOLOGIC AGENTS: IMMUNE CELL RECEPTORS AND SOLUBLE MEDIATORS

Effective immune responses ensue from cooperation between functionally distinct cell types that are antigen-presenting cells (APC), B and T lymphocytes that communicate through an intricate network of cell receptors, and soluble mediators, namely, cytokines. Cell-to-cell cooperation involves a number of surface receptors interacting with their specific ligands as well as with a variety of cytokines mediators (Fig. 7.3). Depending on the context, the stimuli elicited trigger the transduction of intracellular signals leading to immune cell activation, differentiation, functional inactivation (anergy), or programmed cell death (apoptosis).

The allogeneic response of acute rejection is essentially a T-cell mediated immune reaction. In theory, each of the cell actors implicated in this response—namely, the APCs, the $CD4^+$ helper cytokine producers, and $CD8^+$ cytotoxic effectors—and each of their membrane receptors or derived cytokines represent equally good targets for therapeutically relevant immunosuppressants (see Fig. 7.3). In practice,

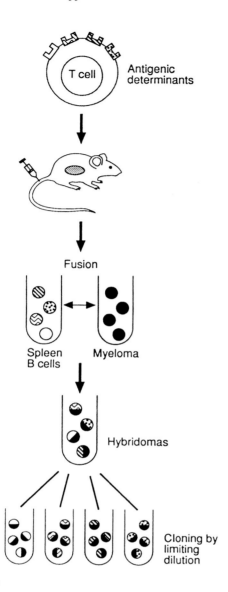

**FIGURE 7.1.** *Production of monoclonal antibodies according to the technique described by Kohler and Milstein (2). Splenocytes from immunized mice are fused with myeloma cells. The hybridomas obtained are cultured by limiting dilution in individual wells. The supernatants are screened for the desired specificity. Large-scale production of selected hybridomas may then be performed either in vitro or in vivo (i.e., ascites).*

however, this is not the case. As a consequence of the very restricted specificity of monoclonal antibodies, it soon became apparent that the in vivo therapeutic capacity of a given antibody was directly correlated with the functional relevance of its molecular target. For instance, all CD3 antibodies used in vivo so far have proved to be excellent immunosuppressants (17). In contrast, this was not the case for most of the CD2 antibodies tested, despite the fact that both specificities are expressed on all mature T cells (18).

## Receptors and Coreceptors Involved in Antigen Recognition

T-cell antigen recognition involves a molecular triad including specialized membrane receptors, some of which are privileged targets for therapeutic biologic agents (see Fig. 7.3). T cells bind peptides presented in the context of major histocompatibility complex (MHC) molecules via specialized dimeric receptors: the T-cell receptor (TCR) α and β chains. The variable regions of the TCR α and β chains dictate antigen specificity. The CD3 molecular complex consists of at least five invariant membrane proteins designated γ, δ, ε, ζ, and η (19). The γ, δ, and ε subunits are expressed as noncovalently linked γ–δ and γ–ε dimers; the ζ and η subunits form disulfide-linked homo-ζζ and heterodimers ζη. CD3 regulates the assembly and expression of TCR and is responsible for transducing TCR αβ signals.

The CD4 and CD8 receptors were initially considered to be simple adhesion molecules interacting with their specific ligands: the MHC class II and I products, respectively. It soon became apparent, however, that upon antigen binding the cross-linking of CD4 and CD3/TCR significantly improved T-cell signaling (20). According to recent data CD4, through its noncovalently associated lymphocyte-specific tyrosine kinase p56$^{lck}$, associates to the "activated" form of the CD3 ζ–ζ chains (tyrosine phosphorylated ζ associated to tyrosine phosphorylated cytoplasmic ZAP-70), thereby stabilizing the CD3/TCR–antigen–MHC interaction and amplifying the signaling process. CD4 thus represents an important "coreceptor" of CD3/TCR that actively participates in the delivery of activation signals (Fig. 7.4) (21).

## Receptors Delivering "Costimulatory" Signals and Adhesion Molecules

T-cell activation is initiated through the CD3/TCR complex, but this signal is not sufficient to sustain full activation of naive T cells. In contrast, a state of unresponsiveness or anergy may result on rechallenge. In order for sustained T-cell activation to occur, CD3/TCR costimulatory signals derived from specialized receptors must be delivered. In the case of naive T cells, CD28 is one important receptor mediating costimulation on interaction with the B7 family (B7.1, B7.2) of ligands expressed on antigen-presenting cells (22–24) (see Fig. 7.3).

The term *adhesin* encompasses a variety of cell receptors that enhance cell contacts and represent interesting targets for immunosuppressive agents (25–27). Two major systems have been investigated: ICAM-1–LFA-1 and CD2–LFA-3 (25–27). There is increasing evidence that, under certain circumstances, several adhesion receptor–ligand pairs can modulate an immune response not simply by enhancing adhesion, but by providing additional activation signals (28). Thus, in the case of memory T cells that possess a lower

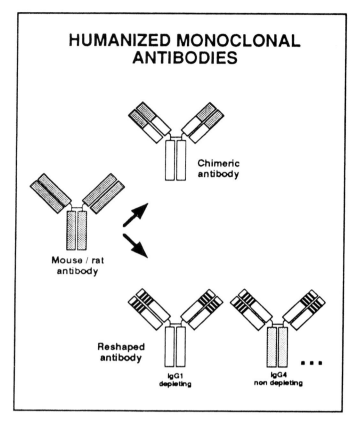

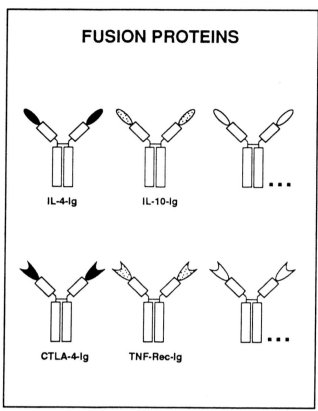

**FIGURE 7.2.**   *Scheme describing the structural characteristics of molecularly engineered monoclonal antibodies and immuno-adhesins (3).*

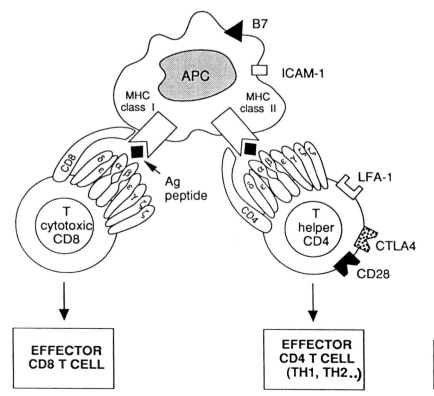

**FIGURE 7.3.**   *Principal targets of therapeutic biologic immunosuppressants expressed at the surface of functionally distinct immune cells.*

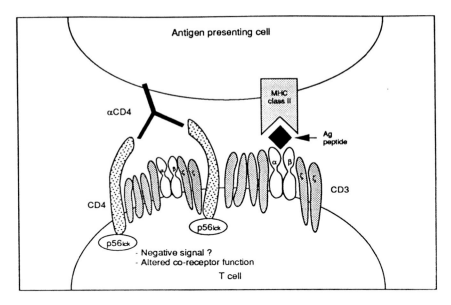

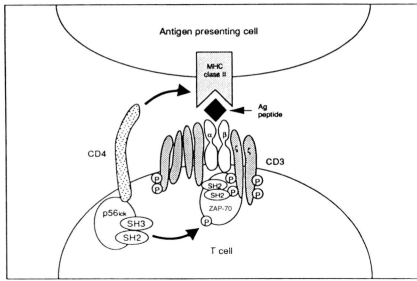

**FIGURE 7.4.** *The intracellular pathways of T-cell activation: the interaction of CD3 and CD4 molecules (20,21). In addition, the top panel illustrates the hypothesis proposed to explain the mode of action of anti-CD4 monoclonal antibodies. (Adapted from Thome M, Duplay P, Guttinger M, et al. Syk and ZAP-70 mediate recruitment of p561ck/CD4 to the activated T-cell receptor/CD3/zeta complex. J Exp Med 1995;181:1997–2006.)*

activation threshold compared to naive T cells, adhesins may enter into play to deliver effective costimulatory signals.

## Receptors Selectively Expressed by Activated Cells

Cytokine receptors probably illustrate the best example of membrane molecules selectively expressed by activated immune cells and used as targets of therapeutic monoclonal antibodies. In transplantation, efforts have been devoted predominantly to the targeting of the interleukin (IL)-2 receptor. Both murine and humanized antibodies directed at the α chain of IL-2 receptor (CD25) have been applied (29). Humanized antibodies to CD25 especially seem to express a potent therapeutic capacity when used for prophylaxis of allograft rejection (29).

## Soluble Mediators of Immunity: Cytokines

Cytokines are essential mediators of immunity and inflammation, two processes that operate to variable extents during each of the three essential phases of the alloimmune response: 1) antigen recognition, 2) proliferation and differentiation of committed cells, and 3) target destruction.

A major concept emerged in the mid 1980s from the work of Mosmann et al (30), who proposed that CD4+ T lymphocytes providing help for humoral (B-cell–dependent) or cellular (T-cell–dependent) responses were in fact distinct and could be differentiated on the basis of the cytokines they produced. Thus, two lymphokine patterns termed $T_H1$ (type 1 helper T cell) and $T_H2$ (type 2 helper T cell) were identified. Activation of the $T_H1$ cells [IL-2 and interferon gamma (IFNγ) producers] supports macrophage activation and cell-mediated delayed-type hypersensitivity responses.

Activation of $T_H2$ cells (IL-4, IL-5, IL-6, IL-10, and IL-13 producers) provides efficient B-cell help, thus favoring humoral responses. Fully differentiated $T_H1$ and $T_H2$ subsets do not preexist in the naive immunologically unprimed host. Among the various factors that direct a naive T helper precursor to differentiate upon antigen encounter into a $T_H1$ or a $T_H2$ cell are the type of antigen and its dose, the nature of the APC, the genetic background (both MHC and non-MHC genes), and, interestingly enough, the environmental cytokines by themselves. $IFN\gamma$, produced by $T_H1$ cells, inhibits the proliferation of $T_H2$ cells; conversely, IL-10, produced by $T_H2$ cells, inhibits the synthesis of cytokines by $T_H1$ cells by acting at least in part on APCs (31,32). IL-12, an APC-derived cytokine, is a key factor driving the differentiation of $T_H1$ cells, at least in part through its capacity to induce $IFN\gamma$. Conversely, IL-4 strongly directs the development of $T_H2$ cells and together with IL-10 shows a strong inhibitory capacity on $T_H1$-type response development (31).

Enormous efforts to delineate the role of a polarization toward a preferential $T_H1$ or $T_H2$ helper T-cell phenotype in the establishment and the control of allogeneic responses have paved the way to developing new therapeutic strategies (31,32). In particular, specific, long-term tolerance to alloantigens and autoantigens in rodent models has been interpreted as resulting from a favoring of a $T_H2$ versus a $T_H1$ response. Depending on the situation considered—transplantation or autoimmunity—this may be achieved by treatment with antibodies to given cytokines (anti-$IFN\gamma$) (33), antibodies to T-cell receptors (CD4, CD4+CD8, CD3, CD28) (34), or with the cytokines themselves (IL-4) (35).

## The Particular Case of Polyclonal Antilymphocyte Sera

Polyclonal antilymphocyte globulins (ALG), which are widely used in transplantation, represent a mixture of a wide spectrum of antibody specificities that probably include, in variable proportions, a large number (if not all) of the cell-related specificities mentioned above. It is the variability in the concentration of each given specificity, to which can be added the isotype and the affinity of antibodies, that probably explains the differences in the batch-to-batch therapeutic potencies (36). Among the various in vitro properties ascribed to ALS preparations, only two are relevant to predicting immunosuppressive capacity in vivo. These are inhibition of the mixed lymphocyte reaction, which correlates, albeit moderately, with in vivo immunosuppression, and inhibition of E-rosette formation resulting from the interaction between the adhesion molecules CD2 (on T cells) and LFA-3 (on sheep erythrocytes) (27).

### CELLULAR MECHANISMS

Although they are not mutually exclusive, three principal mechanisms have been identified through which biologic therapeutic agents affect the immune response: 1) the physical elimination of the target cells, which raises the issue of the turnover of the removed cell population, 2) the inhibition or blockade of the functional capacity of the target cells, and 3) the triggering of cell-mediated immunoregulatory circuits that redirect a destructive alloreactive effector response toward a nondestructive type of alloreactivity (Fig. 7.5). The latter unique capacity is considered at present as one major mechanism underlying the tolerogenic properties of biologic agents in general and anti-T–cell antibodies in particular. This clearly distinguishes biologic agents from chemical immunosuppressants that exclusively act through mechanisms involving the removal and/or the functional inhibition of their targets.

### Cellular Depletion

From the biochemical point of view, the effector functions of an antibody molecule, such as the capacity to interact with Fc receptors and to activate the complement cascade, rely on the structure of the constant region. Cell lysis can occur following direct complement-dependent lysis in the circulation or by means of cell opsonization and removal in the liver and the spleen by reticuloendothelial cells. Trapping in these organs of lymphoid cells preincubated in vitro with polyclonal antilymphocyte antibodies or following their in vivo injection has been shown in both murine and clinical studies (37,38). Only C1, C4, C2, and C3 complement components are needed for effective opsonization. Some data suggest that only C1 and C4 would be sufficient (39).

In contrast, with cell-directed monoclonal antibodies the mechanisms involved in antibody-mediated cell destruction in vivo are more variable and complex. Actually, not only the antibody isotype but also its fine specificity can influence the lytic capacity. Thus, it is not sufficient to select for the adequate antibody isotype to achieve a desired in vivo depleting or nondepleting effect (40,41). When injected into humans, mouse and rat monoclonal antibodies to cell determinants mostly show a rather poor lytic capacity in the presence of human complement. This is due to the now well-characterized membrane-bound factors that inhibit complement activation in a species-restricted manner. Despite this, some antibody specificities, for reasons that are not fully understood, are highly depleting. This was the case for the CAMPATH-1 antibody (CD52) directed to a small GPI-linked protein abundantly expressed on B cells, T cells, and monocytes and extensively used to purge T cells from allogeneic bone marrow prior to transplant for prevention of graft-versus-host disease (GVHD) (40). Using molecular engineering, sets of recombinant antibodies with identical specificities but different constant regions were analyzed and probed for the sequences that determine antibody function (41). These have been used to rank the antibodies with regard to efficiencies in human complement-mediated lysis and also in antibody-dependent cell-mediated cytotoxicity (ADCC) by activated $Fc\gamma RIII$

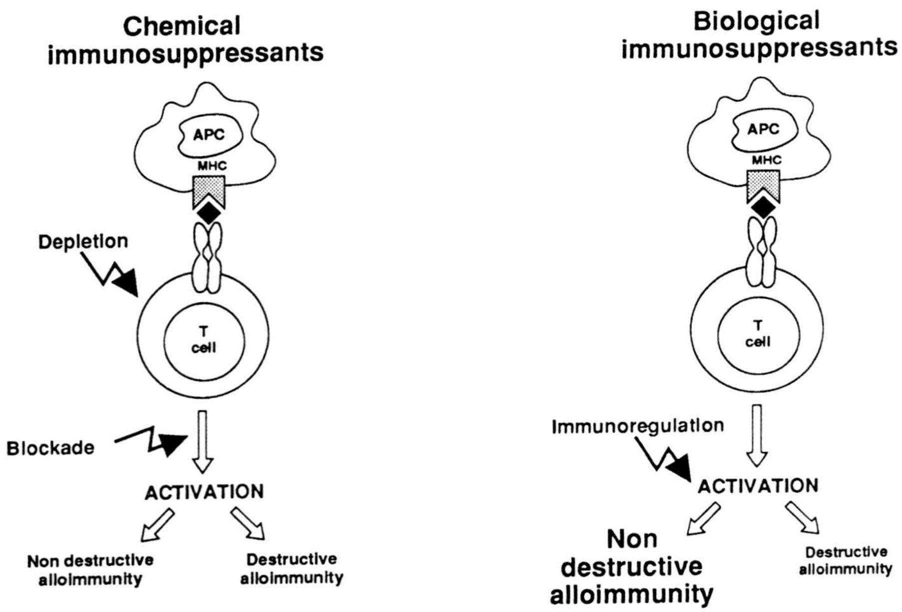

## Chemical immunosuppressants

## Biological immunosuppressants

**FIGURE 7.5.** *Schematic representation of the mechanisms involved in the mode of action of immunosuppressants. The figure highlights the distinct points within an immune response that are the targets for chemical or biologic agents.*

(CD16) expressing effector cells. These studies showed that the lytic capacity of antibodies is greatly influenced by the antibody specificity as well as by the density and the distribution of the antigen on the target cell surface. However, among a given set of monoclonal antibodies sharing the same variable region, a hierarchy in terms of lytic capacity can be established that in the case of human immunoglobulins, for instance, is as follows (from highest to lowest): IgG1, IgG2, IgG3, IgG4.

An antigen may be a poor target for lysis when it easily undergoes antigenic modulation—namely, the disappearance from the cell surface upon binding by a specific ligand (in this case the monoclonal antibody). This is the case for B-cell (surface Ig) and T-cell antigen receptors (CD3/TCR) (see below for more details).

Among the other mechanisms studied and potentially involved in antibody-mediated depletion are redirected T-cell lysis consequent to bridging of cytotoxic T cells to the target (42) and, particularly for antibodies to CD3 and CD4, induction of apoptosis or programmed cell death. Apoptosis is a signal-dependent suicidal process associated with the activation of an endogenous endonuclease that leads to genomic DNA fragmentation. The delivery of apoptotic signals is elicited by the interaction between membrane receptors preferentially expressed at the surface of activated cells, namely, Fas/Fas ligand, TNF/TNF receptor. Apoptosis mediated via CD3/TCR signaling was initially demonstrated in immature thymocytes but it is also triggered in activated mature peripheral T cells (43–45).

To be complete, one may add here immunotoxins that consist of conjugates of a toxin (diphtheria toxin or ricin) coupled to an antibody or to a cytokine (46,47). The immunotoxin is delivered to the target cell by the antibody

or the cytokine, whereupon the toxin kills the target cell after being internalized (46,47).

The immunologic effects of cell depletion will depend on the cellular selectivity of the immunosuppressive agent and on the renewal rate of the target cell population. Depletion may globally affect leukocytes (CD52), T cells (CD3), or T-cell subsets (CD4, CD8). In other cases, only activated T cells may be hit, as is the case for IL-2 receptor (CD25)-specific agents. The renewal rate varies considerably with cellular subsets. Pools of B cells and short-lived T cells will rapidly reappear after initial depletion. Conversely, recirculating long-lived T cells will take several weeks in the mouse and several months in humans to replenish initial cell pools. This very slow turnover of circulating T cells explains the T-cell selectivity of polyclonal ALS (48). The case of depleting monoclonal antibodies to CD4 is intriguing and deserves a word of clinical caution. This is best illustrated by the case of the humanized antibody to CD4 MT-412 (human IgG1) that was used in both transplanted and autoimmune patients. Especially at high doses (700 mg of cumulated dosage), peripheral CD4+ cell counts remained very low for several consecutive months (49).

### Functional Inhibition

Several nonmutually exclusive mechanisms may account for antibody-mediated inhibition of cell function, including: 1) antibody-mediated cell coating that interferes with physiologic cell-to-cell interactions, 2) the antigenic modulation of the target cell receptor, and 3) the induction of cell anergy.

The relevance of antibody-mediated cell coating was initially discussed with polyclonal antilymphocyte antibodies since absolute lymphocytopenia did not appear to be essential for their therapeutic effect. In fact, T cells that reappeared after treatment were functionally impaired both in vitro and in vivo. It was, however, difficult to identify among the various specificities present in polyclonal ALS preparations which targets were the most relevant for cell inactivation.

Several monoclonal antibodies to human, mouse, and rat CD4 have been described that express immunosuppressive and tolerogenic effects but are nondepleting (9,12,34,50,51). It is likely that CD4 coating, given the contribution of CD4 to TCR/CD3-mediated signaling, not only interferes with lymphocyte binding to MHC class II–bearing cells but also triggers therapeutically relevant but still elusive negative "signals" (52). Thus, upon independent ligation of CD3 and CD4, as may occur with the injection of antibodies to CD4, the physiologic stimulation of resting T cells is significantly inhibited (see Fig. 7.4). In addition, a decrease in induced proliferative responses and lymphokine production response to various stimuli, including soluble antigens, alloantigens, lectins, and antibodies to TCR/CD3, is observed but cannot be accounted for by simple blockade of adhesion to MHC class II (53).

Cell-directed antibodies can also induce antigenic modulation, which is the redistribution of the molecules that they bind on the cell surface (54) (Fig. 7.6). The antigen–antibody complex will ultimately cap at a pole of the cell and disappear upon internalization or shedding. If the molecule is central to the cell function, the loss of the membrane receptor expression will render the cell incompetent. This has been well documented in the case of antibodies to CD3 (54–56). In both mice and humans, therapeutic doses produce only partial depletion (in lymphoid organs 30% to 40% of CD3+ cells). Remaining cells

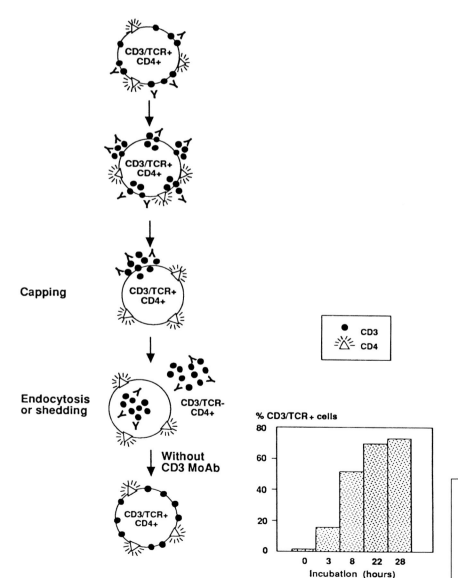

**Capping**

**Endocytosis or shedding**

**FIGURE 7.6.** *Antigenic modulation of the CD3/TCR complex from peripheral blood cells in transplant patients treated with a CD3 antibody. During treatment, cells modulate the CD3/TCR receptor, but within a few hours of in vitro incubation in the absence of the antibody the receptor is re-expressed (54,56).*

undergoing antigenic modulation express a particular phenotype; they are CD3-TCR-CD4+ or CD3-TCR-CD8+ (54,56). The phenomenon is reversible within a few hours (in vitro, 8 to 12 hours) when the antibody is cleared from the surrounding medium. Cells undergoing CD3 antibody-mediated antigenic modulation are completely unresponsive to antigen-specific or mitogen stimulation (54,56). This correlates with the profound in vivo immunosuppression exhibited by these patients, in whom allograft rejection is seldom observed when T cells in the circulation do not express CD3 (17,57).

As mentioned above, sustained T-cell activation upon engagement of CD3/TCR requires the simultaneous delivery of costimulatory signals through specialized receptors, such as CD28 interacting with B7 ligands at the surface of APCs (see Fig. 7.3). Several in vitro models using both murine and human clones showed that occupancy of the TCR alone, in the absence of adequate costimulation, induced a state of unresponsiveness termed *anergy* (58,59). Depending on the system, anergy in vitro is reversible by adding IL-2 either alone or in association with CD2 antibodies (59). The role of anergic cells in physiologic or induced immune tolerance is still debated. At present, only through the injection of superantigens or by using adoptive transfer of TCR transgenic cells can anergic cells be demonstrated in vivo (59).

It is important to mention at this point the very interesting results of using antibodies or fusion proteins that interfere with costimulatory signals in experimental transplantation (11,60,61). Thus, in a mouse heart and skin allograft model, the simultaneous (but not the independent) blockade of the CD28 and CD40 costimulatory pathways promoted long-term allograft survival. Importantly, the technique also inhibited the development of chronic vascular rejection in the grafted hearts (61). Chronic vascular rejection remains a major cause of long-term graft failure for which no effective therapy is available. If confirmed, these data point to selective inhibitors of costimulation as major immunosuppressive tools capable of interfering simultaneously with acute and chronic rejection.

### Acquired Transplant Peripheral Tolerance: The Way to "Nonaggressive" Alloreactivity

Achieving donor-specific tolerance while preserving normal immune responsiveness to other foreign antigens is a major goal in clinical transplantation. A previously long-held tenet was that physiologic immune tolerance could only result from intrathymic, clonal deletion of immunoreactive cells, a concept supported by the direct demonstration of intrathymic negative selection (4). However, it is now extensively documented that, in normal individuals, although deletion mechanisms ensure the elimination of most autoreactive T and B lymphocytes, this purging is far from complete. Thus, autoreactive T and B cells can be found in all normal subjects. In most cases, however, they do not give

rise to clinically evident autoimmune diseases (4). This is because extremely potent, extrathymic nondeletional active mechanisms—cytokine-mediated immune deviation, anergy, suppression, and vetoing—are operative and prevent potentially destructive immunoreactivity (4).

Although transplantation tolerance can be induced through intrathymic deletion of alloreactive T cells (e.g., stable lymphohematopoietic mixed chimerism follows the infusion of allogeneic bone marrow in adequately conditioned recipients), this approach is difficult to apply clinically. Application is limited by its aggressive nature (62,63) as well as by the fact that a loss of functional thymus occurs after puberty.

Peripheral tolerance can be successfully induced and maintained over a long term in adult recipients, even after thymectomy, if the alloantigen is delivered appropriately. Whether antigen presentation is via bone marrow, whole blood, or the allograft itself, the development of tolerance also requires particular biologic agents. As already mentioned, it appears that biologic agents (i.e., natural or biotechnologically engineered antigens, antibodies, receptors, and cytokines) are particularly capable of providing the positive signals required for the reorientation of the immune response leading to peripheral immune tolerance induction.

The groundbreaking experiments by Monaco and Wood in the 1960s (5,64) used a combination of ALS and post-transplantation donor bone marrow infusion to induce specific unresponsiveness to skin allografts (5,64,65). This approach, with modifications, has been successfully used to transplant mismatched renal allografts in nonhuman primates. Prolonged survival of histoincompatible kidney transplants has been achieved in rhesus monkeys with a combination of rabbit ALG plus low-dose lymphoid irradiation and a post-transplantation donor bone marrow (depleted of bright CD3+/DR+ cells) infusion (66–69).

Importantly, monoclonal antibodies can afford the same effect. In the monkey model, a CD3 immunotoxin can also provide the allograft tolerance induced by the ALG + TLI conditioning regimen (70). A nondepleting antibody to CD4 has also been successfully used in this setting.

The unique tolerogenic capacity of antibodies to CD4 has long been known. The first important finding was that rat antibodies to CD4 injected into mice did not trigger an antiglobulin response as was the case with the majority of rodent monoclonal antibodies against other T-cell antigens (6,7). Moreover, specific tolerance to soluble antigens could be induced by delivering them to normal adult euthymic animals under the cover of depleting or nondepleting antibodies to CD4 (6,34,71). Importantly, all that was needed to maintain this immune tolerance was the antigen alone, delivered at regular time intervals, in the absence of any further monoclonal antibody treatment. These findings were rapidly extended to tissue antigens and in particular allo-antigens. This protocol has been recently adapted by Wood's group using as a source of antigen donor-type whole blood in association with depleting or nondepleting antibodies to CD4 (12,14). Thus, specific tolerance to completely mismatched fully vascularized cardiac allografts is achieved. Importantly, through the exclusive administration at regular intervals of donor blood, the time of allograft implantation can be delayed for several months (12,14).

In adult euthymic mice, combinations of antibodies to CD4 and CD8, even if nondepleting, can induce classic transplantation tolerance to skin grafts across partial and fully mismatched combinations (72). This antibody-induced tolerance can also be induced and maintained in thymectomized animals, clearly showing that it is a peripheral event. Not unexpectedly, no evidence for clonal deletion of specific alloreactive T cells was found (9,34).

Antibodies to specificities other than CD4 are also of interest. For instance, antibodies to CD3, to LFA-1 and ICAM-1, and to CD25 (especially in rat transplant models), and agents interfering with costimulatory pathways such as CTLA4Ig have been shown to be effective. Combined administration of LFA-1 and ICAM-1 to mice resulted in permanent engraftment of fully mismatched vascularized heart allografts but also specific tolerance to donor-type skin allografts (10). Similarly, antibodies to CD3 can promote long-term specific unresponsiveness to both alloantigens and autoantigens. In the rat, CD3 antibody induces permanent engraftment of histoincompatible vascularized heart grafts and permanent tolerance (i.e., skin graft acceptance) (73). Moreover, in NOD mice, who develop a spontaneous form of T-cell–mediated autoimmune, insulin-dependent diabetes mellitus, low-dose CD3 treatment applied at the stage of overt disease induces permanent remission and restores self tolerance (16). Finally, in both xenogeneic and allogeneic transplant models, CTLA4Ig was shown to have great potential (74,75).

Apart from their potential therapeutic interest, all these models support the fundamental notion that the organ allograft itself may provide an effective presentation of antigen for induction of transplantation tolerance. Moreover, the major features characterizing these models of monoclonal antibody–induced peripheral immune tolerance are their active (dominant) nature and their strict antigen dependence. This is well illustrated by the fact that tolerant animals resist the transfer of immunocompetent naive and sensitized effectors that could reverse or "break" the tolerant state by eliminating or functionally blocking immune cell subsets—mainly regulatory CD4+ cells—that are known to mediate suppression if adoptively transferred into naive recipients (9,34).

Can all this be explained by an exclusive immune deviation from a $T_H1$ allodestructive response to a $T_H2$ nondestructive or even protective response? Supporting this hypothesis are the data showing dominant $T_H2$ responses in neonatal tolerance models in which establishment is completely blocked by the administration of a monoclonal antibody to IL-4 (76). Moreover, although it is more controversial, in some models of CD4 antibody–induced tolerance, the presence of a dominant $T_H2$ response has been

reported (31). However, when it comes to the phenomenon of transferable suppression, the available data show only a partial blockade upon treatment with anti-IL-4 (34). Another important unresolved question concerns the cellular source of IL-4. Although the assumption is that tolerant or suppressor cells would produce it, there is no firm evidence to show their $T_H2$ origin. Taken together, the present data suggest that diverting to an IL-4–producing phenotype could be but one of the critical factors involved in the tolerance induction phase; whether it is also relevant during the long-term maintenance phase is still unresolved.

An alternate possibility is that tolerant cells might be to some extent anergic, that is, capable of providing no help while competing for APC binding with potentially reactive effectors. There is interesting in vitro and in vivo evidence to support this hypothesis. In vitro, anergic human T-cell clones could suppress the proliferation of potentially reactive cells by nonanergic cells, provided the same APC was presenting the peptides specific for both partners (77). Competition for the APC surface and locally produced IL-2 has been proposed as the mechanism for this effect while excluding a role for "inhibitory" cytokines (i.e., IL-4, IL-10) secreted by the anergic cells (77). Similarly, in vivo, tolerance to a given alloantigen may "spread" to third-party allografts, provided the initially "tolerated" and the third-party alloantigen are presented by the same APC (i.e., usage of organ allografts from F1 donors) (34). This very interesting phenomenon is termed *linked suppression*. Once again, the molecular basis for this "competition" remains obscure and could in principle involve a low cytokine-producing ability (i.e., anergy), the production of cytokines modulating T-cell or APC function (i.e., IL-4, IL-10, TGFβ, etc.), and competition for costimulatory molecules on the APC (34).

In conclusion, although the molecular mechanisms remain to be clarified, T-cell–mediated suppression represents a field that can no longer be ignored by groups attempting to achieve successful clinical immunomodulation.

## CELL ACTIVATION AS A PREREQUISITE FOR ANTI-T-CELL ANTIBODY–INDUCED TOLERANCE

Some recent data emphasize the role of T-cell activation in the induction of immune tolerance by means of biologic agents. Of particular relevance are the studies showing that cyclosporine abrogates the tolerogenic properties of antibodies to CD3 or of agents blocking CD28 and CD40 (61). This is particularly evident when cyclosporine is used with biologic agents at the inception of treatment. It is well established that cyclosporine selectively interferes with TCR/CD3 T-cell activation pathways, leading to the transcription of both $T_H1$ and $T_H2$ cytokine genes. Thus it inhibits the transcription not only of IL-2 and IFNγ mRNA but also of IL-4 and IL-10 mRNA (78,79). The effect of cyclosporine on IL-10 production depends on the cell source of the cytokine; the inhibition is exclusively noted on stimulation with CD3 antibodies and not with bacterial lipopolysaccharide (79).

This may be of relevance for future clinical strategies of tolerance induction in transplant patients. In fact, in clinical protocols, for obvious reasons, drug association is indispensable. However, it is important to develop the best combinations in order to avoid deleterious, potentially antagonistic effects, for example by preventing the induction of antigen-specific long-term hyporesponsiveness. For instance, a recent report from the Collaborative Transplant Study Group shows that the kidney allograft survival in patients who received OKT-3 as part of their prophylactic regimen was significantly lower if cyclosporine was given from the beginning of OKT-3 treatment, as compared to patients in whom the administration of cyclosporine was delayed (80).

## CONCLUSIONS

Most chemical immunosuppressive agents act by promoting cell depletion and/or blockade of cell activation. These therapeutic approaches are nonantigen specific and their major drawback is their relatively long-term ineffectiveness typically resulting in recurrence of the pathogenic immune process at drug cessation. The need to reduce chronic immunosuppression, with its potential for infectious and tumorigenic complications, seems achievable through the use of nontoxic biologic agents.

Moreover, from a more fundamental point of view, an understanding of the molecular basis of the tolerogenic properties of monoclonal antibodies would clear the way for development of more readily applicable therapeutic strategies—simple chemicals or recombinant receptor agonist and/or antagonist ligands that would mimic the desired therapeutic effect. Dissecting the intimate molecular and cellular mechanisms through which antibodies express these subtle modulatory effects certainly promises future exciting challenges for immunopharmacologists.

## REFERENCES

1. Starzl TE. Heterologous antilymphocyte globulin. N Engl J Med 1968;279:700–705.
2. Kohler G, Milstein C. Continuous cultures of fused cells secreting antibody of predefined specificity. Nature 1975;256:495–497.
3. Winter G, Milstein C. Man-made antibodies. Nature 1991;349:293–299.
4. Schwartz RH. Immunological tolerance. In: Paul WE, ed. Fundamental immunology. New York: Raven, 1993:677–731.
5. Monaco AP, Wood ML, Russell PS. Studies on heterologous antilymphocyte serum in mice. III. Immunological tolerance and chimerism produced across the H2-locus with adult thymectomy and antilymphocyte serum. Ann NY Acad Sci 1966;129:190–209.
6. Benjamin RJ, Waldmann H. Induction of tolerance by monoclonal antibody therapy. Nature 1986;320:449–451.
7. Gutstein NL, Seaman WE, Scott JH, Wofsy D. Induction of immune tolerance by administration of monoclonal antibody to L3T4. J Immunol 1986;137:1127–1132.
8. Cobbold SP, Qin S, Leong LY, Martin G, Waldmann H. Reprogramming the immune system for peripheral tolerance with CD4 and CD8 monoclonal antibodies. Immunol Rev 1992;129:165–201.
9. Qin S, Cobbold SP, Pope H, et al. "Infectious" transplantation tolerance. Science 1993;259:974–977.
10. Isobe M, Yagita H, Okumura K, Ihara A. Specific acceptance of cardiac allograft after treatment with antibodies to ICAM-1 and LFA-1. Science 1992;255:1125–1127.
11. Lin H, Bolling SF, Linsley PS, et al. Long-term acceptance of major histocompatibility complex mismatched cardiac allografts induced by CTLA4Ig plus donor-specific transfusion. J Exp Med 1993;178:1801–1806.
12. Pearson TC, Madsen JC, Larsen CP, et al. Induction of transplantation tolerance in adults using donor antigen and anti-CD4 monoclonal antibody. Transplantation 1992;54:475–483.
13. Wofsy D, Seaman WE. Reversal of advanced murine lupus in NZB/NZW F1 mice by treatment with monoclonal antibody to L3T4. J Immunol 1987;138:3247–3253.
14. Wood KJ. Transplantation tolerance with monoclonal antibodies. Semin Immunol 1990;2:389–399.
15. Shizuru JA, Taylor-Edwards C, Banks BA, et al. Immunotherapy of the nonobese diabetic mouse: treatment with an antibody to T-helper lymphocytes. Science 1988;240:659–662.
16. Chatenoud L, Thervet E, Primo J, Bach JF. Anti-CD3 antibody induces long-term remission of overt autoimmunity in nonobese diabetic mice. Proc Natl Acad Sci USA 1994;91:123–127.
17. Cosimi AB, Colvin RB, Burton RC, et al. Use of monoclonal antibodies to T-cell subsets for immunologic monitoring and treatment in recipients of renal allografts. N Engl J Med 1981;305:308–314.
18. Jonker M, Goldstein G, Balner H. Effects of in vivo administration of monoclonal antibodies specific for human T cell subpopulations on the immune system in a rhesus monkey model. Transplantation 1983;35:521–526.
19. Clevers H, Alarcon B, Wileman T, Terhorst C. The T cell receptor/CD3 complex: a dynamic protein ensemble. Annu Rev Immunol 1988;6:629–662.
20. Rudd CE. CD4, CD8 and the TCR-CD3 complex: a novel class of protein-tyrosine kinase receptor. Immunol Today 1990;11:400–406.
21. Thome M, Duplay P, Guttinger M, et al. Syk and ZAP-70 mediate recruitment of p56lck/CD4 to the activated T cell receptor/CD3/zeta complex. J Exp Med 1995;181:1997–2006.
22. Linsley PS, Brady W, Urnes M, et al. CTLA-4 is a second receptor for the B cell activation antigen B7. J Exp Med 1991;174:561–569.
23. Van Den Eertwegh AJ, Noelle RJ, Roy M, et al. In vivo CD40-gp39 interactions are essential for thymus-dependent humoral immunity. I. In vivo expression of CD40 ligand, cytokines, and antibody production delineates sites of cognate T-B cell interactions. J Exp Med 1993;178:1555–1565.
24. Boise LH, Noel PJ, Thompson CB. CD28 and apoptosis. Curr Opin Immunol 1995;7:620–625.
25. Springer TA. Adhesion receptors of the immune system. Nature 1990;346:425–434.
26. Makgoba MW, Sanders ME, Shaw S. The CD2-LFA-3 and LFA-1-ICAM pathways: relevance to T-cell recognition. Immunol Today 1989;10:417–422.
27. Springer TA, Dustin ML, Kishimoto TK, Marlin SD. The lymphocyte function-associated LFA-1, CD2, and LFA-3 molecules: cell adhesion receptors of the immune system. Annu Rev Immunol 1987;5:223–252.
28. Clark EA, Ledbetter JA. How B and T cells talk to each other. Nature 1994;367:425–428.
29. Waldmann TA, O'Shea J. The use of antibodies against the IL-2 receptor in transplantation. Curr Opin Immunol 1998;10:507–512.
30. Mosmann TR, Coffman RL. TH1 and TH2 cells: different patterns of lymphokine secretion lead to different functional properties. Annu Rev Immunol 1989;7:145–173.
31. Nickerson P, Steurer W, Steiger J, et al. Cytokines and the Th1/Th2 paradigm in transplantation. Curr Opin Immunol 1994;6:757–764.
32. Bromberg JS. IL-10 immunosuppression in transplantation. Curr Opin Immunol 1995;7:639–643.
33. Bach JF. Anti-gamma interferon (IFN-gamma) monoclonal antibodies. In: Bach JF, ed. Monoclonal antibodies and peptide therapy in autoimmune diseases. New York: Marcel Dekker, 1993:319–391.
34. Cobbold SP, Adams E, Marshall SE, et al. Mechanisms of peripheral tolerance and suppression induced by monoclonal antibodies to CD4 and CD8. Immunol Rev 1996;149:5–33.
35. Rapoport MJ, Jaramillo A, Zipris D, et al. Interleukin 4 reverses T cell proliferative unresponsiveness and prevents the onset of diabetes in nonobese diabetic mice. J Exp Med 1993;178:87–99.
36. Balner H, Eysvoogel VP, Cleton FJ. Testing of anti-human lymphocyte sera in chimpanzees and lower primates. Lancet 1968;1:19–22.
37. Greaves MF, Tursi A, Playfair JH, et al. Immunosuppressive potency and in vitro activity of antilymphocyte globulin. Lancet 1969;1:68–72.
38. Martin WJ, Miller JF. Cell to cell interaction in the immune response. IV. Site of action of antilymphocyte globulin. J Exp Med 1968;128:855–874.
39. Bach JF, Gigli I, Dardenne M, Dormont J. Mechanism of complement action

in rosette inhibition and lymphocytotoxicity of antilymphocyte serum. Immunology 1972;22:625–635.

40. Bindon CI, Hale G, Waldmann H. Importance of antigen specificity for complement-mediated lysis by monoclonal antibodies. Eur J Immunol 1988;18:1507–1514.

41. Isaacs JD, Clark MR, Greenwood J, Waldmann H. Therapy with monoclonal antibodies. An in vivo model for the assessment of therapeutic potential. J Immunol 1992;148:3062–3071.

42. Wong JT, Colvin RB. Selective reduction and proliferation of the CD4+ and CD8+ T cell subsets with bispecific monoclonal antibodies: evidence for inter-T cell-mediated cytolysis. Clin Immunol Immunopathol 1991;58:236–250.

43. Smith CA, Williams GT, Kingston R, et al. Antibodies to CD3/T-cell receptor complex induce death by apoptosis in immature T cells in thymic cultures. Nature 1989;337:181–184.

44. Wesselborg S, Janssen O, Kabelitz D. Induction of activation-driven death (apoptosis) in activated but not resting peripheral blood T cells. J Immunol 1993;150:4338–4345.

45. Choy EH, Adjaye J, Forrest L, et al. Chimaeric anti-CD4 monoclonal antibody cross-linked by monocyte Fc gamma receptor mediates apoptosis of human CD4 lymphocytes. Eur J Immunol 1993;23:2676–2681.

46. Kronke M, Schlick E, Waldmann TA, et al. Selective killing of human T-lymphotropic virus-I infected leukemic T-cells by monoclonal anti-interleukin 2 receptor antibody-ricin A chain conjugates: potentiation by ammonium chloride and monensin. Cancer Res 1986;46:3295–3298.

47. Walz G, Zanker B, Brand K, et al. Sequential effects of interleukin 2-diphtheria toxin fusion protein on T-cell activation. Proc Natl Acad Sci USA 1989;86:9485–9488.

48. Lance EM. The selective action of antilymphocyte serum on recirculating lymphocytes: a review of the evidence and alternatives. Clin Exp Immunol 1970;6:789–802.

49. Moreland LW, Pratt PW, Bucy RP, et al. Treatment of refractory rheumatoid arthritis with a chimeric anti-CD4 monoclonal antibody. Long-term followup of CD4+ T cell counts. Arthritis Rheum 1994;37:834–838.

50. Powelson JA, Knowles RW, Delmonico FL, et al. CDR-grafted OKT4A monoclonal antibody in cynomolgus renal allograft recipients. Transplantation 1994;57:788–793.

51. Darby CR, Bushell A, Morris PJ, Wood KJ. Nondepleting anti-CD4 antibodies in transplantation. Evidence that modulation is far less effective than prolonged CD4 blockade. Transplantation 1994;57:1419–1426.

52. Bank I, Chess L. Perturbation of the T4 molecule transmits a negative signal to T cells. J Exp Med 1985;162:1294–1303.

53. Emmrich F, Kanz L, Eichmann K. Cross-linking of the T cell receptor complex with the subset-specific differentiation antigen stimulates interleukin 2 receptor expression in human CD4 and CD8 T cells. Eur J Immunol 1987;17:529–534.

54. Chatenoud L, Bach JF. Antigenic modulation: a major mechanism of antibody action. Immunol Today 1984;5:20–25.

55. Hirsch R, Eckhaus M, Auchincloss H Jr, et al. Effects of in vivo administration of anti-T3 monoclonal antibody on T cell function in mice. I. Immunosuppression of transplantation responses. J Immunol 1988;140:3766–3772.

56. Chatenoud L, Baudrihaye MF, Kreis H, et al. Human in vivo antigenic modulation induced by the anti-T cell OKT3 monoclonal antibody. Eur J Immunol 1982;12:979–982.

57. Vigeral P, Chkoff N, Chatenoud L, et al. Prophylactic use of OKT3 monoclonal antibody in cadaver kidney recipients. Utilization of OKT3 as the sole immunosuppressive agent. Transplantation 1986;41:730–733.

58. Schwartz RH. A cell culture model for T lymphocyte clonal anergy. Science 1990;248:1349–1356.

59. Schwartz RH. Models of T cell anergy: is there a common molecular mechanism? Comment. J Exp Med 1996;184:1–8.

60. Lenschow DJ, Zeng Y, Thistlethwaite JR, et al. Long-term survival of

xenogeneic pancreatic islet grafts induced by CTLA4Ig. Science 1992;257:789–792.

61. Larsen CP, Elwood ET, Alexander DZ, et al. Long-term acceptance of skin and cardiac allografts after blocking CD40 and CD28 pathways. Nature 1996;381:434–438.

62. Sykes M, Sheard M, Sachs DH. Effects of T cell depletion in radiation bone marrow chimeras. I. Evidence for a donor cell population which increases allogeneic chimerism but which lacks the potential to produce GVHD. J Immunol 1988;141:2282–2288.

63. Sykes M, Sachs DH. Bone marrow transplantation as a means of inducing tolerance. Semin Immunol 1990;2:401–417.

64. Wood ML, Monaco AP, Gozzo JJ, Liegeois A. Use of homozygous allogeneic bone marrow for induction of tolerance with antilymphocyte serum: dose and timing. Transplant Proc 1971;3:676–679.

65. Maki T, Gottschalk R, Wood ML, Monaco AP. Specific unresponsiveness to skin allografts in anti-lymphocyte serum-treated, marrow-injected mice: participation of donor marrow-derived suppressor T cells. J Immunol 1981;127:1433–1438.

66. Thomas JM, Carver FM, Foil MB, et al. Renal allograft tolerance induced with ATG and donor bone marrow in outbred rhesus monkeys. Transplantation 1983;36:104–106.

67. Thomas J, Carver M, Cunningham P, et al. Promotion of incompatible allograft acceptance in rhesus monkeys given posttransplant antithymocyte globulin and donor bone marrow. I. In vivo parameters and immuno-histologic evidence suggesting microchimerism. Transplantation 1987;43:332–338.

68. Thomas JM, Carver FM, Cunningham PR, et al. Kidney allograft tolerance in primates without chronic immunosuppression—the role of veto cells. Transplantation 1991;51:198–207.

69. Thomas J, Alqaisi M, Cunningham P, et al. The development of a posttransplant TLI treatment strategy that promotes organ allograft acceptance without chronic immunosuppression. Transplantation 1992;53:247–258.

70. Harawy MM, Knechtle SJ. Strategies for tolerance induction in nonhuman primates. Curr Opin Immunol 1998;10:513–517.

71. Wofsy D, Mayes DC, Woodcock J, Seaman WE. Inhibition of humoral immunity in vivo by monoclonal antibody to L3T4: studies with soluble antigens in intact mice. J Immunol 1985;135:1698–1701.

72. Qin SX, Cobbold S, Benjamin R, Waldmann H. Induction of classical transplantation tolerance in the adult. J Exp Med 1989;169:779–794.

73. Nicolls MR, Aversa GG, Pearce NW, et al. Induction of long-term specific tolerance to allografts in rats by therapy with an anti-CD3-like monoclonal antibody. Transplantation 1993;55:459–468.

74. Lenschow DJ, Zeng Y, Thistlethwaite JR, et al. Long-term survival of xenogeneic pancreatic islet grafts induced by CTLA4Ig. Science 1992;257:789–792.

75. Lin H, Bolling SF, Linsley PS, et al. Long term acceptance of major histocompatibility complex mismatched cardiac allografts induced by CTLA4Ig plus donor-specific transfusion. J Exp Med 1993;178:1801–1806.

76. Schurmans S, Heusser CH, Qin HY, et al. In vivo effects of anti-IL-4 monoclonal antibody on neonatal induction of tolerance and on an associated autoimmune syndrome. J Immunol 1990;145:2465–2473.

77. Lombardi G, Sidhu S, Batchelor R, Lechler R. Anergic T cells as suppressor cells in vitro. Science 1994;264:1587–1589.

78. Granelli-Piperno A, Keane M, Steinman RM. Evidence that cyclosporine inhibits cell-mediated immunity primarily at the level of the T lymphocyte rather than the accessory cell. Transplantation 1988;46:53S–60S.

79. Durez P, Abramowicz D, Gerard C, et al. In vivo induction of interleukin 10 by anti-CD3 monoclonal antibody or bacterial lipopolysaccharide: differential modulation by cyclosporin A. J Exp Med 1993;177:551–555.

80. Opelz G. Efficacy of rejection prophylaxis with OKT3 in renal transplantation. Collaborative Transplant Study. Transplantation 1995;60:1220–1224.

# Chapter

8

# Biologic Immunosuppressive Agents

JAMES D. EASON    A. BENEDICT COSIMI

Organ transplantation has become the treatment of choice for many patients with end-stage kidney, liver, heart, or lung disease. Much of the clinical success that has been achieved has relied on life-long administration of pharmacologic agents that rather nonselectively block immune responsiveness. Since the cellular interactions involved in the recipient's reaction to an allograft are mediated through T-cell subsets bearing distinctive cell surface molecules, one approach to providing a more selective immunosuppressive strategy might be through the use of antibodies targeted to specific sites involved in the immune response.

The initial effort to achieve this goal was through the use of polyclonal antilymphocyte sera (ALS). These preparations were designed to attack principally the infiltrating mononuclear cells observed in allograft biopsies coincident with allograft rejection. Such suppression conceptually could retain much of the host's response to bacterial infection, since this is more dependent on B-cell–mediated humoral processes. Following the introduction of antilymphocyte globulin (ALG) by Starzl et al in 1967 (1), extensive clinical studies established the efficacy of these polyclonal preparations for both prophylaxis and treatment of rejection and they continue to be used today in many clinical situations (2–5). However, with the use of classic techniques to immunize animals that generate these polyclonal products, a heterogeneous group of antibodies is produced not only to most T-cell populations, but also to B cells and even nonlymphoid cells. Thus, global suppression can result from the administration of polyclonal antilymphocyte antibodies, not infrequently resulting in opportunistic infections. Hence, the search for even more specific agents has continued.

Another milestone toward this goal occurred when cell hybridization techniques were developed that could yield monoclonal antibodies (MAbs) to single-cell membrane determinants (6). This Nobel Prize–winning technology provided reagents that are reactive only with T cells or, even more importantly, with specific T-cell subsets or other molecular targets. Monoclonal antibody therapy was introduced into clinical protocols in 1981, when Cosimi reported the rapid reversal of acute rejection in renal allograft recipients treated with OKT-3 MAb without the use of increased steroid dosages (7). This MAb has since become the treatment of choice for steroid-resistant rejection in recipients of all types of allografts. As detailed below, its role in induction therapy has been less well established.

With the addition of OKT-3 to therapeutic protocols, it seemed a new clinical era had been entered in which monoclonal ALS would be extensively used to manipulate selected T-cell populations while leaving intact most of the host's other immune competence. Like the polyclonal antilymphocyte preparations, OKT-3 is a pan-T-cell antibody and therefore affects all aspects of cell-mediated immunity. The successful clinical application of this MAb, however, emphasized that this technology could provide further designer proteins targeting less broadly expressed cell surface markers that are important components of the effector pathways of rejection. Unfortunately, progress in defining clinically effective MAbs that provide more selective suppression of immunologic responses than OKT-3 has been frustratingly limited. Undoubtedly, this is due to the complexity of the rejection reaction, which must include alternate pathways that can be utilized to mount an effective response following highly selective blocking of known mechanisms.

Some of the most promising agents currently under investigation are directed toward the integrins or adhesion molecules, the costimulatory pathways, and the cytokine receptors. In addition to the use of MAbs to inhibit the function of these molecules, the use of soluble receptors [e.g., tumor necrosis factor receptor (TNFR), interleukin 2 receptor (IL-2R)] as immunosuppressive agents is being explored. The constantly expanding identification of new molecules involved in the rejection process promotes continuing opportunities for targeting specific components of the immune system. This chapter traces the evolution of antilymphocyte antibodies (both polyclonal and monoclonal) in the context of their preparation, their prophylactic administration, and their abolition of the rejection reaction as well as the possible future role some of these agents may play in the development of conditioning regimens that may even induce donor-specific tolerance.

## POLYCLONAL ANTILYMPHOCYTE SERA

ALS, ALG, and antithymocyte globulin (ATG) are xenotypic polyclonal antibody preparations with differing degrees of immunoglobulin purity produced by immunizing animals with different source lymphocytes (see below).

### Production of ALS Preparations

Polyclonal antibodies are produced by immunizing animals with human lymphoid cells. The immunized animal produces numerous antibodies, each from an individual cell clone, in response to the various antigens contained on the immunogen. Cultured lymphoblasts (producing ALG) or human thymocytes (producing ATG) are the most commonly employed immunogens. Cultured lymphoblasts have the advantage of being free of contaminants such as erythrocytes, platelets, or stromal elements that induce unwanted antibodies. However, stable cultured clones are typically B cells, so thymocytes remain the immunogen of choice for many commercial preparations (Table 8.1). Thymocytes are obtained from cadaver donors or patients undergoing open heart surgery. The selection of specific animals for immunization is based on practical considera-

tions including cost, animal size, and availability (8). The most commonly used preparations are of equine or rabbit origin. These two species have been demonstrated to produce large volumes of potent antilymphocyte antibodies. Sera from multiple animals are usually pooled in the attempt to achieve batch-to-batch consistency.

Following immunization of the selected animals, sera are harvested and processed to obtain purified globulin. This generally involves extensive absorption with nonlymphoid cells in order to remove contaminating antibodies (e.g., hemolysins) and fractionation, thus obtaining the IgG portion of the serum that contains the immunosuppressive component. Nevertheless, over 95% of the final product is made up of irrelevant equine or rabbit globulin, and it is estimated that only about 2% of the administered antibodies are specifically reactive with human T lymphocytes (9). The steps involved in the production of a typical polyclonal ALS are summarized in Figure 8.1.

### Administration

The initial reports of antilymphocyte antibody use involved intramuscular or subcutaneous administration. However, local inflammatory reactions and the increased immunogenicity associated with these approaches plus the need for relatively large volumes of polyclonal agents make intravenous administration the preferred approach. A painful chemical phlebitis can be associated with peripheral administration through low-flow veins, and so antilymphocyte antibodies are sometimes given via central venous access lines or an arteriovenous fistula. Central venous administration also allows for more concentrated individual doses in patients unable to tolerate large volume infusions. The currently available commercial preparations include ATG-Fresenius and Thymoglobulin (Pasteur Merieux; in the

**Table 8.1.** Comparison of Polyclonal Antilymphocyte Preparations

| | ATGAM (Upjohn) | Lymphoglobuline (Merieux) | Thymoglobuline (Merieux) | ATG (Fresenius) | MALG (U. Minn) | RATG (12) |
|---|---|---|---|---|---|---|
| **Immunogen** | Thymus | Thymus | Thymus | Jurkat Cell Line | Cultured Lymphoblasts | Thymus |
| **Species** | Equine | Equine | Rabbit | Rabbit | Equine | Rabbit |
| **Dosage (mg/kg/d)** | 10–30 | 10 | 1.25–2.5 | 1–5 | 15–20 | 1–5 |
| **Reactivity Against*:** | | | | | | |
| CD2 | ++ | ++++ | + | ± | + | + |
| CD3 | ++ | + | + | 0 | + | ± |
| CD4 | +++ | + | ± | 0 | + | + |
| CD8 | ++ | +++ | ++ | 0 | + | + |
| CD11a | ++ | + | ± | 0 | + | + |
| CD18 | ++ | ++ | + | 0 | ++ | ++++ |
| CD28 | + | ++ | ± | ± | ++ | ++++ |
| TCR | ++ | + | + | 0 | + | N/A |

* Comparative in vitro reactivity to specific CD antigens (11–13).

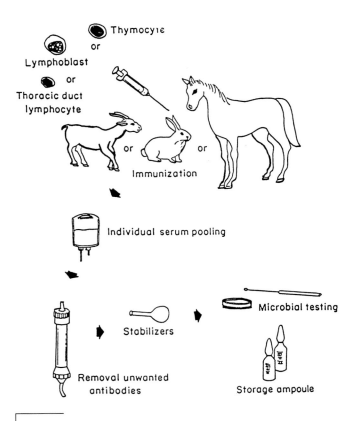

Thymocyte
or
Lymphoblast
or
Thoracic duct
lymphocyte

Immunization

Individual serum pooling

Stabilizers

Removal unwanted
antibodies

Microbial testing

Storage ampoule

**FIGURE 8.1.** *Production of polyclonal ALS preparations for human use. Selected animals are immunized with human thymocytes, thoracic duct lymphocytes, or cultured lymphoblasts. Harvested sera are pooled, extensively absorbed to remove unwanted antibodies, and processed to obtain the IgG portion.*

U.S.A., Sangstat Medical Corp.), which are of rabbit origin and are given in doses of 1.25–5.0 mg/kg/day, and ATGAM (Upjohn) and Lymphoglobuline (Pasteur Merieux), which are of equine origin and are given at doses of 10–30 mg/kg/day. Minnesota ALG (MALG), which is currently not available (10), has been administered at a dose of 15–20 mg/kg/day. In addition, some transplant centers continue to produce their own individual products. Since no single agent has been defined as most efficacious, ALS, ATG, and ALG preparations can be considered under the single heading of ALS.

### Mechanisms of Action

Polyclonal ALS contain antibodies reactive with multiple common T-cell surface molecules (see Table 8.1). Probably most relevant are antibodies targeting the cluster designation (CD) determinants CD2, CD3, CD4, CD8, CD11a, CD25, CD40, and CD54 (11–13). There appear to be at least three mechanisms of action by which polyclonal antibodies exert their effects. In vivo administration of ALS often results in profound lymphopenia. One mechanism for this lymphopenia appears to be classic complement-mediated cell

lysis. Another likely mechanism for the lymphopenia and its resultant immunosuppressive effect is uptake of opsonized T cells by the reticuloendothelial system. ALS-coated T cells can be found sequestered in the reticuloendothelial system of the spleen, liver, lungs, thymus, and lymph nodes of treated animals. A third mechanism by which ALS could exert its immunosuppressive properties is through masking or modulation of essential surface receptors on lymphocytes that remain in the circulation but whose function is blocked. After cessation of ALS therapy, repopulation of peripheral blood lymphocytes usually occurs within 3 to 10 days. However, the proliferative response of these lymphocytes often remains impaired. This phenomenon may result from the development of nonspecific suppressor cells (14).

### CLINICAL APPLICATIONS OF POLYCLONAL ANTIBODIES

Polyclonal ALS preparations for intravenous administration are typically diluted in isotonic saline to concentrations not exceeding 4 mg/cc. Dextrose- or heparin-containing solutions are generally avoided because they may result in protein aggregation. Infusion is by slow intravenous administration over approximately four hours in order to minimize toxicity. An in-line filter is recommended to prevent infusion of precipitates that may develop during storage. Corticosteroids along with acetaminophen and antihistamines are often given prior to administration of ALS to limit the side effects resulting from the rapid release of cytokines that is associated with initial infusions (see below). A skin test or a slowly infused test dose has been recommended for exclusion of preexisting type I sensitivity to equine or rabbit serum. Most clinicians, however, have discontinued skin testing since little correlation with allergic reactions has been demonstrated (15). The duration of ALS therapy is generally 5 to 14 days, depending on the specific indication for treatment as well as center preferences.

### ALS Rejection Prophylaxis (Induction Therapy)

While there is little disagreement about the efficacy of polyclonal preparations in rejection reversal, the role of these agents for induction therapy is more controversial. Early studies demonstrated a significant delay in the onset of first rejection episodes in renal allograft recipients treated with ALS in conjunction with azathioprine and steroids compared to patients on azathioprine and steroids alone. After cessation of ALS therapy, however, a high incidence of rejection episodes occurred and significant improvement in long-term allograft or patient survival was difficult to demonstrate (16,17). Many of these early studies suggested an improvement in graft survival of approximately 10%, but the low numbers of patients in individual reports, the nonstandardized products being used, and the multiple other variables involved in such clinical trials made it difficult to provide statistically significant conclusions.

The subsequent addition of cyclosporine (CsA) to immunosuppressive protocols clearly improved survival for recipients of all types of allografts, suggesting induction ALS therapy might no longer be a consideration (see also Chapter 1). However, the apparent nephrotoxic synergism between CsA and the physiologic factors associated with acute tubular necrosis (ATN), which are frequently encountered in the early postoperative period especially after renal transplantation, has raised concerns that irreversible renal damage may occur if CsA is being administered when the kidney is in the initial recovery phase. This has prompted many centers to replace CsA with an antilymphocyte preparation until satisfactory renal function is restored (18–22). Observations in patients treated with such protocols have been encouraging, including a lower incidence of delayed graft function, minimally increased risks of viral infections, and a rejection-free early course in the majority of recipients. Improved long-term allograft survival has been achieved only in some individual center reports (23,24). Retrospective analyses of large databases (Table 8.2), however, have documented an advantage of induction antilymphocyte therapy in conjunction with delayed CsA therapy, particularly for recipients of older donor kidneys, highly sensitized patients, retransplant recipients, and those with delayed graft function (25,26). Concerns regarding the costs and potential risks of ALS immunosuppression have led many centers to recommend ALS induction therapy only for these high-risk recipients (27) or to reduce the dosage administered based on T-cell monitoring of individual patients (28). The continuing lack of consensus regarding the most cost-effective approach for induction therapy is emphasized by a recent survey of US transplant programs (29) (Table 8.3).

While most of the early studies using ALS involved renal transplantation, polyclonal antibody induction therapy has more recently been evaluated in recipients of extrarenal allografts. Sequential ALS-CsA induction therapy in hepatic transplant recipients has been reported from some centers to limit renal dysfunction, improve allograft survival and thus require fewer retransplants, and reduce the incidence of rejection. These benefits were achieved without an increased incidence of infectious complications or malignancy. Survival rates of over 90% have been reported using this approach (30,31). A recent study comparing ATG–CsA quadruple immunosuppression to tacrolimus and prednisone showed improved graft and patient survival in the ATG–CsA group with similar rejection rates (32). ALS induction has also been reported to increase survival rates in pediatric recipients of major blood group (ABO)-incompatible liver allografts (33). Some centers, however, caution that ATG therapy is an increased risk factor for subsequent cytomegalovirus (CMV) infection and recommend such induction only in selected high-risk hepatic allograft recipients (34).

ALS has also been considered an important induction agent in pancreatic transplantation (35). A lower incidence of rejection episodes, along with a delay in onset to first rejection, and pancreatic graft survival rates of over 80% have been reported using sequential ALS–CsA quadruple induction therapy in combined kidney–pancreas transplantation.

ALS was used almost universally in cardiac transplantation prior to the introduction of CsA. In contrast to the observations in recipients of renal allografts, the efficacy of ALS had been felt to be conclusive for cardiac transplantation (36,37). With the addition of CsA to

**Table 8.2.** The Effect of Induction Therapy with ALS or OKT-3 on CD Renal Allograft Survival

| | No Antibody | | ALG/OKT-3 | | |
|---|---|---|---|---|---|
| | % 1-Yr Survival | Recipients (*n*) | % 1-Yr Survival | Recipients (*n*) | *P* value |
| **Primary Transplant** | 78 | 14,450 | 80 | 4820 | <0.001 |
| Donor age >55 | 68 | 92 | 76 | 350 | 0.006 |
| DGF | 64 | 3690 | 70 | 1185 | <0.0001 |
| PRA >50% | 72 | 1345 | 77 | 550 | 0.02 |
| Diabetic | 76 | 2830 | 80 | 1025 | 0.004 |
| **Retransplant** | 70 | 2680 | 74 | 1050 | 0.006 |
| Donor age >55 | 52 | 160 | 65 | 65 | 0.04 |
| DGF | 53 | 965 | 60 | 390 | 0.01 |
| PRA >50% | 63 | 770 | 72 | 415 | 0.002 |
| Diabetic | 69 | 310 | 77 | 100 | NS |

NS = not stated.
Source: Adapted from Cecka JM, Terasaki PI. The UNOS Scientific Renal Transplant Registry. In: Teraski PI, Cecka JM, eds. Clinical transplants 1991. Los Angeles: UCLA Tissue Typing Laboratory, 1992:6.

**Table 8.3.**    Preferred Immunosuppressive Approaches of US Transplant Programs

| | Kidney | | Heart | | Liver | | Pancreas | |
|---|---|---|---|---|---|---|---|---|
| | I[a] | II[b] | I[a] | II[b] | I[a] | II[b] | I[a] | II[b] |
| **Induction Therapy** | | | | | | | | |
| Polyclonal Ab | 54% | 25% | 54% | 28% | 37% | 42% | 76% | 12% |
| Monoclonal Ab | 51% | 26% | 55% | 28% | 35% | 40% | 72% | 8% |
| **Rejection Therapy** | | | | | | | | |
| Monoclonal Ab | 94% | 2% | 92% | 3% | 95% | 0% | 92% | 0% |
| IV Steroids | 90% | 4% | 97% | 0% | 91% | 5% | 80% | 0% |
| Polyclonal Ab | 73% | 12% | 82% | 5% | 67% | 7% | 68% | 4% |

[a]   Proportion of programs regarding the approach as important or essential to successful patient outcome.
[b]   Proportion of programs regarding the approach as unnecessary or undesirable.
Adapted from Evans RW, Manninen DL, Dong FB, et al. Immunosuppressive therapy as a determinant of transplantation outcomes. Transplantation 1993;55:1297–1305.

immunosuppressive protocols, many centers discontinued the use of ALS induction. As in renal transplant recipients, however, the severe nephrotoxic effects of CsA that became apparent following heart transplantation have led some centers to replace CsA with ALS during the immediate post-transplant period (38,39). This approach is reported to reduce the incidence and severity of rejection and improve long-term outcome and renal function in cardiac transplant recipients (40–42). Again, however, this practice is far from universal (see Table 8.3).

Since steroids have been shown to inhibit bronchial healing in lung transplant recipients (43), ALS in conjunction with CsA and azathioprine induction has been used for induction therapy that withholds steroids for up to three weeks in these patients (44).

## ALS Rejection Therapy

The first randomized trial comparing ALS to high-dosage steroids for the treatment of established rejection was conducted in 1979 (45). The patients in that study were living–related donor renal allograft recipients who had received induction immunosuppressive therapy with azathioprine and prednisone. With the onset of biopsy-proven rejection, the patients were randomized to receive either high-dose steroids or ALS. ALS proved to be as effective as high-dosage steroids, with the added benefit of more rapid rejection reversal and fewer subsequent rejection episodes. Long-term follow-up indicated that a one-year allograft survival of over 90% could be achieved in azathioprine–steroid–treated recipients of haploidentical renal allografts if rejection was reversed with ALS, versus a survival of only 74% following rejection treatment with steroids (46). The efficacy of ALS in reversing rejection in CsA-treated patients has also been demonstrated (47,48). ALS has even been used

to reverse steroid-resistant rejection in patients who had previously received ALS induction, with no increase in infectious morbidity being observed (3,49). The value of ALS, particularly for treating steroid-resistant rejection in renal transplant recipients, is therefore widely acknowledged (see Table 8.3), although, as discussed below, OKT-3 MAb is now usually preferred. Nevertheless, ALS provides a useful option in rejection therapy, especially for patients who may have been sensitized to murine protein after a previous course of MAb therapy.

ALS has also been used to treat primary or steroid-resistant rejection in liver transplantation (50,51). Again, however, with the availability of tacrolimus and OKT-3, current use of ALS in hepatic transplantation is primarily as an induction agent given to patients with perioperative renal dysfunction. ALS has also been used to treat steroid-resistant rejection in pancreatic, cardiac, and pulmonary transplant recipients. The choice of polyclonal versus MAb therapy in each of these situations remains unresolved and will be discussed further below.

## ALS Induction of Transplant Tolerance

The feasibility of inducing allograft tolerance in adult recipients has been established in a number of rodent models, many of which, interestingly, have required ALS as part of the T-cell–depleting conditioning protocol (52,53). In murine models, highly specific unresponsiveness to donor antigens can be consistently produced using donor blood or bone marrow infusions and ALS. Long-term allograft survival without the requirement for chronic immunosuppression has been much more difficult to achieve in large animal models, but a similar protocol has been extended to non-human primates (54). With a brief course of post-transplant ALS therapy, donor bone marrow infusion, and no further immunosuppression after the fifth day following transplant, indefinite renal allograft survival was observed in about one-third of these recipients (55). On the basis of these observations, a pilot trial in humans was undertaken in which cadaveric renal allograft recipients received ALS followed by the transfusion of donor-specific bone marrow. Control patients received the contralateral kidney without bone marrow transfusion (56). Both groups of patients received CsA, azathioprine, and prednisone. The allograft survival rate for the bone marrow group was significantly improved at 12 months, and it was possible to withdraw steroids completely from a number of these patients. No attempt was made to withdraw all immunosuppression as had been done in the nonhuman primate trials.

Recent data have demonstrated that a state of multilineage mixed chimerism and donor-specific tolerance to renal allografts can be produced in the majority of nonhuman primates that have undergone a brief period of T-cell depletion with a conditioning regimen that also requires ALS (57,58). The mechanism of tolerance in these recipients, in contrast to what has been felt to represent peripherally mediated "anergy" in the previous models, appears to involve clonal deletion. Because of the highly durable donor-specific unresponsiveness associated with this type of tolerance, this approach is quite attractive for clinical application, although no trials have yet been undertaken. Nevertheless, these demonstrations of donor-specific hyporesponsiveness in large animal models emphasize that transplant tolerance induction in human recipients should be possible and that initial therapeutic protocols are likely to include ALS.

## In Vitro Monitoring of ALS Therapy

Since different ALS preparations, and even the same preparation in different individuals, may produce variable immunosuppressive effects, a number of in vitro assays have been utilized in the attempt to both standardize different batches of ALS and monitor the level of suppression that is being achieved during treatment. For quality control and standardization purposes, the lymphocytotoxicity of each preparation may be determined by adding decreasing concentrations of ALS to lymphocytes in order to determine the lowest concentration at which more than 50% of lymphocytes are killed (59). Preparations are also assayed for their ability to inhibit the formation of rosettes by sheep erythrocytes with human T lymphocytes. Rosette inhibition results from the anti-CD2 antibodies contained in the ALS preparations.

Clinical activity has been evaluated by monitoring T-cell numbers in peripheral blood with the use of MAbs (60). Interestingly, some of the T-cell subset alterations have been documented to persist for periods as long as five years after ALS treatment (61). Depression of CD2- or CD3-positive cells (mature T lymphocytes) to less than 10% of pretreatment values has generally been correlated with rejection

control (62,63). In contrast, persistent elevation of this cell population is often associated with unresolved rejection, requiring either increased ALS dosages or the addition of other immunosuppressants. Since most of these preparations are contaminated with antibodies reactive with human erythrocytes and thrombocytes, serial hematocrits and platelet counts must also be monitored during therapy and dosages of the administered product adjusted to prevent unacceptable anemia or thrombocytopenia.

## Immunogenicity of Polyclonal Preparations

During or following a course of ALS therapy, serum antibodies reactive with rabbit or equine immunoglobulin can be detected in 10% to 30% of patients (49,64). Such antibodies, if present in sufficient titer during therapy, could neutralize the beneficial effects of the agent and might explain why peripheral blood T cells are not effectively depleted in some patients. However, no consistent correlation has been demonstrated between circulating levels of ALS and allograft survival.

The major immunologic concern associated with infusions of heterologous antibodies is the possibility of producing serum sickness. As noted above, pretreatment skin testing has not proved to be useful for predicting the likelihood of reactions to the foreign protein. Fortunately, anaphylactic reactions and serum sickness have been surprisingly infrequent (65), generally being noted in 1% to 3% of treated patients. Furthermore, many patients have been treated with ALS on repeated occasions without adverse effects. This apparent lack of a clinically relevant immune response to the foreign protein is presumably due to multiple factors, including careful deaggregation of the products prepared for clinical infusion, the intravenous route of administration, and the large dosages employed that should provide a significant antigen excess and favor the development of small and highly soluble complexes. In addition, because these polyclonal antisera react with a variety of lymphocyte populations, the ALS may, in combination with the concomitant pharmacologic immunosuppression being administered, suppress the recipient's response to the foreign protein as well (8). Cessation of ALS therapy and administration of high-dosage steroids has effectively controlled the signs and symptoms of serum sickness in the few patients who have developed this condition.

## Side Effects of Polyclonal Preparations

The reported incidence and severity of adverse clinical reactions following ALS administration have varied with the preparation used (Table 8.4). Fever, often in association with significant chills and sometimes diarrhea, develops during the initial infusion in the majority of patients. Intensive evaluation of these "first-dose reactions" following either polyclonal or monoclonal antibody therapy has established that increased serum cytokine levels including TNF, IL-1 and IL-

**T a b l e   8 . 4 .**     Clinical Toxicity of ALS Administration

| Reported Incidence >10% | | Reported Incidence 5% to 10% | | Reported Incidence ≤5% | |
|---|---|---|---|---|---|
| **Early Reactions** | | | | | |
| Chills, Fever (d1) | 15–60% | Nausea, diarrhea | 1–10% | Hypotension | 2–5% |
| (d2) | 4–25% | Neutropenia | 1–10% | Dyspnea | 2–5% |
| Thrombocytopenia | 1–30% | (<2000/mm³) | | Seizures | 0–1% |
| (<50,000/mm³) | | Serum sickness | 1–8% | Anaphylaxis | 0–1% |
| Rash/pruritus | 1–20% | Arthralgia | 1–7% | | |
| Anemia | 5–15% | | | | |
| Local phlebitis | 2–15% | | | | |
| | | | | | |
| **Late Side Effects** | | | | | |
| CMV infection | | Herpes simplex reactivation | | PTLD | |
| | | EBV reactivation | | | |

6, and interferon gamma (IFN-γ) are highly correlated with the side effects (66,67). To limit the morbidity of this cytokine release, patients are usually premedicated with antipyretics, antihistamines, and intravenous steroids. There is also evidence that anti-TNF antibodies or TNF soluble receptors may limit the cytokine release syndrome (68,69). Such approaches have generally been employed only with MAb therapy where the syndrome has been more severe (see below). During ALS treatment, pruritic skin eruptions (Fig. 8.2) have been noted in approximately 20% of recipients. Although this presumably represents a type of hypersensitivity to the agent, most patients can complete the therapeutic protocol without the development of more significant problems with only antihistamine administration being required for symptomatic relief.

Thrombocytopenia and/or anemia of varying severity have been reported in up to 30% of patients. This is generally dose-related, occurring in patients who require maximum dosages to depress T-cell levels adequately. A modest reduction in ALS dosage, or further reduction in the concomitantly administered azathioprine or mycophenolate mofetil dose, usually resolves this problem without the need for discontinuing ALS therapy (see also Chapter 5). Although thrombocytopenia primarily results from low levels of contaminating antiplatelet antibodies, reversible platelet aggregation within the pulmonary microcirculation in the absence of antiplatelet antibodies has also been demonstrated (70). These aggregates release vasoactive substances that could induce interstitial pooling and hypotensive reactions, even in the absence of hypersensitivity. Such a sequence of events could explain the observation of occasional hypotensive episodes associated with rapid infusions of ALS.

An increased incidence of infectious complications has been reported in many trials of ALS therapy. Of particular importance was the early observation that CMV infection seemed to be disproportionately more frequent and more severe in allograft recipients treated with ALS (8,51). One

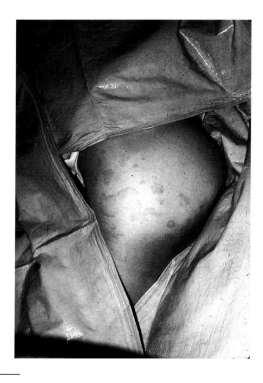

**FIGURE 8.2.**     *Skin rash in an ATG-treated patient. The maculopapular, blotchy eruption developed primarily over the recipient's thighs and buttocks six days after initiating ATG therapy. The 12-day course of treatment, required to reverse the patient's acute rejection episode, was completed without complications following administration of antihistamines for symptomatic relief.*

group observed the incidence of CMV infection to be twice as high in liver allograft recipients treated with ALS compared to those treated with conventional immunosuppression (34). Similar observations were reported in ALS-treated renal and cardiac allograft recipients. Further experience has established that reducing the dosages of concomitantly administered pharmacologic agents, in conjunction with the steroid-sparing effect achieved by ALS, results in infectious complication rates similar to those observed using conventional immunosuppression (17,71). Unfortunately, if concomitantly administered pharmacologic agents are withdrawn completely during ALS therapy, the incidence of sensitization to the heterologous protein is markedly increased. Routine ganciclovir administration during the period of ALS therapy has therefore also been recommended to further limit the incidence of CMV infection (72).

As with any potent immunosuppression, administration of ALS is associated with an increased incidence of malignancy (73), particularly post-transplant lymphoproliferative disease (PTLD). This lymphoma-like process results from primary infection (in children) or reactivation (in adults) of Epstein-Barr virus (EBV). This complication is seen most frequently in allograft recipients who have had multiple courses of antirejection therapy, especially if this included ALS.

## MONOCLONAL ANTIBODIES

The production of MAbs is based on two well-established observations. First, each B lymphocyte and its expanded clone in an immunized animal produce a single specific antibody but have a very short life span when cultured ex vivo; and second, malignant myeloma cells can be grown permanently in culture but produce antibodies with no predefined specificity. The key breakthrough in MAb technology occurred in 1975 when Kohler and Milstein succeeded in fusing these two cell types, thus combining the essential properties of specific antibody secretion and permanent cell growth (6). Each fusion-derived hybridoma cell line secretes a single antibody of predefined reactivity plus the irrelevant myeloma protein. This methodology allows the production of essentially unlimited quantities of the desired MAb, which can be selected to target virtually any cell surface antigen or circulating molecule. As a result, major advances in both identifying and manipulating cell surface antigens and other immune mediators have occurred.

The previous success of polyclonal ALS in immunosuppressive regimens strongly suggested that MAbs might be even more effectively employed as immunosuppressive agents. This was confirmed when OKT-3, which targets the CD3 complex associated with the T-cell receptor (TCR) expressed on all mature T lymphocytes, was first used clinically (7).

### Production of Monoclonal Antibodies

Monoclonal antibody production begins with immunization of mice using human T lymphocytes or selected membrane fragments (Fig. 8.3). After approximately four to six weeks, splenocytes are harvested from the immunized mice. The antibody-producing cells are then mixed with mouse myeloma cells and polyethylene glycol to promote fusion. The hybridomas obtained are assayed and those hybridomas

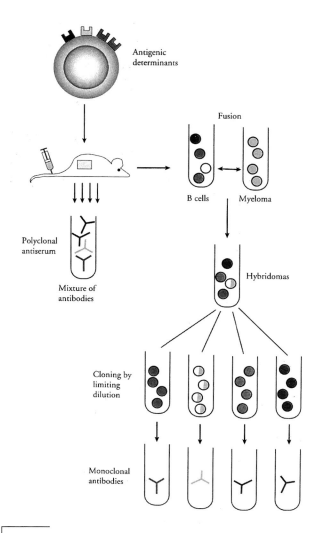

**FIGURE 8.3.** *Production of monoclonal antibodies for human use. Splenocytes (B cells) from immunized mice are fused with myeloma cells to produce the "immortalized" antibody-producing hybridoma. The desired hybridoma is isolated and expanded by random cloning. (Reprinted with permission. Copyright 1995, Hoffman-La Roche Inc. All rights reserved.)*

demonstrating positive antibody activity are subsequently grown in a hypoxanthine, aminopterin, and thymidine (HAT)-containing medium that kills parental cells but allows the hybridomas to survive. By random cloning, the desired hybridomas are then isolated and expanded. The selected clones are maintained in vitro by mass tissue culture or in vivo by intraperitoneal injection into mice, which results in the formation of an ascites-producing tumor. From these sources, large volumes of tissue culture supernatant or antibody-containing ascites can be sequentially collected for clinical use.

More recent refinements have led to the development of "humanized" monoclonal antibodies (74). Humanized antibodies have been developed in an attempt to overcome the human antimouse antibody (HAMA) response observed in most patients receiving MAbs of murine origin. These HAMAs cause rapid clearance of the murine antibody from the recipient's circulation, thereby reducing the therapeutic efficacy and possibly precluding sequential courses of MAb therapy. As a first step in the production of humanized agents, the mouse variable region is joined to a human constant region (see Chapter 7, Fig. 7.2). Using gene recombinant techniques, the chimeric MAb is further modified so that only the essential antigen-combining sequences of mouse origin are retained (75,76). These segments, termed the *complementary determining regions (CDRs)*, continue to confer antigenic specificity to the antibody. However, since the CDR-grafted antibodies differ from human immunoglobulin only at the epitope-combining site, the HAMA response to these agents is both reduced and predictably anti-idiotypic (77). As a result, the therapeutic course of one humanized MAb should not prevent subsequent treatment with other MAbs bearing different idiotypes. Furthermore, humanized MAbs are less likely to induce the cytokine release syndrome (78,79), and the effective half-life of the administered agent is greatly prolonged in the recipient's circulation (80).

Most recently, MAb immunoconjugates with striking immunosuppressive potency have been developed through fusion technology (81,82). These MAbs allow delivery of drugs or toxins to selected target cells that have surface components reactive with the antibody portion of the conjugate. The immunotoxin portion, which is then internalized by receptor-mediated endocytosis, has proved to be highly efficacious for inducing T-cell depletion in these studies.

## Administration

The initial clinical trial using OKT-3 without additional steroids demonstrated the efficacy of this intravenously administered MAb in reversing established renal allograft rejection with dosages as low as 1–2 mg/day (7). However, in some patients, daily T-cell monitoring revealed incomplete depletion or modulation of circulating CD3+ cells. This led to the currently recommended adult dosage of 5 mg/day in order to reduce the need for frequent monitoring. The optimal dosage, however, remains undefined (83) and undoubtedly could be tailored to individual patient requirements by serial monitoring of circulating T lymphocytes (see below). The dosage in children is typically 1.0–2.5 mg/day depending on the size of the child. The duration of therapy may vary depending on whether the drug is being given as an induction agent or as therapy for steroid-resistant rejection. The usual course of OKT3 treatment for rejection is 10 to 14 days, depending on the clinical response, while the course for induction may be shortened depending on the degree of ATN. OKT-3 is injected as a single intravenous bolus and may be given through a peripheral vein. Because OKT-3 may contain particulate protein matter, the drug should be drawn through a 0.22-micron filter prior to infusion. Before initiating therapy, the patient's

volume status should be assessed carefully to avoid precipitation of pulmonary edema (see side effects, below).

As with the polyclonal preparations, antihistamines, acetaminophen, and corticosteroids should be given prior to administration of the first one or two OKT-3 doses to alleviate the "first-dose response" (84,85). Concomitant pharmacologic immunosuppression should be reduced to decrease the risks of infection; however, maintenance of at least low-dose CsA may be beneficial to limit the recipient's immune response and prevent recurrent rejection (86). Dosages of other MAbs used in clinical protocols have been widely variable, ranging from as little as 0.5 mg/kg given every two weeks (80) to 1 mg/kg/day (87). As with OKT-3, sequential monitoring of the degree of depletion or modulation of the targeted cell population that is being achieved during therapy has been used to define the appropriate dosage for each preparation.

## Mechanisms of Action

Monoclonal antibodies may exert their immunosuppressive effects by several mechanisms (see Chapter 7) including cell depletion (Fig. 8.4), cell coating, and antigenic modulation (88). True T-cell depletion is suggested by a decrease in the number of lymphocytes expressing CD determinants other than the targeted antigen (e.g., absence of cells expressing CD2 following anti-CD3 therapy). Opsonizing antibodies clear T lymphocytes via complement fixation or interaction with Fc receptors that results in reticuloendothelial uptake and lysis in the spleen, liver, and lymph nodes (89). Direct lysis of lymphocytes in the circulation, particularly if a toxin has been conjugated to the MAb, may also contribute to T-cell depletion. Whether opsonization and lymphocyte clearance is more likely from the peripheral circulation or from

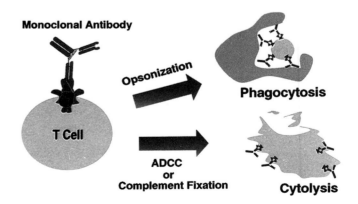

**FIGURE 8.4.**     *T-cell clearance by monoclonal antibodies. Depleting monoclonal antibodies may trigger complement activation through their Fc portion or produce cell cytolysis via antibody-dependent cell cytotoxicity (ADCC). Opsonization and phagocytosis of the antibody-coated cell may contribute to cell clearance in the reticuloendothelial system.*

the transplant itself may be determined by the subclass of administered antibody (90).

Monoclonal antibodies may also exert immunosuppressive activity by coating cell surface antigens. This process may block the function of the cell by interfering with cell-to-cell interactions, by transducing signals that result in inactivation or activation of particular cells, or by cross-linking different cells (91,92). Cells coated with murine MAb can be detected in vitro using antimurine-immunoglobulin–fluoresceinated antibodies. Antigenic coating appears to be the primary mechanism of action for many of the MAbs directed against adhesion molecules (90).

Antigenic modulation (see Chapter 7, Fig. 7.6) is a phenomenon that results in redistribution of antigen–antibody complexes on the cell surface forming a "cap" (88,93). These "caps" of antibody–antigen complexes are then internalized or shed from the cell surface. This process renders the cell unresponsive if the molecule is functionally relevant as in the TCR–CD3 complex, which is targeted by OKT-3 (94). Antigenic modulation may be reversible as demonstrated by reexpression of the molecule if the cells are cultured in vitro or after MAb therapy is withdrawn.

## Molecular Targets of Monoclonal Antibodies

While MAbs could be produced against virtually any cell surface or secreted antigen, immunosuppressive activity requires that the antibody be directed against a functionally important molecule. Target antigens for immunosuppressive MAbs are typically expressed on the surface of cells that are known to be involved in the immune response, particularly T cells (see Chapter 2). T cells are equipped with an array of such cell surface molecules (Fig. 8.5) that mediate interactions between nonactivated T cells and antigen-presenting cells (APCs), or between cytotoxic T cells and their targets (e.g., allograft endothelium). Interference with the molecules mediating these interactions therefore represents an attractive approach to selectively interrupting the immune response to an allograft. The important antigens that have been targeted for clinical trials or appear to have significant clinical promise are listed in Table 8.5.

**CD2,** also known as the E-rosette receptor or lymphocyte function associated antigen-2 (LFA-2), functions as an adhesion and signal transduction molecule. It is expressed on T cells and natural killer (NK) cells. CD2 is physically

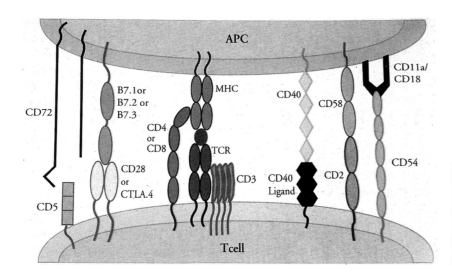

**FIGURE 8.5.** *Schematic depiction of some of the cell surface molecules involved in T-cell activation. Monoclonal antibodies that are specifically targeted to any one of these determinants can be utilized to selectively interrupt essential intercellular reactions. (Reprinted with permission. Copyright 1995, Hoffman-La Roche Inc. All rights reserved.)*

**Table 8.5.**  Promising Targets for MAb Immunomodulation

| Specificity | Distribution | Ligand | Function |
|---|---|---|---|
| CD2 (E-Rosette R) | T cells, NK cells | LFA3 | Adhesion with TCR/MHC |
| CD3 | Mature T cells | — | Activation, ↑IL-2 |
| CD4 | 50–65% T cells | MHC class II | Stabilize TCR/MHC |
| CD7 | T cells, blasts | — | T-cell proliferation |
| CD8 | 30–35% T cells | MHC class I | Stabilize TCR/MHC |
| CD25 (IL-2R) | Activated cells | IL-2 | T-cell proliferation |
| CD28/CTLA4 | T cells | B7.1 (CD80), B7.2 (CD86) | Costimulation |
| CD40L (CD154) | T cells | CD40 | APC maturation, ↑IL-12 |
| CD45 | BM-derived cells | — | Regulate phosphorylation |
| CD54 (ICAM) | Endothelium, activated cells | LFA1 | Leukocyte adhesion |
| TCR | T cells | MHC 1 or 2 + peptide | Ag specificity |

and functionally linked to TCR and CD3 and enhances their binding to major histocompatibility complex (MHC) antigen. Its ligand is LFA-3 (CD58), found on APCs. Inhibition of CD2 signaling has been shown to result in apoptosis (95) or induction of an anergic state (96). Anti-CD2 MAbs, therefore, could be useful in controlling rejection. Early preclinical studies, however, suggested poor immunosuppressive efficacy of these agents (97). Recently, evaluation of a new anti-CD2 MAb (LO-CD2a) produced from rat ascites has been undertaken in Brussels (98). This agent has been shown to produce prolonged depletion of CD2 reactive cells when administered to chimpanzees and to be minimally mitogenic in vitro. Predictably, therefore, "first dose reactions" should be less severe than those encountered with OKT-3. Initial clinical evaluation of LO-CD2a as treatment for graft-versus-host disease (GVHD) and renal allograft rejection has been encouraging and is continuing.

**CD3,** a cell-surface immunoglobulin found on mature T cells, is associated with the antigen-recognition site of the T-cell receptor. This molecule is believed to be responsible for T-cell activation and upregulation of IL-2 production along with mitogenesis. OKT-3, which targets this molecule, is the prototype MAb that, to date, has been most widely used for immunosuppression in transplantation (see below).

**CD4,** a glycoprotein that belongs to the immunoglobulin family, is found on the majority of mature thymocytes and the 55% to 60% of peripheral T cells that bind MHC class II antigens. Historically, these cells were termed *helper/inducer T lymphocytes*. Similarities between human and lower animal CD4 molecules illustrate evolutionary conservation of this component, suggesting its essential role in T-cell function. This molecule is believed to be essential for alloactivation when MHC class II antigen is presented to CD4-bearing T cells. It is an accessory cell adhesion molecule that stabilizes the interaction of the TCR–CD3 complex with the antigen–MHC class II complex. Monoclonal antibodies directed against CD4 block MHC class II–dependent cell proliferation in vitro and block production of IL-2 by T cells in the presence of antigen and thus have been extensively evaluated for clinical use (see below).

**CD5,** an adhesion molecule found on all T cells and some B cells, apparently plays a role in costimulatory signal transduction. Its importance, however, remains unclear. Xomazyme-65, a ricin-conjugated MAb, is the only preparation directed against CD5 that has been evaluated clinically. Its immunosuppressive efficacy has been difficult to establish (94), and this agent has not been approved for human use.

**CD6,** an integrin found on all T lymphocytes and some B cells, is apparently involved in costimulatory signal transduction modulating TCR-mediated T-cell activation (99). Monoclonal antibodies directed against CD6 inhibit its interaction with a recently identified ligand, activated leukocyte cell adhesion molecule (ALCAM). Anti-T12, the only anti-CD6 MAb to be evaluated clinically, has not demonstrated consistent efficacy (100).

**CD7** is a T-cell surface antigen present on most mature and immature T cells, whose expression is quantitatively increased on T-cell blasts such as those generated by alloactivation. This molecule is an attractive target for selective immunosuppression because of the possibility of removing donor-reactive T-cell blasts without removing resting cells from the circulation (see below).

**CD8** is a glycoprotein expressed on the approximately 20% to 40% of peripheral T cells that bind MHC class I antigens. These cells have also been termed *cytotoxic/ suppressor T lymphocytes*. CD8 is an important accessory molecule for antigen-dependent T-cell activation and direct adhesion with MHC class I proteins. Leu-2a, an MAb reactive with CD8, has been shown to deplete T cells from the circulation in humans; however, it had limited efficacy as an immunosuppressive agent (101).

**CD25,** previously known as the IL-2 receptor or Tac, is found on virtually all activated T cells, B cells, and macrophages, plus approximately 15% of resting cells. There are now known to be three IL-2R subunits, $\alpha$ (55 kd), $\beta$ (75 kd), $\gamma$ (64 kd). Although the $\beta$ and $\gamma$ subunits have been given separate CD designations (CD122 and CD132, respectively), MAbs targeting IL-2R are generally referred to as anti-CD25 reagents. They prevent expansion of CD4 and CD8 cells in mixed lymphocyte reactions (MLRs) and block the generation of cytotoxic T cells in vitro and are thus attractive candidates for selective modulation of immune responses. A number of these MAbs have been evaluated and several have now become available for clinical protocols (see below).

**CD40L** (CD154), is the T-cell ligand for the CD40 complex on antigen-presenting cells. The CD40/CD40L pathway appears to have a central role in the T-cell helper effector functions governing acute rejection (102). Interaction of CD40 with its ligand leads to APC maturation, increased secretion of the inflammatory cytokine IL-12, and upregulation of other costimulatory pathways including **CD28/B7.** Blocking this pathway with anti-CD40L MAbs results in dramatic prolongation of heart and kidney allograft survival in nonhuman primates (103). No clinical trials have been reported to date. (See further discussion in accompanying Commentary to this chapter.)

**CD54,** also known as intercellular adhesion molecule (ICAM), is a member of the immunoglobulin supergene family. CD54 is found on endothelial cells, fibroblasts, epithelial cells, and activated lymphocytes. Lymphocyte function associated antigen-1 (LFA-1 or CD11a/CD18), a member of the integrin family, is a ligand for CD54. The interaction of these molecules is involved in the adhesion of leukocytes to blood vessel walls and in their transendothelial migration. The ICAM–LFA-1 interaction is also believed to provide costimulatory signals during antigen presentation and to mediate adhesion between cytotoxic T lymphocytes and target cells (105). Monoclonal antibodies targeting this interaction may be efficacious in limiting reperfusion injury as well as in the prophylaxis and treatment of allograft rejection (see below).

**T-cell receptor (TCR)** is a heterodimeric polypeptide of the immunoglobulin supergene family closely associated with CD3. The majority (95%) of T cells express the TCR composed of an α and β chain that appear to be responsible for determining the antigen specificity of all cytotoxic and helper T cells. The remaining 5% of T cells express a γ/δ dimer whose function is unknown. The dramatic immunosuppressive efficacy of the anti-CD3 MAb, OKT-3, suggests anti-TCR MAbs could also be useful clinically (see below).

**Tumor necrosis factor (TNF)** is a cytokine produced by macrophages and activated T lymphocytes. TNF is believed to play a role in the immune response to allografts by stimulating IL-1 production, MHC class I expression on endothelial cells, T-cell proliferation, and initiation of procoagulant activity. TNF is also believed to be one of the primary cytokines responsible for the "first-dose syndrome" observed in recipients of antilymphocyte antibodies. Monoclonal antibodies to TNF and TNF-soluble receptors may be beneficial in limiting the immune response to allografts as well as the cytokine release syndrome (69).

## CLINICAL APPLICATIONS OF MONOCLONAL ANTIBODIES

The MAbs that currently have defined clinical efficacy or seem likely to be useful are listed in Table 8.6.

### Anti-CD3 Monoclonal Antibodies

OKT-3 is the prototype MAb with demonstrated efficacy particularly for reversal of steroid-resistant rejection in every field of organ transplantation (106). It has been in clinical use for over 15 years and remains the "gold standard" to which newer MAbs are compared for both efficacy and toxicity. While the efficacy of OKT-3 is without question, there are several limitations to its use. Among its limitations are the adverse effects related to the massive cytokine release associated with initial infusions, its immunogenicity, and the not infrequent occurrence of subsequent rejection episodes after discontinuation of OKT-3. Another drawback to OKT-3 is its pan-T-cell suppression that increases the risk of infectious complications and PTLD.

### *Mechanism of Action*

OKT-3, a murine IgG2a MAb, binds the epsilon portion of the human CD3 molecular complex on mature T lymphocytes. Cross-reactivity with other species is limited to the chimpanzee. Consequently, the in vivo evaluation of this MAb has been primarily in humans, where dramatic immunosuppressive effects have been observed (7,107). The CD3 complex is closely associated with the TCR and plays a vital role in T-cell activation and proliferation following presentation of antigen. OKT-3 exerts its effects through opsonization with subsequent complement-mediated cytolysis or reticuloendothelial uptake and destruction of T cells. This initially results in profound T-cell depletion as evidenced by a fall in the total peripheral lymphocyte count, absence of cells expressing other T-cell markers, and a lack of detectable cells coated with mouse immunoglobulin. With continued therapy, antigenic modulation demonstrated by the reappearance of T cells expressing other surface markers (CD4, CD8), but not CD3, occurs. This process involves redistribution of the OKT-3–CD3 complex on the T-cell surface and removal of the complex by internalization or shedding. Since the CD3 antigen is critical for MHC antigen recognition and T-cell–mediated cytotoxicity, the absence of CD3 on the cell surface renders the lymphocytes

**Table 8.6.**   Clinically Useful or [Promising] Monoclonal Antibodies

| Specificity | MAb | Therapeutic Indication | | |
| --- | --- | --- | --- | --- |
| | | Induction | Rejection | Other |
| CD2 | [BTI-322] | X | X | GVHD |
| CD3 | OKT-3 | X | X | |
| | [CD3-Immunotoxin] | Preclinical | | |
| CD4 | [cMT-412] | X | | |
| CD7 | [SDZCHH380] | X | | |
| CD11a/CD18 | [Odulimomab] | X | | |
| CD25 | BT563 | X | | |
| | Zenapax (HAT or daclizumab) | X | | |
| | [33B3.1] | X | | |
| | Simulect (basiliximab) | X | | |
| CD40L | [5C8] | Preclinical | | |
| CD54 | [BIRR1] | | | Autoimmune ?Reperfusion injury |
| TCR | [T10B9.1A-31] | | X | |

immunoincompetent. In addition to depletion and antigenic modulation, OKT-3 also causes activation or mitogenesis. While this may seem paradoxical to its immunosuppressive effect, the activated cells are receptorless, as a result of modulation, and do not respond to antigen. It has been suggested that this mechanism of activation may contribute to the induction of suppressor cells (108).

Immunopathologic examination of allograft biopsies following OKT-3 treatment for rejection reveals variable degrees of CD3+ T-cell depletion. A persistent infiltrate, however, has not been reliably correlated with recurrent rejection. Modulation of the CD3 complex, which is observed in circulating lymphocytes, is less pronounced on cells within the allograft. In fact, intragraft T cells appear to be activated as indicated by the expression of IL-2 receptors. The exact mechanism by which OKT-3 reverses rejection at the tissue level therefore remains unclear.

### OKT-3 Rejection Prophylaxis (Induction Therapy)

Because OKT-3 inhibits the ability of T cells to recognize antigen, it became a logical choice for prophylaxis in clinical trials. When used as the sole immunosuppressive agent in renal allograft recipients, a vigorous HAMA response was found to rapidly neutralize the effect of OKT-3 (109). Acute rejection occurred in most of these recipients within two weeks of transplantation. A subsequent randomized clinical trial comparing azathioprine and steroids with or without OKT-3 in renal allograft recipients demonstrated a delay in the HAMA response for approximately three weeks (110). Allograft survival of 89% at two years with fewer rejection episodes was observed in the OKT-3 group compared to a 70% graft survival in the control arm. More recently, multicenter trials of renal transplant recipients, comparing induction triple drug therapy including CsA, azathioprine, and steroids with or without OKT-3, demonstrated a significant delay to first rejection, a decreased incidence of rejection, and fewer patients with multiple rejection episodes in the OKT-3–treated group (111,112). As in the previous polyclonal trials, a significant improvement in patient or allograft survival has been difficult to demonstrate in these relatively small studies. Large databases, such as those provided by the Collaborative Transplant Study, however, have demonstrated a survival advantage following OKT-3 induction in conjunction with delayed CsA therapy (113). This approach, in addition to avoiding CsA nephrotoxicity, essentially eliminates the development of early rejection episodes. A disadvantage to the use of OKT-3 as an induction agent is the development of HAMA in some recipients that might preclude later treatment with OKT-3, which could be indicated if severe rejection is encountered. Another concern has been related to the agent's procoagulant activity, which has been implicated in cases of graft thrombosis (114).

OKT-3 induction therapy has been evaluated in liver, cardiac, lung, and pancreatic transplant recipients as well. In liver transplantation, the primary rationale for OKT-3 induction is to avoid renal dysfunction associated with CsA

or tacrolimus in the immediate post-transplant period, especially since other perioperative factors such as prolonged vena cava clamping, preexisting hepatorenal syndrome, and hemodynamic instability could also enhance the nephrotoxicity of these drugs. As in renal transplantation, liver recipients treated prophylactically with OKT-3 have had a lower incidence of rejection, a delay in onset of first rejection, and a decreased incidence of steroid-resistant rejection (115,116).

Attempts to limit the severity of early postoperative renal dysfunction have also been the impetus for OKT-3 induction in cardiac transplantation. Delay in onset of rejection along with fewer rejection episodes have been observed. In addition, some have reported a reduction in late deaths resulting from graft atherosclerosis in patients who had received OKT-3 induction (117). Recent evidence also suggests that these patients may be more easily weaned off of steroids without adverse consequences. Some groups, however, have warned of an increased incidence of clinically significant hemodynamic instability associated with early post-heart transplant administration of OKT-3 (118).

OKT-3 has also been used effectively for induction therapy in lung and heart–lung transplant recipients. A recent survey revealed that 52.4% of heart–lung transplant programs favored the use of OKT-3 or other MAb preparations for the prevention of rejection (29). Induction therapy is especially attractive in these patients as an approach that minimizes steroid requirements during the early postoperative period, thereby promoting healing of the bronchial anastomosis. The intensity of the suppression provided by OKT-3 must be recognized, and it is clear that concomitant application of carefully designed infection control measures are required in these MAb-treated patients (119).

In the same survey noted earlier (see Table 8.3), 72% of transplant directors suggested that OKT-3 plays an important role in induction therapy for pancreas allograft recipients. A retrospective review of United Network for Organ Sharing (UNOS) data, however, suggested that OKT-3 induction may be associated with a lower graft survival rate than that achieved with ALS induction in pancreas alone and pancreas-after-kidney transplants (120).

### OKT-3 Rejection Therapy

OKT-3 was first evaluated as treatment for established rejection at a time when azathioprine and steroids still constituted the foundation of immunosuppressive induction protocols (7). The initial pilot trial demonstrated that renal allograft rejection could be reversed with as little as 1–2 mg of OKT-3 administered daily. This led to the design of a multi-institutional randomized study in which OKT-3 was compared to conventional therapy for reversal of rejection. In that study, OKT-3 reversed 94% of initial rejection episodes, in contrast to a reversal rate of approximately 70% in conventionally treated patients (121). A number of reports later confirmed the efficacy of OKT-3 in reversing renal allograft rejection that developed in patients on azathioprine and steroids.

A significant limitation in these early trials was the occurrence of subsequent rejection episodes in over 50% of patients, usually within the first eight weeks after OKT-3 had been discontinued. The introduction of CsA partially addressed this limitation. In CsA-based immunosuppressive protocols, about 20% of renal allograft recipients have been found to require OKT-3 therapy if its use is reserved for treatment of acute rejection episodes initially unresponsive to high-dosage steroids (122,123). In 80% to 85% of these patients, a 10- to 14-day course of OKT-3 reverses the steroid-resistant rejection episode, and recurrent rejection has been observed in only 20% of patients receiving maintenance CsA (107,124).

The rather dramatic success of OKT-3 as "rescue" therapy that has been reported even in patients with severe "vascular" rejection (125) has been confirmed in many centers. In a group of nearly 300 patients treated by a number of different investigators, rejection that had failed to respond to CsA, high-dosage steroids, and in many instances ALS, was reversed in 65% of patients. Fifty-six percent of these allografts that were at the point of abandonment under conventional therapy remained functional with a minimum of six months follow-up (122,123).

A meta-analysis of the overall clinical experience published in the English and French literature indicates that OKT-3–treated patients have a threefold higher rate of resolution of the acute episode than do control patients (126). These observations suggest that excessive delay of OKT-3 therapy is probably ill advised. The hazards of prolonged steroid treatment, followed by a course of antilymphocyte antibody therapy, have been well documented. Thus, many clinicians currently recommend limiting the administration of high-dosage methylprednisolone to two or three doses. In those patients with persisting rejection, OKT-3 treatment is then added in preference to more prolonged courses of steroid administration. In fact, some centers advise even earlier institution of OKT-3 as a primary treatment approach for rejection (127), especially in patients with evidence of more severe immunologic injury on histopathologic examination (128).

OKT-3 has also been widely used for steroid-resistant rejection in liver transplantation. Successful allograft rescue can be expected in 75% to 85% of patients treated with OKT-3, with rapid improvement in liver function and resolution of the histologic findings of rejection (129). Failure of OKT-3 treatment in these patients may result from humorally mediated rejection similar to that encountered in ABO-incompatible grafts, which appears to be more resistant to OKT-3 suppression. In a prospective randomized trial, hepatic allograft recipients with first rejection episodes that had failed to respond to one or two boluses of steroids were randomized to receive 10 days of OKT-3 therapy or continued high-dose steroids. This study demonstrated that the results with OKT-3 are significantly better than can be achieved with steroids alone (130). OKT-3 has also been evaluated as first-line therapy for hepatic allograft rejection, where it again proved to be more effective than steroids. However, the incidence of infectious complications was noted to be higher in the patients receiving OKT-3. For this reason, OKT-3 is probably best reserved for patients with steroid-resistant rejection (131).

OKT-3 is typically used to treat steroid-resistant rejection in pancreas transplant recipients as well. In patients who have received simultaneous pancreas and kidney transplants, rejection therapy is usually instituted based on renal dysfunction or biopsy. In pancreas alone or pancreas-after-kidney transplantation, pancreatic biopsy may be necessary to differentiate suspected rejection from other causes of pancreatic dysfunction. OKT-3 has been demonstrated to be efficacious even in cases of pancreatic rejection with histopathologic features of chronic rejection (132).

OKT-3 has also proved effective in the treatment of rejection in cardiac and lung transplant recipients. As with other allografts, severe cases of rejection that do not respond to therapy with high-dose steroids or ATG have been effectively reversed with OKT-3 (133,134). The steroid-sparing effect of OKT-3 is of particular benefit in treating rejection in lung transplantation because of concerns of bronchial integrity.

### Immunogenicity and Monitoring of OKT-3 Therapy

Because OKT-3 is of murine origin, use of this agent is associated with xenosensitization. The HAMA response occurs in approximately 25% to 30% of patients following initial treatment (135) and in a further similar proportion of patients who were HAMA-negative after initial treatment but then required retreatment (136). The probability of a HAMA response, therefore, appears to be relatively constant per exposure and not strongly influenced by intrinsic differences in the patient's immune responsiveness. However, as suggested above, concomitant immunosuppression does influence the likelihood of HAMA formation that decreased from 36% in patients receiving double drug immunosuppression to 21% in those receiving triple drug suppression (137).

Two classes of anti-OKT-3 antibodies have been identified (138). Anti-isotypic antibodies cross-react with all murine IgG2a immunoglobulins (Fig. 8.6). These HAMA therefore could interfere with subsequent therapy using either OKT-3 or any other IgG2a murine MAb. In contrast, anti-idiotypic antibodies react specifically with the antigen-binding region of OKT-3 and, therefore, may preclude the subsequent administration of OKT-3 but not of other murine MAbs (139). As described above, administration of humanized MAbs has been found to greatly reduce the magnitude of the HAMA response. Clinical trials using a humanized OKT-3 preparation are just being initiated.

In most patients, anti-OKT-3 antibodies first become detectable 7 to 10 days after discontinuing therapy, and therefore do not interfere with the initial therapeutic effect.

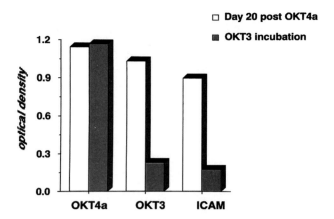

□ Day 20 post OKT4a

■ OKT3 incubation

M 4593

**FIGURE 8.6.** *Human antibody response to murine mono-clonal antibodies. Anti-OKT-4a reactivity [increased optical density in ELISA assay (139)] was detectable in the patient's serum 20 days following initial treatment with this IgG2a MAb. Incubation of the serum sample with OKT-3 resulted in removal of reactivity (anti-isotypic) to OKT-3 and anti-ICAM (both IgG2a), but retention of anti-OKT-4A reactivity (anti-idiotypic).*

Occasionally, the antibody response becomes detectable during the course of OKT-3 therapy, resulting in neutralization of the immunosuppressive effect and in resurgence of rejection. Since the development of HAMA is heralded by the reappearance of CD3+ T cells in peripheral blood, flow cytometric monitoring has been recommended every two to three days during OKT-3 administration (136,140). A rise in detectable CD3+ T cells may be overcome by increasing the OKT-3 dose, thereby re-establishing CD3 clearance or modulation and continued control of the rejection episode. It has been suggested that T-cell monitoring may also be useful in predicting the likelihood of rejection after discontinuing OKT-3, since a correlation between early rejection and the rapidity of recovery of CD3+ T-cell counts has been observed (141,142). On the other hand, because of the costs associated with sequential T-cell monitoring, some centers have adopted an escalating dose regimen to ensure adequate OKT-3 serum levels without the need for frequent in vitro monitoring (143).

### Retreatment with OKT-3

Since approximately 20% of CsA-treated patients in whom rejection is successfully reversed with OKT-3 subsequently develop further rejection episodes, multiple courses of high-dosage suppression are sometimes required. As with the initial episode, recurrent rejection may be treated with steroids, another antilymphocyte preparation such as ALS, or a second course of OKT-3. Unfortunately, the risks of opportunistic infections or PTLD are greatly increased by sequential courses

of antilymphocyte antibody therapy. This approach should therefore be used sparingly.

Before re-treating with OKT-3, the patient's HAMA level should be assayed to rule out the presence of high titers of anti-OKT-3 antibody (139). Interestingly, low levels of reactive endogenous antibodies to murine MAbs can be detected in a small proportion of individuals even before initial therapy. However, clinically evident reactions suggesting anaphylaxis have been distinctly unusual in these OKT-3–treated allograft recipients, and the presence of these preexisting antibodies does not seem to alter the efficacy of therapy or predict the likelihood of subsequent rejection episodes (144).

### Side Effects of OKT-3

The side effects of OKT-3 therapy can be categorized into direct toxic effects and the consequences of overimmunosuppression. The common side effects of OKT-3 therapy are summarized in Table 8.7. The "cytokine-release syndrome," manifested by fever and chills typically beginning within one to two hours after the initial injection, may also include nausea, vomiting, diarrhea, dyspnea, headaches, arthralgias, and myalgias. Aseptic meningitis and pulmonary edema may occur infrequently. Seizures have been reported, but these are rare. As noted earlier, TNF appears to be the primary cytokine responsible for these adverse events (145), although complement activation has also been implicated recently (146,147). High-dosage corticosteroid administration prior to initiation of OKT-3 therapy has been shown to inhibit the release of the cytokines responsible for this syndrome and decrease the severity of the reactions (67,84). Anti-TNF therapy with MAb or TNF-soluble receptors has also been shown to decrease the severity of this syndrome (68,69). TNF-soluble receptors may also inhibit the frequently observed temporary rise in serum creatinine that presumably results from cytokine-induced nephrotoxicity (148,149). Since respiratory symptoms may be more severe in patients with significant fluid retention, the patient's volume status should be assessed carefully and treated with diuretics or ultrafiltration if volume overload is present prior to initiation of OKT-3 therapy. The use of OKT-3 has also been reported to be associated with arterial thrombosis in renal allografts (114). It has been suggested that this complication could result from the procoagulant (endothelial activation) consequences of increased cytokine levels.

As with any agent, overimmunosuppression can result in opportunistic infections (particularly viral). An increased incidence of Herpes group virus infections including CMV and the EBV-associated PTLD has been reported in recipients of every type of organ allograft following treatment with OKT-3 (150,151). Clinical presentation may range from annoying, but easily controllable, herpes simplex stomatitis to life-threatening lymphoproliferative disease. CMV infections were frequent complications of the early ALS trials, until the need for reducing concomitant immunosuppression and the importance of the serologic status of donor

**Table 8.7.**     Clinical Toxicity of OKT-3 Administration

| Cytokine Release Syndrome | | Overimmunosuppression | | Immunogenicity | |
|---|---|---|---|---|---|
| **Reaction** | **Incidence** | **Reaction** | **Incidence** | **Reaction** | **Incidence** |
| Chills, fever | | CMV infection | 20–60% | Rash/Pruritus | 0–5% |
| d1 | 70–90% | Fungal infection | 15–35% | Anaphylaxis | <1% |
| d2 | 10–20% | Herpes simplex | 5–25% | | |
| Nephrotoxicity | 30–40% | PTLD | 0–8% | | |
| Vomiting, diarrhea | 15–30% | | | | |
| Dyspnea | 10–20% | | | | |
| Pulmonary edema | 0–4% | | | | |
| Aseptic meningitis | 0–3% | | | | |
| Arterial thrombosis | <1% | | | | |

and recipient were recognized (151). The risk for CMV infection has proved to be highest (58%) in seronegative recipients of allografts from a seropositive donor, intermediate in seropositive recipients (36%), and negligible when both donor and recipient are seronegative (3%). Preemptive therapy with ganciclovir, particularly for seronegative recipients (72), has greatly reduced these risks.

Latent EBV is reactivated by OKT-3, leading to the outgrowth of virally transformed B cells. These proliferating cells may then evolve from benign EBV-dependent polyclonal B-cell lines to a malignant EBV-independent monoclonal B-cell lymphoma (73), particularly in children previously unexposed to EBV (152). The progression to lymphoma is related to the intensity of the immunosuppression rather than specifically to any particular agent. For example, an increased PTLD incidence was noted retrospectively among 154 heart transplant patients after two weeks of OKT-3 prophylaxis was introduced without reduction of the concomitantly administered triple drug therapy (150). In contrast, one month of OKT-3 prophylaxis, in combination with azathioprine and steroids but without CsA, resulted in no lymphomas in 150 renal transplant patients (110). These observations emphasize the importance of decreasing the dosages of concomitant immunosuppressive therapy during the period that any antilymphocyte antibody is being administered. We recommend at least a 50% reduction in the daily CsA and azathioprine dosages during the period of OKT-3 or ALS administration. A further drastic reduction in immunosuppression or even complete elimination, if possible, should be instituted if the diagnosis of PTLD is made (153).

### Choice of Polyclonal ALS versus OKT-3 MAb

Both ALS and OKT-3 are directed against T cells, admittedly with a differing degree of selectivity. Nevertheless, the indications for their uses overlap, and the preferred clinical circumstances for one versus the other preparation remain controversial (154–158). A comparison of some of the

**Table 8.8.**     Comparison of Monoclonal Versus Polyclonal Antilymphocyte Antibodies

| Characteristic | Monoclonal vs. Polyclonal (Superiority) |
|---|---|
| Ease of production | Monoclonal |
| Cost | Monoclonal |
| Antibody variability | Monoclonal |
| Specificity | Monoclonal |
| Ease of administration | Monoclonal |
| Rejection reversal (early) | Monoclonal |
| Rejection reversal (overall) | Equal |
| Viral infection | Equal |
| PTLD | Equal |
| Recipient survival | Equal |
| Side effects | Polyclonal |
| Immunogenicity | Polyclonal |
| Retreatment possibility | Polyclonal |

important features that distinguish these two generations of antilymphocyte preparations is summarized in Table 8.8. OKT-3 administration is simpler but with more pronounced side effects following the initial infusions. This drawback is countered by the general impression that OKT-3 is somewhat more reliable for treatment of severe acute rejection, since it has been successfully used to rescue allografts in recipients who failed to respond to ALS.

When used as induction agents, ALS and OKT-3 have virtually indistinguishable low rates of rejection and delayed graft function. Conflicting observations regarding the incidence of infection have been reported with some studies indicating that ALS is associated with a significantly increased incidence of CMV infections (157) while others found OKT-3 resulted in symptomatic side effects and more infections (158).

How then does a clinician choose between ALS and OKT-3? One approach is to use pharmacologic therapy

(CsA or tacrolimus plus MMF and/or steroids) for initial baseline induction immunosuppression. In kidney recipients with delayed graft function or extrarenal allograft recipients with renal dysfunction, the introduction of CsA or tacrolimus is delayed in favor of ALS prophylaxis. This allows for subsequent rejection treatment with OKT-3 if it is required. For initial acute rejection episodes, two high-dosage steroid boluses are administered. If rejection is not reversed, OKT-3 therapy is usually begun. This approach attempts to take advantage of the relatively equivalent efficacy of either pharmacologic or antilymphocyte antibody induction therapy in patients with adequate renal function, the apparent heightened susceptibility to CsA or tacrolimus nephrotoxicity during periods of ATN, and the greater reliability of OKT-3 for treatment of acute rejection.

## Anti-CD4 Monoclonal Antibodies

While OKT-3 has proven to be effective for both induction therapy and treatment of rejection, its nonselective suppression of all T lymphocytes can result in increased risks of infection and malignancy. This has naturally stimulated evaluation of MAbs more specifically targeted to T-cell subsets or other molecules crucial for rejection. One such molecule is the CD4 antigen, which is important during the initial stages of alloactivation, when presentation of MHC class II alloantigen to CD4 results in increased avidity with the TCR and releases cytokines that amplify the rejection process (159). Because CD4+ T cells play an important role in this initial activation and amplification of the alloresponse, anti-CD4 MAbs were predicted to be most effective before effector mechanisms become self-sustaining (160). Multiple studies have confirmed this supposition. For example, rats treated with an anti-CD4 MAb for seven days prior to transplantation have been observed to have marked prolongation of allograft survival in contrast to animals treated with the same protocol beginning on the day of transplantation (161). With this type of early treatment, donor-specific unresponsiveness has been achieved in many experimental models using anti-CD4 MAbs, again suggesting that these MAbs may be more effective when used in induction immunosuppressive regimens than for rejection reversal (159).

### Mechanism of Action

Anti-CD4 MAbs may be classified as depleting or nondepleting based on their effect on peripheral blood CD4+ cells. Monoclonal antibodies that are depleting in nature trigger complement activation through the Fc portion of the molecule with resultant target cell lysis (159,162). The depletion of CD4+ cells in peripheral blood and graft infiltrates has correlated in most experimental models with the immunosuppressive activity of these antibodies. Rejection has been observed to occur promptly upon the return of CD4+ cells to the circulation. One disadvantage of depleting antibodies can be the longevity of their effects. CD4+ cells may remain depressed to levels as low as 60% of baseline for up to six months after treatment is discontinued in nonhuman primates (163). Similar results have been reported in patients with depletion persisting for up to two years in one case (164). Precursor lymphocyte depletion could theoretically explain this phenomenon, since immature T cells co-express CD4 and CD8 (165). The clinical consequences of this persistent depletion are unclear.

Nondepleting anti-CD4 MAbs may exert their effect through CD4 modulation or blockade. Modulation presumably removes any contribution of the CD4 molecule to T-cell activation, either as an adhesion molecule or as a signal-transducing molecule. This can lead to significant delay of rejection in rats (166). Similarly, modulation of the CD4 molecule in monkeys was associated with prolonged renal allograft survival. In these animals, intragraft cells were found to be unresponsive to IL-2, suggesting that CD4 modulation prevents T-cell sensitization even in the absence of depletion (167).

CD4 blockade may result from interference with interactions between CD4 and MHC, or between CD4 and the TCR–CD3 complex. Like modulation, this interference might prevent the CD4 molecule from contributing to T-cell activation. Interestingly, CD4 blockade appears even more immunosuppressive than modulation in some models (168). It is possible that CD4 bound by MAb, in contrast to modulation of the CD4 molecule, actually transduces a negative signal to the T cell, thereby suppressing its activation (169).

Since CD4+ T cells are pivotal in the initial activation of the alloresponse, anti-CD4 MAbs have been particularly targeted for their potential to direct the alloresponse toward donor-specific tolerance rather than sensitization. As noted above, striking results have been obtained in rodent models (170–172). Most of these tolerance models have relied on depleting MAbs. Although nondepleting anti-CD4 MAbs may also induce specific tolerance (168), the hyporesponsive state achieved with these agents has usually been to relatively weak antigens or has been confined to limited strain combinations (171). In these models, the CD4+ T cells are presumably rendered anergic when they bind donor antigen without a complete activation signal (173). Interestingly, thymectomy prevents tolerance induction in some anti-CD4 MAb models. It is possible that an intact thymus is necessary for the development of suppressor T cells or that CD4-depleted cells must migrate through the thymus in order to then be rendered anergic when engaging antigen in the periphery (174).

### Preclinical Studies

The first anti-CD4 MAb to be evaluated in a nonhuman primate model was OKT-4 in 1980. OKT-4, as the sole immunosuppressive agent, prolonged allograft survival for as long as 42 days, while control animals developed terminal rejection between 8 and 11 days. Multiple epitopes of the CD4 molecule were identified during these initial studies, and population surveys revealed the absence of the OKT-4 reactive site in some human subjects. Subsequently, OKT-4A, a murine IgG2a immunoglobulin, was produced. OKT-4A binds to a universally expressed epitope of the human CD4 antigen that is separate and noncompeting from the epitope recognized by OKT-4. Prolonged renal allograft survival was observed in nonhuman primate preclinical studies of OKT-4A as well (175). Since there was minimal CD4+ T-cell depletion, the mechanism involved appeared to be through antigenic modulation with interference of signal transduction, blocking of the MHC class II–CD4 interaction, or suppressor cell induction.

Despite the efficacy of these murine anti-CD4 MAbs in monkeys, two significant differences from the earlier rodent observations were apparent. First, allograft rejection, though delayed, eventually occurred in all anti-CD4 MAb treated nonhuman primates; and, second, all monkey recipients developed antimouse antibodies. To address these problems, humanized versions of OKT-4A and other murine MAbs were developed. In the modified OKT-4A, only the original murine CDRs were preserved (see Chapter 7). Since these regions bind the target antigen on CD4, the original specificity of OKT-4A was preserved while the remainder of the molecule was completely humanized. To accomplish this, the murine CDRs were grafted onto a human variable region framework, and the resultant structure was then combined with either a human IgG1 or IgG4 constant region (176). These isotypes were selected because of documented differences in their effector functions: human IgG1 antibodies activate complement, with resultant target cell lysis, whereas IgG4 antibodies do not (177). The CDR-grafted OKT-4A preparations retained only 8% of the murine sequence but had comparable binding affinity for the CD4 molecule.

As anticipated, in vivo monkey studies revealed only MAb coating of CD4+ T cells with the IgG4 preparation but consistent and prolonged CD4+ T-cell depletion following IgG1 administration (178). Both MAbs retained the immunosuppressive potency of the parent murine preparation; however, their immunogenicity was reduced and recipient serum levels were maintained for a longer period than following treatment with the murine preparation (179). Moreover, the antibody response was only anti-idiotypic, presumably restricted to the original CDR, and thus would

not preclude sequential therapy with MAbs targeting another epitope, such as OKT-3.

### Anti-CD4 Rejection Prophylaxis (Induction Therapy)

Based on the encouraging preclinical results, a number of clinical trials have been undertaken mostly in cadaveric renal allograft recipients (159) (Table 8.9). The murine preparation OKT-4A has been well tolerated without first-dose side effects, but the immunosuppressive efficacy has proved inconclusive. A HAMA response occurred in 82% of recipients of this MAb. A subsequent trial evaluating the CDR-grafted OKT-4A was encouraging, with no graft failures; however, the dose used was insufficient to consistently prevent rejection. Two other murine anti-CD4 MAb preparations of the IgG2a isotype, designated BL4 and MT151, have been evaluated in renal allograft recipients. These patients had a discouragingly high incidence of early rejection episodes (180). Recently, B-F5, a murine IgG1 anti-CD4 MAb, was reported to provide significant CD4+ cell depletion in renal allograft recipients and excellent transplant survival. However, one-half of the treated patients experienced an episode of acute rejection within the first three postoperative months (181). The chimeric anti-CD4 MAb, cMT-412, has been evaluated in conjunction with CsA-based triple drug induction therapy in heart and heart–lung recipients (182). This antibody is a combination of the CD4-reactive murine hypervariable regions with human IgG1 constant region. Comparable depletion of CD4+ cells in cMT-412–treated patients and ATG-treated controls was observed. All MAb-treated patients had a benign postoperative course with significantly fewer rejection episodes and fewer infectious complications despite long-lasting T-cell depletion. Despite the partial humanization of the MAb, however, a HAMA response was detected in 64% of patients treated with this agent. Nevertheless, the promising immunosuppressive observations have stimulated continued clinical investigation of this MAb.

### Anti-CD4 Rejection Therapy

Since reversal of established rejection would not be predicted to be likely using anti-CD4 MAbs (see above), there have been limited clinical trials for this indication. The anti-CD4 MAb, Max.16H5, which was also initially studied in

**Table 8.9.** Clinical Trials Using Anti-CD4 Monoclonal Antibodies

| Study | MAb | Report | Outcome | Isotype |
|---|---|---|---|---|
| Kidney Induction | OKT-4A | Delmonico (159) | Variable efficacy | Murine IgG2a |
| Kidney Induction | OKT-cdr4A | Delmonico (159) | Inconclusive | Humanized IgG4 |
| Kidney Induction | BL4 | Land (180) | Ineffective | Murine IgG2a |
| Kidney Induction | MT151 | Land (180) | Ineffective | Murine IgG2a |
| Kidney Induction | BF5 | Dantal (181) | Ineffective | Murine IgG1 |
| Kidney Rejection | Max.16H5 | Reinke (183) | Reversed rejection | Murine IgG1 |
| Heart Induction | cMT-412 | Meiser (182) | ↓Rejection | Humanized IgG1 |

patients with rheumatoid arthritis, has been administered to renal allograft recipients suffering late-onset rejection (183). This MAb was shown to dramatically deplete CD4+ T cells, improve allograft function, and eliminate the histopathologic features of rejection in the majority of treated patients. In addition, neither anti-isotypic nor anti-idiotypic antibodies to Max.16H5 were detected in any of the recipients. Despite these compelling results, further trials with this MAb have not yet been reported.

## Anti-CD7 Monoclonal Antibodies

The anti-CD7 MAb, SDZCHH380, which has been produced through recombinant DNA technology, is composed primarily of human IgG1 with murine hypervariable regions that determine its binding specificity (184). In vitro studies have revealed marked inhibition of T-cell proliferation by this agent. A prospective randomized trial comparing SDZCHH380 to OKT-3 induction in conjunction with CsA-based conventional therapy was performed in cadaveric renal allograft recipients. In this study, the time to first rejection was comparable in both groups of patients; the anti-CD7 MAb was well tolerated with induction of lower levels of TNF and IL-6 than detected in recipients of OKT-3; and no patients produced antibody to SDZCHH380 in contrast to the 70% of OKT-3 recipients with a HAMA response. The investigators concluded that SDZCHH380 could play an important role in induction protocols in renal transplantation. Further trials, however, have not been reported.

## Anti-CD25 Monoclonal Antibodies

The interaction between IL-2 and its receptor is required for the proliferation of T cells and the generation of cytotoxic effector T cells. Since IL-2 receptor expression is upregulated on the T-cell surface during lymphocyte activation, the use of anti-CD25 MAbs to block the interac-

tion between IL-2 and its receptor or to eliminate cells expressing CD25 could presumably limit clonal expansion at this critical stage of the immune response (185). The validity of this hypothesis has been established in some murine models where anti-CD25 MAb therapy provided indefinite survival of vascularized allografts (186).

### Anti-CD25 Rejection Prophylaxis (Induction Therapy)

A number of randomized trials evaluating the efficacy of anti-CD25 MAb induction therapy have been reported (Table 8.10). Use of the murine anti-Tac MAb in human renal allograft recipients in combination with CsA, azathioprine, and prednisone provided a modest decrease in frequency of rejection episodes and delay in onset of rejection compared to controls, but no improvement in graft or patient survival was achieved (187). Two rat anti-CD25 MAbs have been similarly evaluated. One of these antibodies, 33B3.1, was compared in a randomized trial to ATG as an induction agent in cadaveric renal allograft recipients (188). This trial demonstrated that 33B3.1 was well tolerated but somewhat less effective than ATG in preventing acute rejection. Similar results were observed in renal–pancreas recipients (189). The second rat anti-CD25 MAb, Lo-Tact-1, was compared in liver allograft recipients to two other induction protocols: an OKT-3–treated group and a triple drug (CsA-steroid-azathioprine) control group (190). After two years, patient survival in the Lo-Tact-1 group was significantly higher than in the control group, but not higher than in the OKT-3–treated group. The overall rejection rates in the two MAb-treated groups were similar and both were significantly lower than that observed in the control group.

The most extensively studied anti-CD25 MAb has been the murine agent, BT563, which has been evaluated in randomized trials in kidney (191), liver (192,193), and heart (194) allograft recipients. The incidence of rejection was reduced in the kidney and liver trials, although no significant improvement in allograft or patient survival was achieved. In the heart recipient trial, the frequency of rejection was similar in patients

**Table 8.10.**    Randomized Clinical Trials Evaluating Anti-CD25 Induction Therapy

| Allograft | MAb | Control | Report | Efficacy vs. Control |
|---|---|---|---|---|
| Kidney | Tac | (1) | Kirkman (187) | Equivalent |
| | 33B3.1 | ATG + (1) | Soulillou (188) | Equivalent |
| | BT563 | (2) | van Gelder (191) | ↓Rejection |
| | Simulect (basiliximab) | (2) | Nashan (197) | ↓Rejection |
| | Zenapax (HAT or daclizumab) | (1) | Vincenti (198) | ↓Rejection, ↑Survival |
| Liver | Lo-Tact-1 | OKT-3 + (1) | Reding (190) | Equivalent |
| | BT563 | ATG + (2) | Nashan (192) | Equivalent |
| | BT563 | ATG + (1) | Langrehr (193) | ↓Rejection |
| Heart | BT563 | OKT-3 + (3) | van Gelder (194) | Earlier rejection |

(1) CsA-steroids-azathioprine.
(2) CsA-steroids.
(3) CsA (delayed)-steroids-azathioprine.

treated with either BT563 or OKT-3, but rejection occurred earlier in the BT563-treated recipients.

In all of these trials, two major problems were identified that appeared to contribute to the relatively limited effectiveness of the anti-CD25 MAbs in preventing allograft rejection. First, their immunogenicity and short circulating half-life may not have induced adequate periods of immunosuppression. Second, because of their murine or rat structure, the MAbs are less effective than human antibodies in recruiting immune effector functions. To circumvent these limitations, genetic engineering has been used to prepare humanized agents. Initial studies of this approach in nonhuman primates were more promising (195), as was a phase I clinical trial in renal allograft recipients (80). In these patients, the half-life of the humanized agent was extended to over 270 hours in contrast to the 40 hours observed with the parent murine MAb. Similar observations have been made using another humanized anti-CD25 MAb that had a mean half-life in renal allograft recipients of 8.1 days (196). Initial reports of the efficacy and safety of these anti-CD25 MAbs are quite encouraging (197–200). Administration of these agents has been greatly simplified since in vitro monitoring revealed effective depletion of the targeted cell population even with doses given at bi-weekly intervals (201). Both of these agents have recently received FDA approval for clinical use in renal transplant recipients.

### Anti-CD25 Rejection Therapy

As with the anti-CD4 agents, there has been limited experience with the use of anti-CD25 MAbs for treatment of ongoing acute rejection. In a report of 33B3.1 MAb treatment for acute renal allograft rejection, only 2 of 10 patients responded immediately to the MAb and 4 others had a delayed response (202). Possible explanations for this limited efficacy might include insufficient MAb reaching the allograft to provide neutralization of the high levels of IL-2 that are undoubtedly present at the rejection site. It is also possible that the immune response that leads to graft destruction is no longer completely under IL-2 control by the time of MAb treatment and that alternative pathways produce continued cytotoxic effects despite IL-2R blockade. Interestingly, anti-CD25 therapy, using the MAbs BT563 or HAT, has been successful in the treatment of steroid-resistant GVHD (203,204).

## Anti-CD54 and Other Adhesion Molecule Monoclonal Antibodies

The rapid infiltration by inflammatory cell populations that is characteristic of acute rejection is also the histologic hallmark of ischemic reperfusion injury (205). As a barrier between blood and parenchyma, the endothelium is well positioned to regulate cellular migration from the circulation into tissues (206). The endothelial cell apparently recruits infiltrating cells by expressing adhesion molecules on its surface. These adhesion molecules also play an essen-

tial role in providing the accessory signals required for optimal activation of antigen-stimulated cells. Accordingly, disabling these adhesion molecules should limit the inflammatory phenomena associated with cell infiltration, thereby possibly interrupting both the alloresponse and the effects of ischemic injury.

Cell surface adhesion molecules have been grouped into three classes: selectins, integrins, and immunoglobulins. Selectins are small glycoproteins with a lectin domain and an epidermal growth factor (EGF)-like motif. This structure is well adapted for binding surface carbohydrate ligands (207). These molecules are primarily expressed on activated endothelium, platelets, or leukocytes, where they are designated E-, P-, or L-selectin, respectively. In general, selectins mediate the initial weak binding between endothelial cells and leukocytes, setting the stage for stronger binding by other adhesion molecules (208). To date, there has been minimal large animal or clinical evaluation of antiselectin MAbs as immunosuppressive agents.

Integrins are much larger molecules, composed of two noncovalently linked polypeptide chains, each of which has a CD designation. Because they span the cellular membrane, integrins are well adapted to coordinate extracellular contacts with intracellular events (208). As a result, integrins play an important role in regulating the sequential adhesion and deadhesion required for cellular migration into tissues. The integrin LFA-1 (CD11a/CD18), expressed on lymphocytes, granulocytes, and monocytes, is the ligand for CD54. Both of these molecules have been of particular interest as possible targets for MAb therapy.

The immunoglobulin supergene family includes the TCR, MHC classes I and II, CD3, CD4, CD8, and the intercellular adhesion molecules (ICAM-1 or CD54, ICAM-2, and ICAM-3). Resting cells express only limited amounts of these ligands on their surface, but inflammation or early antigen recognition leads to a dramatic upregulation. In general, adhesion molecules in this family bind either integrins or other members of the immunoglobulin supergene family.

### Preclinical Studies

Anti-adhesion molecule MAbs have been remarkably effective in some rodent models. For example, MAb combinations targeting T-cell and APC receptor–ligand pairs, such as LFA-1 (CD11a/CD18) and its ligand CD54 (209) or LFA2 (CD2) and its ligand CD48 (210), have induced permanent allograft survival. With such therapy, the TCR presumably interacts with processed antigen within the context of the MHC on the APC, but without concomitant adhesion molecule costimulation. This results in an incomplete activation signal and T-cell hyporesponsiveness rather than activation (211).

The immunosuppressive efficacy of anti-adhesion molecule immunotherapy in the rodent allograft models has prompted further preclinical evaluation of both anti-CD54 and anti-LFA-1 MAbs in monkey allograft recipients. Renal allograft survival in monkeys that were treated with the anti-CD54 MAb, BIRR1, as the sole immunosuppressive agent was prolonged from 9.2 ± 0.6 days in controls to 24 ± 2.4 days (105). Similar prolongation of skin allograft survival was observed in monkeys treated with anti-LFA-1 MAb (212). Recently, an alternative approach to the interruption of adhesion molecule interactions has been reported in which an entirely human fusion protein rather than the MAb was administered to monkey allograft recipients with encouraging prolongation of allograft survival (213). The mechanism of action involved in the anti-CD54–mediated immunosuppression appears to be through inhibition of ICAM-1–mediated functions, including antigen-independent interactions necessary for leukocyte adhesion and recruitment and antigen-dependent functions such as MHC peptide presentation and effector cytotoxicity (214). Of potential relevance for recipients, particularly of cadaver donor organs, has been the observation that reperfusion injury is also attenuated by the MAbs targeting these adhesion molecules (215–217). As noted above, ischemia activates the endothelium, resulting in adhesion molecule upregulation. This causes circulating neutrophils to adhere to vascular endothelium and infiltrate the reperfused ischemic tissues. There, they release toxic proteases and reactive oxygen metabolites resulting in damage to the ischemic organ. Apparently, this process can be inhibited by anti-adhesion molecule therapy.

### Anti-CD54 Rejection Prophylaxis (Induction Therapy)

The encouraging observations in nonhuman primates led to a phase I clinical study to evaluate the toxicity, dosage requirements, and potential efficacy of BIRR1 in cadaver donor renal allograft recipients (87). Patients with a high risk of acute graft rejection (because of prolonged allograft preservation time or highly sensitized recipient) were included. At 36 months, 78% of the allografts were functional versus 56% of the contralateral kidneys transplanted in a noncontrolled group that received conventional immunosuppression. Subsequently, over 600 cadaver donor renal allograft recipients were enrolled into three randomized, double-blinded, multi-institution trials conducted in European and North American transplant centers. In one of the studies, there was significantly reduced ($P < 0.05$) severity of rejection and a trend ($P = 0.07$) toward decreased rejection in the MAb-treated group, but neither of the other trials confirmed these observations. As a result, further clinical evaluation of this MAb in renal allograft recipients has been discontinued. A similar protocol using BIRR1 has been conducted in a phase I study in liver transplant recipients (218). Patients who maintained therapeutic levels of BIRR1 had a 40% incidence of rejection compared to a 70% incidence of rejection in conventionally treated liver recipients. All of these trials indicated that relatively large doses of this MAb were necessary to achieve therapeutic levels.

Clinical trials of MAbs targeting LFA-1, the ligand for the CD54 molecule, have also been undertaken. Bone marrow transplant patients were the first recipients of MAb 25.3, which is directed against the CD11a epitope of LFA-1. This agent appeared to improve engraftment in a group of pediatric recipients that was compared to historical controls. However, the same MAb administered to adult leukemic bone marrow recipients was unable to prevent rejection of T-cell–depleted HLA-matched transplants (219). A MAb directed against the CD18 epitope on LFA-1 provided results comparable to those observed in a historical group of renal allograft recipients receiving ATG. A subsequent randomized trial has confirmed this observation (220).

A single report using anti-LFA-1 MAb to treat established rejection in renal allograft recipients noted unsatisfactory reversal of the rejection episode (221).

### Anti–TCR Monoclonal Antibodies

The TCR is essential for antigen recognition that, in conjunction with costimulatory signals, leads to T-cell activation. T10B9.1A-31 (T10B9), an antihuman T-cell MAb of murine IgM isotype, is reactive with the α/β chain of the TCR and, thus, is a pan-T-cell antibody with the exception of γ/δ T-cell sparing. Approximately 99% of mature CD3+ cells are lysed by T10B9. This MAb is not mitogenic and therefore does not induce the first-dose reactions associated with cytokine release (222). T10B9 has been evaluated in a prospective randomized trial of renal allograft recipients comparing it to OKT-3 for treatment of acute rejection (148). The trial included 76 evaluable renal allograft recipients treated with conventional immunosuppression until rejection occurred. At this point, therapy with one of the MAbs was initiated. Graft survival was excellent in both groups with a trend toward improved survival at three and four years in the T10B9 group. Recurrent rejection and the requirement for crossover to the other agent were essentially the same in both groups. The incidence and severity of "first-dose" symptoms were decreased in the T10B9-treated patients. The explanation for this difference is the observation that plasma levels of TNF and IFN were much lower following treatment with T10B9 than with OKT-3. In addition, there was no cytokine-induced nephropathy in the T10B9 patients, who therefore had a more rapid reversal of renal dysfunction. There was no statistically significant difference in the incidence of infectious complications between the two groups. The development of a HAMA response was similar in the two groups, but most importantly, there was no cross-reactivity of the HAMA of one MAb with those produced in response to treatment by the other agent. Thus, an alternative therapy would be available should the first MAb fail or if re-rejection occurs.

## CONCLUSIONS

Over the last two decades, new and more specific immunosuppressive agents have increased the one-year survival of transplanted organs to the 70% to 90% range. With the current availability of CsA, tacrolimus, mycophenolate mofetil, ALS, and OKT-3, clinicians can devise individualized, multifaceted strategies that provide effective induction therapy and treatment of acute rejection, while limiting the nephrotoxicity of CsA and tacrolimus. A newer pan-T-cell MAb, T10B9.1A-31, could provide even more flexible immunosuppressive strategies, because it could be used in patients who fail to respond to, or have been previously sensitized to, OKT-3. It has not yet been approved for clinical use, however.

Despite these many advances, it remains evident that none of these therapeutic combinations lead reliably to donor-specific tolerance. Thus, the longer-term surviving transplant recipient is continuously threatened by a relentless attrition in allograft survival and continuing morbidity from the chronically administered immunosuppressive agents. The successful clinical application of OKT-3 has emphasized that MAbs could be a potential solution to many of the limitations of conventional immunosuppression. It is now possible to reliably design MAbs to essentially any molecular component essential to the immune response, rather than relying on serendipity for the discovery of new immunosuppressive agents.

There is much current interest in immunotoxin conjugates of MAbs (81,223,224) and in MAbs targeting costimulatory molecules such as CD4, CD25, CD28, and CD40L, since the accessory signals provided by these molecules are essential for immune activation (225,226). Based on the encouraging observations of tolerance induction by such agents in preclinical models, it is hoped that these agents may play an important role in future clinical protocols.

One of the most promising additions to MAb technology is the recombinant DNA technology that is used to "humanize" murine or rat preparations. With these methods, novel antibody molecules that retain only short sequences from the rodent variable region can be consistently constructed. The initial clinical trials using these designer molecules are highly encouraging and have already provided sufficient evidence of immunosuppressive efficacy to justify regulatory approval for several of these agents (197–200). The development of these new molecular agents, more effectively directed to specific cellular targets, should play an increasingly important role in future clinical protocols and perhaps finally provide a means to achieve long-term tolerance in human transplant recipients.

## COMMENTARY

*Jean-Paul Soulillou*

James D. Eason and A. Benedict Cosimi have thoroughly reviewed many of the bioreagents, defined as "biologic immunosuppressive agents," that have entered clinical trials or are expected to be soon available to patients. Although the gap between experiments in test tubes,

first clinical trials, and the actual drug registration is extremely long (for instance, 10 years between the first clinical report on the effect of anti-IL-2 receptor in humans and the first double-blind phase II/III trial of modified MAb) (1,2), the high specificity of action and low level of side effects associated with biologic agents (with the exception of the commercial OKT-3) may open new avenues in the treatment of graft recipients and maybe of autoimmune diseases. Moreover, humanized/chimeric forms of these agents may make longer or repeated usage possible and suggest that they could be used for induction therapy during the first months after transplantation, instead of only the first weeks. These agents might thus become popular drugs and the repeated assessment that has restricted them to marginal usage might be a lack of vision for the future!

In this short commentary I would like to elaborate on several issues that could further increase the usefulness of these reagents. However, the number of potentially interesting molecules itself acts as a self limitation, owing to the cost of clinical studies and their rather restricted application as compared to conventional drugs, at least as used currently.

Early phases after grafting are crucial for long-term graft function, principally because of the occurrence of two major events: delayed graft function and acute rejection, both of which are associated with inferior long-term graft function. Therefore, owing to the usual restricted period of time of administration, antilymphocyte antibodies have been mostly devoted to overcoming ongoing rejection and preventing very early rejection and, more recently, reperfusion injuries. The strategy of restricting powerful immunosuppressive treatments to short intervals of time after grafting has recently received some support by the demonstration that—at least for kidney recipients—even "normal" long-term immunosuppression might have overall detrimental effects and, that the current paradigm attributing most overimmunosuppression hazards to induction treatment may be wrong (3). Instead, the intensity of early treatment might be crucial, after which long-term treatment might be reduced. Therefore, the use of bioreagents at the time of transplantation could be the method of choice for treating graft recipients.

### TARGETING SECOND SIGNAL MOLECULES

Experimental data, including preliminary results in monkeys (4,5), suggest that inhibiting second signal molecules could be extremely effective. So far, besides recently recognized new targets (CD40L, CD28/B7 interaction, see below), several encouraging reports are already available on the effect of anti-CD2 or anti-LFA-1 (6,7). Interestingly, anti-LFA-1, which is considered to primarily inhibit the interaction between recipient immunocompetent cells and donor endothelial cells, could also act by inhibition of secondary signals (8). This is also suggested—although not well documented yet—by a recent randomized study where anti-LFA-1 administration was associated with the same rate of early rejection as observed in controls, despite no CsA being given during the first 10 days in the anti-LFA-1 arm of the trial (7). This is more suggestive of an action on early rejection than a major effect of ischemia reperfusion (the rate of delayed graft function was not significantly affected). Whether anti-ICAM-1 could be placed on the same level in terms of both efficacy and mechanism of action is still undetermined. The causal events that have been responsible for the interruption of the clinical trials have not yet been released. One can, however, mention the predictable activation on endothelial cells that express high levels of this inducible target molecule after various stimuli such as ischemia and surgical stress.

The use of agents blocking another major second signal, anti-CD40 ligand (CD40L), alone or in association with anti-B7, have produced extremely interesting preliminary results in animals. Long-term allograft acceptance was first observed in rodents, when associated with inhibition of the CD28 pathway (9) [although combined anti-LFA-1 and anti-ICAM-1 were reported to have similar effects (10)]. Similar results were more recently achieved in primates (4). A very promising possibility, which has also been claimed but not confirmed for anti-CD4 and anti-LFA-1, is that agents inhibiting CD40L/CD40 or B7/CD28 pathways might also inhibit help to B cells and the resulting antibody formation, including against their own determinants (4,5). In primates, inhibition of CD40L/CD40 pathway could be even more efficient than that of CD28/B7. The manipulation of CD28/B7 interaction is so far mostly related to the use of CTLA4 Ig fusion molecules or anti-B7 antibody usage. However, this approach might not be optimal and could even be harmful in patients with underlying autoimmune disorders. Indeed, both agents inhibit, without discrimination, the CD28/B7 costimulatory signal *and* the regulatory signal CTLA4/B7. The importance of this negative signal has been—as for CD40L signal in a mirror representation—exemplified by the lethal phenotype due to severe inflammatory processes of the CTLA4 Knock Out (KO) mice (11). The nondiscriminative blocking of these two B7 ligands could also—as for CsA (9)—inhibit the induction of tolerance that appears to require CTLA4 (12). A more adequate option would therefore be to selectively inhibit B7/CD28 interaction that provides a powerful and CsA-insensitive signal for $T_H1$ cytokine production, without interfering with CTLA4/B7 interaction that is likely to provide regulatory signals after the CTLA4 upregulation that follows TCR ligation. As all described MAbs against CD28 are agonists, such aims would require a more sophisticated design avoiding CD28 cross-linking. Nev-

ertheless, these preliminary results, particularly with combinations of reagents, make imaginable a control of early rejection (without mention of the possibility of tolerance induction). Owing to their well-identified targets, the combination of such reagents is likely to be as efficient as presently available therapies, but with fewer side effects and the opportunity for more precise monitoring.

Interestingly, recent data have also raised the possibility that the inhibition of the CD28/B7 pathway could have some utility in preventing the damage of reperfusion syndrome (13). Indirectly, these data reinforce the hypothesis that anti-LFA-1 (see above) could also act on reperfusion syndrome by an inhibitory effect on T-cell activation rather than through the blockade of leukocyte/endothelial cell interaction only.

## TARGETING THE IL-2 RECEPTOR

Although KO mice for various cytokines can develop almost normal rejection, inhibition of a single signal, such as that controlled by the inducibe IL-2R required for T-cell growth, has proven to be highly effective in animals and humans. The possibility of increasing effectiveness by reducing redundancy (such as IL-15, IL-4, IL-7, IL-2 for T-cell growth) is nevertheless suggested by the behavior of KO mice. This could be achieved on the IL-2R target of activated T cells by using a combination of antibodies blocking different epitopes [e.g., IL-2R α-chain for IL-2, IL-2R β chain for IL-15 (14,15)]. Even more efficient would be the possibility of interaction on the γ-chain of the IL-2R involved in multiple cytokine-mediated signals (IL-2, IL-4, IL-7), the mutation of which has been associated with severe immunodeficiencies in humans. This possibility of having both a rather specific effect and a decreased redundancy, drawn from the IL-2/IL-2R pathway, is not the only example. Molecular interactions governing the binding of leukocytes and endothelial cells of various integrins, selectins, and chemokine receptors are also characterized by an extremely high level of redundancy evidenced by both the effect of the corresponding KO gene and the high efficiency of the association of blocking antibodies, suggesting again that multiple interactions also could be strongly beneficial to a "biologic" activity (16). Newly designed antibodies reacting at two epitopes could be useful in the future (17).

## BEYOND MONOCLONAL ANTIBODIES

Antibodies or fusion molecules that use parts of immunoglobulins, such as CTLA4 Ig, do not summarize all biologic immunosuppressive agents. There is a diversity of molecules that could be used, including competing soluble receptors (such as soluble TNFR, soluble CR1 complement receptor, or inhibitory cytokines). These agents could be used to inhibit nonspecific inflammation, immune response, or endothelial cell activation in hyperimmunized patients or to prevent reperfusion injury. This field, currently being actively explored in the test tube and in the rodent model, has not yet reached clinical application. Moreover, there is also the possibility to introduce some immunoregulatory cytokines [through recombinant viruses, such as adenoviruses or adenovirus-associated viruses (AAV) for the corresponding molecule] in organs before transplantation. This gene-therapy–derived device for "treating" the organ's microenvironment, rather than the recipient's, may be applicable in the future.

Bioreagents, owing to their property to specifically target functional molecules, used alone or in combination, are also likely to be the tools for inducing tolerance. In this regard, donor MHC expressed by non-APC recipient cells (18) or soluble MHC molecules (19) are interesting. These "biologic agents" might mimic the signals that induce peripheral tolerance following donor blood infusion, a model that has been one of the most efficient in animals.

In conclusion, although long considered to be marginal, bioreagents have gained solid reliability with ATG and OKT-3 and now appear as unique tools as we imagine the future of immunointervention. Interestingly, for instance, two injections (day 0 and day 4 following transplantation) of an antibody directed at the α–chain of IL-2 receptor have been shown to provide about the same level of effect on prevention of early graft rejection, without side effects, as six months of treatment with MMF (20). This example could foreshadow a new paradigm in immunointervention.

## CHAPTER REFERENCES

1. Starzl TE, Porter KA, Iwasaki Y, et al. The use of heterologous antilymphocyte globulins in human homotransplantation. In: Wolstenholme GEW, O'Connor M, eds. Antilymphocyte Serum. Boston: Little, Brown, 1967:1.
2. Gantenbein H, Bachmann P, Huynh U, et al. Comparison of two antilymphocyte globulins replacing cyclosporine A after first kidney allotransplantation and prolonged graft ischemia. Clin Transplant 1996;10:384–385.
3. Malinow L, Walker J, Klassen DK, et al. Antilymphocyte induction immunosuppression in the post-Minnesota antilymphocyte globulin era: incidence of renal dysfunction and delayed graft function. A single center experience. Clin Transplant 1996;10:237–242.
4. Guttmann RD, Fleming C. Sequential biological immunosuppression. Induction therapy with rabbit antithymocyte globulin. Clin Transplant 1997;11:185–192.
5. Gaber AO, First MR, Tesi RJ, et al. Results of the double blind randomized multicenter phase III clinical trial of thymoglobulin versus ATGAM in the treatment of acute graft rejection episodes after renal transplantation. Transplantation 1998;66:29–37.
6. Kohler G, Milstein C. Continuous cultures of fused cells secreting antibody of predefined specificity. Nature 1975;256:495.
7. Cosimi AB, Burton RC, Colvin RB, et al. Treatment of acute renal allograft rejection with OKT3 monoclonal antibody. Transplantation 1981;32:535.
8. Cosimi AB, Delmonico FL. Antilymphocyte antibody therapy. In: Burdick JF, Racusen LC, Solez K, eds. Kidney transplant rejection. 2nd ed. New York: Marcel Dekker, 1992:541–565.
9. Simpson MA, Monaco AP. Clinical uses of polyclonal and monoclonal antilymphoid sera. In: Chatenoud L, ed. Monoclonal antibodies in transplantation. Austin, TX: RG Landes, 1995:1–19.
10. Lum CT, Umen AJ, Kasiske B, et al. Clinical impact of replacing Minnesota antilymphocyte globulin with ATGAM. Transplantation 1995;59:371–376.
11. Bonnefoy-Berard N, Vincent C, Revillard JP. Antibodies against functional leukocyte surface molecules in polyclonal antilymphocyte and antithymocyte globulins. Transplantation 1991;51:669–673.
12. Rebellato LM, Gross U, Verbanac KM, et al. A comprehensive definition of the major antibody specificities in polyclonal rabbit antithymocyte globulin. Transplantation 1994;57:685–694.
13. Bourdage JS, Hamlin DM. Comparative polyclonal antithymocyte globulin and antilymphocyte/antilymphoblast globulin anti-CD antigen analysis by flow cytometry. Transplantation 1995;59:1194–1200.
14. Thomas JM, Carver FM, Halsch CE, et al. Suppressor cells in Rhesus monkeys treated with antithymocyte globulin. Transplantation 1982;34:83–89.
15. Brooks CD, Karl KJ, Francom SF. ATGAM Skin Test Standardization: comparison of skin testing techniques in horse-sensitive and unselected human volunteers. Transplantation 1994;58:1135–1137.
16. Wechter WJ, Broodie JA, Morrell RM, et al. Antithymocyte globulin (ATGAM) in renal allograft recipients. Transplantation 1979;28(4):294–307.
17. Cosimi AB. The clinical value of antilymphocyte antibodies. Transplant Proc 1981;13(1):462–468.
18. Novick AC, Ho-Hsieh H, Steinmuller D, et al. Detrimental effect of cyclosporine on initial function of cadaver renal allografts following extended preservation. Transplantation 1986;42:154.
19. Sommer BG, Henry M, Ferguson RM. Sequential antilymphoblast globulin and cyclosporine for renal transplantation. Transplantation 1987;43(1):85–90.
20. Grundmann R, Hesse U, Wienand P, et al. Graft survival and long-term renal function after sequential conventional cyclosporin A therapy in cadaver kidney transplantation—a prospective randomized trial. Klin Wochenschr 1987;65:879–884.
21. Ferguson RM. A multicenter experience with sequential ALG/cyclosporine therapy in renal transplantation. Clin Transplant 1988;2:285–290.
22. Stratta RJ, D'Alessandro AM, Armbrust MJ, et al. Sequential antilymphocyte globulin/cyclosporine immunosuppression in cadaveric renal transplantation. Transplantation 1989;47:96–102.
23. Stratta RJ, Mason B, Lorentzen DF, et al. Cadaveric renal transplantation with quadruple immunosuppression in patients with a positive antiglobulin crossmatch. Transplantation 1989;47(2):282–286.
24. Hariharan S, Alexander JW, Schroeder TJ, First MR. Outcome of cadaveric renal transplantation by induction treatment in the cyclosporine era. Clin Transplant 1996;10:186–190.
25. Cecka JM, Terasaki PI. The UNOS Scientific Renal Transplant Registry. In: Terasaki PI, Cecka JM, eds. Clinical transplants 1991. Los Angeles: UCLA Tissue Typing Laboratory, 1992:6.
26. Shield CF, Edwards EB, Davies DB, Daily OP. Antilymphocyte induction therapy in cadaver renal transplantation. Transplantation 1997;63:1257–1263.
27. Slakey DP, Johnson CP, Callaluce RD, et al. A prospective randomized comparison of quadruple versus triple therapy for first cadaver transplants with immediate function. Transplantation 1993;56:827–831.
28. Abouna GM, Al-Abdullah IH, Kelly-Sullivan D, et al. Randomized clinical trial of antithymocyte globulin induction in renal transplantation comparing a fixed daily dose with dose adjustment according to T cell monitoring. Transplantation 1995;59:1564–1568.
29. Evans RW, Manninen DL, Dong FB, et al. Immunosuppressive therapy as a determinant of transplantation outcomes. Transplantation 1993;55:1297–1305.
30. McVicar JP, Kowdley KV, Emond MJ, et al. Induction immunosuppressive therapy is associated with a low rejection rate after liver transplantation. Clin Transplant 1997;11:328–333.
31. Langrehr JM, Nussler NC, Neumann U, et al. A prospective randomized trial comparing interleukin-2 receptor antibody versus antithymocyte globulin as part of a quadruple immunosuppressive induction therapy following orthotopic liver transplantation. Transplantation 1997;63:1772–1781.
32. Jonas S, Kling N, Bechstein WO, et al. Rejection episodes after liver transplantation during primary immunosuppression with FK506 or a cyclosporin-based regimen: a controlled, prospective randomized trial. Clin Transplant 1995;9:406–414.
33. Renard TH, Andrews WS. An approach to ABO-incompatible liver transplantation in children. Transplantation 1992;53(1):116–121.
34. Stratta RJ, Shaeffer MS, Pharm D, et al. Cytomegalovirus infection and disease after liver transplantation: an overview. Digest Dis Sci 1992;37(5):673–688.

35. Sollinger HW, Stratta RJ, Kalayoglu M, et al. Pancreas transplantation with pancreaticocystostomy and quadruple immunosuppression. Transplantation 1987;102(4):674–679.

36. Griepp RB, Stinson EB, Dong EJ, et al. Use of antithymocyte globulins in human heart transplantation. Circulation Suppl 1972;15:147.

37. English TAH, McGregor C, Wallwork J, et al. Aspects of immunosuppression for cardiac transplantation. Heart Transplant 1981;4:281.

38. Devi333i R, McKenzie N, Keown P. Cyclosporine in cardiac transplantation. Transplantation 1984;27:252–254.

39. Deeb MG, Kolff J, McClurken JB, et al. Antithymocyte gamma globulin, low-dose cyclosporine, and tapering steroids as an immunosuppressive regimen to avoid early kidney failure in heart transplantation. J Heart Transplant 1987;6:406–414.

40. Kormos RL, Armitage JM, Stephen AJ, et al. Optimal perioperative immunosuppression in cardiac transplantation using rabbit antithymocyte globulin. Transplantation 1990;49(2):306–311.

41. Menkis AH, Powell AM, Novick RJ, et al. A prospective randomized controlled trial of initial immunosuppression with ALG versus OKT3 in recipients of cardiac allografts. J Heart Lung Transplant 1992;11:569–576.

42. Carrier M, Pelletier G, Cartier R, et al. Induction of immunosuppression with rabbit antithymocyte globulin: five-year experience in cardiac transplantation. Can J Cardiol 1993;9(2):171–176.

43. Cooper JD. Lung Transplantation. Ann Thorac Surg 1989;47:28–44.

44. Stuart S, Griffith B. Single and double lung transplantation. In: Starzl TE, Shapiro R, Simmons RI, eds. Atlas of organ transplantation. New York: Gower Medical, 1992:1–29.

45. Shield III CF, Cosimi AB, Tolkoff-Rubin N, et al. Use of antithymocyte globulin for reversal of acute allograft rejection. Transplantation 1979;28(6):461–464.

46. Nelson PW, Cosimi AB, Delmonico FL, et al. Antithymocyte globulin as the primary treatment for renal allograft rejection. Transplantation 1983;36:587–589.

47. Richardson AJ, Higgins RM, Liddington M, et al. Antithymocyte globulin for steroid resistant rejection in renal transplant recipients immunosuppressed with triple therapy. Transplant Int 1989;2:27–32.

48. Gaber AO, First MR, Tesi RJ, et al. Results of the double-blind randomized multicenter phase III clinical trial of Thymoglobulin versus ATGAM in the treatment of acute graft rejection after renal transplantation. Transplantation 1998;66:29–37.

49. Bock HA, Gallati H, Zurcher RM, et al. A randomized prospective trial of prophylactic immunosuppression with ATG-Fresenius versus OKT3 after renal transplantation. Transplantation 1995;59(6):830–840.

50. Starzl TE, Iwatsuki S, Van Thiel DH, et al. Evolution of liver transplantation. Hepatology 1982;2(5):614–636.

51. Ascher NL, Freese DK, Paradis K, et al. Rejection of the transplanted liver. In: Maddrey WC, ed. Transplantation of the liver. New York: Elsevier, 1988:167–169.

52. Monaco AP, Wood ML. The potential for induction of specific unresponsiveness to organ allografts in clinical transplantation. Heart Transplant 1982;1:257–260.

53. Cosimi AB. Antilymphocyte globulin—a final (?) look. In: Morris PJ, Tilney NL, eds. Progress in transplantation. Vol. 2. Edinburgh: Churchill Livingston, 1986:167–188.

54. Thomas JM, Carver FM, Foil MB, et al. Renal allograft tolerance induced with ATG and donor bone marrow in outbred rhesus monkeys. Transplantation 1983;36:104–106.

55. Thomas JM, Carver FM, Kasten-Jolly J, et al. Further studies of veto activity in rhesus monkey bone marrow in relation to allograft tolerance and chimerism. Transplantation 1994;57:101–115.

56. Barber WH, Mankin IA, Laskow DA, et al. Long-term results of a controlled prospective study with transfusion of donor-specific bone marrow in 57 cadaveric renal allograft recipients. Transplantation 1991;51:70.

57. Kawai T, Cosimi AB, Colvin RB, et al. Mixed allogeneic chimerism and renal allograft tolerance in cynomolgus monkeys. Transplantation 1995;59(2):256–262.

58. Kimikawa M, Sachs DH, Colvin RB, et al. Modifications of the conditioning regimen for achieving mixed chimerism and donor-specific tolerance in cynomolgus monkeys. Transplantation 1997;64:709–716.

59. Terasaki P. Microdroplet assay of human serum cytotoxins. Nature 1964;204:998–1000.

60. Delmonico FL, Auchincloss H, Rubin RH, et al. The selective use of antilymphocyte serum for cyclosporine treated patients with renal allograft dysfunction. Ann Surg 1987;206:649–654.

61. Muller TF, Grebe SO, Neumann MC, et al. Persistent long-term changes in lymphocyte subsets induced by polyclonal antibodies. Transplantation 1997;64:1432–1437.

62. Kreis H, Mansouri R, Descamps J-M, et al. Antithymocyte globulin in cadaver kidney transplantation: a randomized trial based on T-cell monitoring. Kidney Int 1981;19:438–444.

63. Clark K. Monitoring antithymocyte globulin in renal transplantation. Ann Royal College Surgeons Eng 1996;78(6):536–540.

64. Tatum AH, Bollinger RR, Sanfilippo F. Rapid serologic diagnosis of serum sickness from antilymphocyte globulin therapy using enzyme immunoassay. Transplantation 1984;38:582–586.

65. Lawley TJ, Bielovy L, Gascon P, et al. A prospective clinical and immunologic analysis of patients with serum sickness. N Engl J Med 1984;311:1407.

66. Debets JMH, Leunissen KML, van Hooff HJ, et al. Evidence of involvement of tumor necrosis factor in adverse reactions during treatment of kidney allograft rejection with antithymocyte globulin. Transplantation 1989;47:487.

67. Chatenoud L, Ferran C, Legendre C, et al. In vivo cell activation following OKT3 administration. Systemic cytokine release and modulation by corticosteroids. Transplantation 1990;49:697.

68. Charpentier B, Hiesse C, Lantz O, et al. Evidence that antihuman tumor necrosis factor monoclonal antibody prevents OKT3-induced acute syndrome. Transplantation 1993;54:997.

69. Eason JD, Wee SL, Kawai T, et al. Inhibition of the effects of TNF in renal allograft recipients using recombinant human dimeric tumor necrosis factor receptors. Transplantation 1995;59(2):300–305.

70. Henricsson A, Husberg B, Bergentz SE. The mechanism behind the effect of ALG on platelets in vivo. Clin Exp Immunol 1977;29:515–522.

71. Rubin RH, Cosimi AB, Hirsch MS, et al. Effects of antithymocyte globulin on cytomegalovirus infection in renal transplant recipients. Transplantation 1981;31:143.

72. Rubin RH. Preemptive therapy in immunocompromised hosts. N Engl J Med 1991;324:1057.

73. Malatack JF, Gastner JC, Urbach AH, Zitelli BJ. Orthotopic liver transplantation, Epstein Barr virus, cyclosporine, and lymphoproliferative disease: a growing concern. J Pediatr 1991;118:667–673.

74. Winter G, Milstein C. Man-made antibodies. Nature 1991;349:293–299.

75. Boulianne GL, Hozumi N, Shulman MI. Production of functional chimeric mouse-human antibody. Nature 1984;312:643.

76. Heinrich G, Gram H, Kocher HP, et al. Characterization of a human T cell-specific chimeric antibody (CD7) with human constant and mouse variable regions. J Immunol 1989;143:3589.

77. Delmonico FL, Cosimi AB, Kawai T, et al. Nonhuman primate responses to murine and humanized OKT4A. Transplantation 1993;55:722–728.

78. Alegre M-L, Peterson LJ, Xu D, et al. A non-activating "humanized" anti-CD3 monoclonal antibody retains immunosuppressive properties in vivo. Transplantation 1994;57:1537–1543.

79. Alegre ML, Lenschow DJ, Bluestone JA. Immunomodulation of transplant rejection using monoclonal antibodies and soluble receptors. Digest Dis Sci 1995;40(1):58–64.

80. Vincenti F, Lantz M, Birnbaum J, et al. A phase I trial of humanized anti-interleukin 2 receptor antibody in renal transplantation. Transplantation 1997;63:33–38.

81. Knechtle SJ, Vargo D, Fechner J, et al. FN18-CRM9 immunotoxin promotes tolerance in primate renal allografts. Transplantation 1997;63:1–6.

82. Mottram PL, Han W-R, Murray-Segal LJ, et al. Idarubicin-anti-CD3: a new immunoconjugate that induces alloantigen-specific tolerance in mice. Transplantation 1997;64:684–690.

83. Midtvedt K, Tafjord AB, Hartmann A, et al. Half dose of OKT3 is efficient in treatment of steroid-resistant renal allograft rejection. Transplantation 1996;62:38–42.

84. Chatenoud L, Legendre C, Ferran C, et al. Corticosteroid inhibition of the OKT3-induced cytokine-related syndrome-dosage and kinetics prerequisites. Transplantation 1991;51:334–338.

85. Pescovitz MD, Milgrom ML, Leapman SB, Filo RS. Corticosteroid inhibition of the OKT3-induced febrile and nephrotoxic responses during treatment of renal allograft rejection. Clin Transplant 1993;7:529–536.

86. Thistlethwaite JR Jr, Stuart JK, Mayes JT, et al. Complications and monitoring of OKT3 therapy. Am J Kid Dis 1988;11:112–119.

87. Haug CE, Colvin RB, Delmonico FL, et al. A phase I trial of immunosuppression with anti-ICAM-1 (CD54) mAb in renal allograft recipients. Transplantation 1993;55:766–773.

88. Bach JF, Chatenoud L. Immunology of monoclonal antibodies in solid organ transplantation: yesterday, today and tomorrow. Transplant Sci 1992;2(2)suppl:4–8.

89. Janossy G. Purging of bone marrow and immunosuppression. Br Med Bull 1984;40:247.

90. Burdick JF. Biology of immunosuppression mediated by antilymphocyte antibodies. In: Burdick JF, Racusen LC, Solez K, eds. Kidney transplant rejection. 2nd ed. New York: Marcel Dekker, 1992:505–539.

91. Jonker M, Goldstein G, Balner H. Effect of in vivo administration of monoclonal antibodies specific for human T cell subpopulations on the immune system in a rhesus monkey model. Transplantation 1983;35:521–526.

92. Tite JP, Sloan A, Janeway CJ. The role of L3T4 in T cell activation L3T4 may be both an Ia-binding protein and a receptor that transduces a negative signal. J Mol Cell Immunol 1986;2:179.

93. Kerr PG, Atkins RC. The effects of OKT3 therapy on infiltrating lymphocytes in rejecting renal allografts. Transplantation 1989;48:33.

94. Cosimi AB. The future of monoclonal antibody immunosuppression in solid organ transplantation. Transplant Sci 1992;2(2)suppl:28–34.

95. Rouleau M, Mollereau B, Bernard A, et al. Mitogenic monoclonal antibody pairs predispose peripheral T cells to undergo apoptosis on interaction with a third CD2 monoclonal antibody. J Immunol 1994;152:4861–4872.

96. Boussiotis VA, Freeman GJ, Griffin JD, et al. CD2 is involved in maintenance and reversal of human allo antigen–specific clonal anergy. J Exp Med 1994;180:1665–1673.

97. Thurlow PJ, Lovering E, D'Apice AJF, et al. A monoclonal anti-pan-T-cell antibody. Transplantation 1983;36:293–298.

98. Giovino-Barry VC, Latinne D, Xu Y, et al. Perturbation of CD2 can induce alloantigen specific hyporesponsiveness in naive T cells. FASEB 1995;9:A1345.

99. Starling GC, Whitney GS, Siadak AW, et al. Characterization of mouse CD6 with novel mAbs which enhance the allogeneic mixed leukocyte reaction. Eur J Immunol 1996;26(4):738–746.

100. Kirkman RL, Araujo JL, Busch GJ, et al. Treatment of acute renal allograft rejection with monoclonal anti-T12 antibody. Transplantation 1983;36(6):620–626.

101. Wee SL, Phelan JM, Preffer FI, et al. Anti-Leu2a (anti-CD8) monoclonal antibody therapy: antibody-mediated cell clearance in vivo requires Fc-FcRII interaction. Transplant Proc 1989;21:117.

102. Larsen CP, Elwood ET, Alexander DZ, et al. Long-term acceptance of skin and cardiac allografts after blocking CD40 and CD28 pathways. Nature 1996;381:434–438.

103. Kirk AD, Harlan DM, Davis TA, et al. CTLA 4 Ig and anti-CD40 ligand prevent renal allograft rejection in primates. Proc Natl Acad Sci 1997;94:8789–8794.

104. Goldberg LC, Bradley JA, Connolly J, et al. Anti-CD45 monoclonal antibody perfusion of human renal allografts prior to transplantation. Transplantation 1995;59:1285–1293.

105. Cosimi AB, Conti D, Delmonico FL, et al. In vivo effects of monoclonal antibody to ICAM-1 (CD54) in nonhuman primates with renal allografts. J Immunol 1990;144:4604–4612.

106. Kreis H, Legendre C, Chatenoud L. OKT3 in organ transplantation. Transplant Rev 1991;5:181–199.

107. Delmonico FL, Cosimi AB. Monoclonal antibody treatment of human allograft recipients. Surg Gynecol Obstet 1988;166:89–98.

108. Kunicka JE, Platsoucas CD. Induction of suppressor cells to T- and B-cell proliferative responses and immunoglobulin production by monoclonal antibodies recognizing CD3 T-cell differentiation antigen. Cell Immunol 1988;116:195–215.

109. Vigeral P, Chkoff N, Chatenoud L, et al. Prophylactic use of OKT3 monoclonal antibody in cadaver kidney recipients. Transplantation 1986;41:730–733.

110. Debure A, Chkoff N, Chatenoud L, et al. One-month prophylactic use of OKT3 in cadaver kidney transplant recipients. Transplantation 1988;45:546–553.

111. Norman DJ, Kahana L, Stuart FP, et al. A randomized clinical trial of induction therapy with OKT3 in kidney transplantation. Transplantation 1993;55:44–50.

112. Abramowicz D, Goldman M. OKT3 for induction of immunosuppression in renal transplantation. Transplantation 1993;43:91–95.

113. Opelz G, for the Collaborative Transplant Study. Efficacy of rejection prophylaxis with OKT3 in renal transplantation. Transplantation 1995;60:1220–1224.

114. Abramowicz D, Pradier O, Marchant A, et al. Induction of thromboses within renal grafts by high-dose prophylactic OKT3. Lancet 1992;339:777–778.

115. Millis JM, McDiarmid SV, Hiatt JR, et al. Randomized prospective trial of OKT3 for early prophylaxis of rejection after liver transplantation. Transplantation 1989;47:82.

116. Farges O, Ericzon B-G, Bresson-Hadni S, et al. A randomized trial of OKT3-based versus cyclosporine-based immunoprophylaxis after liver transplantation. Transplantation 1994;58:891–898.

117. Robbins RC, Oyer PE, Stinson EB, Starnes VA. The use of monoclonal antibodies after heart transplantation. Transplant Sci 1992;2:22–27.

118. Griffith BP, Kormos RL, Armitage JM, et al. Comparative trial of immunoprophylaxis with RATG versus OKT3. J Heart Transplant 1990;9:301–305.

119. Kramer MR, Stoehr C, Lewiston NJ, et al. Trimethoprim-sulfamethoxazole prophylaxis for *Pneumocystisis carinii* infections in heart-lung and lung transplantation—how effective for how long? Transplantation 1992;53:586–589.

120. Gruessner A, Sutherland DE. Pancreas transplantation in the United States and non-US. In: Terasaki PI, Cecka JM, eds. Clinical transplants 1996. Los Angeles: UCLA Tissue Typing Laboratory, 1996:47–68.

121. Ortho Multicenter Transplant Study Group. A randomized clinical trial of OKT3 monoclonal antibody for acute rejection of cadaveric renal transplants. N Engl J Med 1985;313:337–342.

122. Ponticelli C, Rivolta E, Tarantino A, et al. Treatment of severe rejection of kidney transplants with Orthoclone OKT3. Clin Transplant 1987;1:99–103.

123. Norman DJ, Barry JM, Bennett WM, et al. The use of OKT3 in cadaveric renal transplantation for rejection that is unresponsive to conventional anti-rejection therapy. Am J Kid Dis 1988;11:90–93.

124. First MR, Schroeder TJ, Melvin DB, et al. OKT3 therapy in kidney, liver, heart, and pancreas transplantation. Clin Transplantation 1988;2:185–189.

125. Gaber LW, Gaber AO, Vera SR, et al. Successful reversal of hyperacute renal allograft rejection with the anti-CD3 monoclonal OKT3. Transplantation 1992;54:930–932.

126. Carrier M, Jenicek M, Pelletier LC. Value of monoclonal antibody OKT3 in solid organ transplantation: a meta-analysis. Transplant Proc 1992;24:2586–2591.

127. Tesi RJ, Elkhammas EA, Henry ML, Ferguson RM. OKT3 for primary therapy of the first rejection episode in kidney transplants. Transplantation 1993;55:1023–1029.

128. Kamath S, Dean D, Peddi VR, et al. Efficacy of OKT3 as primary therapy for histologically confirmed acute renal allograft rejection. Transplantation 1997;64:1428–1432.

129. Woodle ES, Thislethwaite JR, Emond JC, et al. OKT3 therapy for hepatic allograft rejection. Transplantation 1991;51:1207–1212.

130. Cosimi AB, Cho SI, Delmonico FL, et al. A randomized clinical trial comparing OKT3 and steroids for treatment of hepatic allograft rejection. Transplantation 1987;43:91–95.

131. Solomon H, Gonwa TA, Mor E, et al. OKT3 rescue for steroid-resistant rejection in adult liver transplantation. Transplantation 1993;55:87–91.

132. Nakhleh RE, Sutherland DE. Pancreas rejection: significance of histopathologic findings with implications for classification of rejection. Am J Surg Pathol 1992;16:1098–1107.

133. Gilbert EM, DeWitt CW, Eisworth CC, et al. Treatment of refractory cardiac allograft rejection with OKT3 monoclonal antibody. Am J Med 1982;82:202.

134. Shennib H, Massard G, Reynaud M, Noirclerc M. Efficacy of OKT3 therapy for acute rejection in isolated lung transplantation. J Heart Lung Transplant 1994;13:514–519.

135. Carey G, Lisi PJ, Schroeder TJ. The incidence of antibody formation to OKT3 consequent to its use in organ transplantation. Transplantation 1995;60:151–158.

136. Colvin RB, Preffer FI. Laboratory monitoring of therapy with OKT3 and other murine monoclonal antibodies. Clin Lab Med 1991;11:693.

137. Nelson PW, Jaffers GJ, Fuller TC, et al. Reduction of immune response to OKT3 monoclonal antibody. Transplant Proc 1985;17:644–645.

138. Chatenoud L, Jonker M, Villemain F, et al. The human immune response to the OKT3 monoclonal antibody is oligoclonal. Science 1986;232:1406–1408.

139. Legendre CM, Kreis H, Bach J, Chatenoud L. Prediction of successful allograft rejection retreatment with OKT3. Transplantation 1992;53:87–90.

140. Cosimi AB, Colvin RB, Burton RC, et al. Use of monoclonal antibodies to T-cell subsets for immunologic monitoring and treatment in recipients of renal allografts. N Engl J Med 1981;305:308–314.

141. Stephen RN, Munschauer CE, Kohli RK, et al. Post-OKT3 induction therapy CD complex response predicts renal allograft rejection. Transplantation 1997;63:1183–1186.

142. Sheiner PA, Guarrera JV, Grunstein E, et al. Increased risk of early rejection correlates with recovery of CD3 cell count after liver transplant in patients receiving OKT3 induction. Transplantation 1997;64:1212–1216.

143. Woodle ES, Bruse DS, Josephson M, et al. OKT3 escalating dose regimens provide effective therapy for renal allograft rejection. Clin Transplant 1996;10:389–395.

144. Jaffers GJ, Fuller TC, Cosimi AB, et al. Monoclonal antibody therapy: anti-idiotypic and non-anti-idiotypic antibodies to OKT3 arising despite intense immunosuppression. Transplantation 1986;41:572–578.

145. Chatenoud L, Ferran C, Reuter A, et al. Systemic reaction to the monoclonal antibody OKT3 in relation to serum levels of tumor necrosis factor and interferon γ. N Engl J Med 1989;320:1420.

146. Buysmann S, Hack CE, van Diepen FNJ, et al. Administration of OKT3 as a 2-hour infusion attenuates first dose side effects. Transplantation 1997;64:1620–1623.

147. Vallhonrat H, Williams WW, Cosimi AB, et al. In vivo generation of C4d, Bb, iC3b and SC5b-9 after OKT3 administration in kidney and lung transplant recipients. Transplantation 1999 (in press).

148. Waid TH, Lucas BA, Thompson JS, et al. Treatment of renal allograft rejection with T10B9.1A31 or OKT3. Transplantation 1997;64:274–281.

149. Eason JD, Pascual M, Wee S, et al. Evaluation of recombinant human soluble dimeric tumor necrosis factor receptor for prevention of OKT3-associated acute clinical syndrome. Transplantation 1996;61:224–228.

150. Swinnen LJ, Costanzo-Nordin MR, Fisher SG, et al. Increased incidence of lymphoproliferative disorder after immunosuppression with the monoclonal antibody OKT3 in cardiac transplant recipients. N Engl J Med 1990;323:1723–1728.

151. Hibberd PL, Tolkoff-Rubin NE, Cosimi AB, et al. Symptomatic cytomegalovirus disease in the cytomegalovirus antibody seropositive renal transplant recipient treated with OKT3. Transplantation 1992;53:68–72.

152. Andrews W, Sommerauer J, Roden J, et al. 10 years of pediatric liver transplantation. J Pediatr Surg 1996;31:619–624.

153. Chen JM, Barr ML, Chadburn A, et al. Management of lymphoproliferative disorders after cardiac transplantation. Ann Thorac Surg 1993;56:527–538.

154. Steinmuller DR, Hayes JM, Novick AC, et al. Comparison of OKT3 with ALG for prophylaxis for patients with acute renal failure after cadaveric renal transplantation. Transplantation 1991;52:67–71.

155. Frey DJ, Matas AJ, Gillingham KJ, et al. Sequential therapy—a prospective randomized trial of MALG versus OKT3 for prophylactic immunosuppression in cadaver renal allograft recipients. Transplantation 1992;54:50–56.

156. Cole EH, Cattran DC, Farewell VT, et al. A comparison of rabbit antithymocyte serum and OKT3 as prophylaxis against renal allograft rejection. Transplantation 1994;57:60–67.

157. Hanto DW, Jendrisak MD, So SKS, et al. Induction immunosuppression with antilymphocyte globulin or OKT3 in cadaver kidney transplantation. Transplantation 1994;57:377–384.

158. Block HA, Gallati H, Zurcher RM, et al. A randomized prospective trial of prophylactic immunosuppression with ATG-fresenius versus OKT3 after renal transplantation. Transplantation 1995;59:830–840.

159. Delmonico FL, Cosimi AB, et al. Anti-CD4 monoclonal antibody therapy. Clin Transplant 1996;10:397–403.

160. Powelson JA, Cosimi AB. The experimental and clinical use in transplantation of monoclonal antibodies to CD4 and other adhesion molecules. In: Chatenoud L, ed. Monoclonal antibodies in transplantation. Austin, TX: RG Landes, 1995:21–52.

161. Sablinski T, Sayegh MH, Kut JP, et al. The importance of targeting the CD4+ T cell subset at the time of antigenic challenge for induction of prolonged vascularized allograft survival. Transplantation 1992;53:219–221.

162. Sablinski T, Hancock WW, Tilney NL, Kupiec-Weglinski JW. CD4 monoclonal antibodies in organ transplantation—a review of progress. Transplantation 1991;52:579–589.

163. Powelson JA, Knowles RW, Delmonico FL, et al. CDR-grafted OKT4A monoclonal antibody in cynomolgus renal allograft recipients. Transplantation 1994;57:788–793.

164. Horneff G, Emmrich F, Reiter C, et al. Persistent depletion of CD4+ T cells and inversion of the CD4/CD8 T cell ratio induced by anti-CD4 therapy. J Rheumatol 1992;19:1845–1850.

165. Sprent J. T lymphocytes and the thymus. In: Paul WE, ed. Fundamental immunology. 3rd ed. New York: Raven, 1993:75–109.

166. Lehmann M, Sternkopf F, Metz F, et al. Induction of long-term survival of rat skin allografts by a novel, highly efficient anti-CD4 monoclonal antibody. Transplantation 1992;54:959–962.

167. Wee SL, Stroka DM, Preffer FI, et al. The effects of OKT4A monoclonal antibody on cellular immunity of nonhuman primate renal allograft recipients. Transplantation 1992;53:501–507.

168. Darby CR, Morris PJ, Wood KJ. Evidence that long-term cardiac allograft survival induced by anti-CD4 monoclonal antibody does not require depletion of CD4+ T cells. Transplantation 1992;54:483–490.

169. Darby CR, Bushell A, Morris PJ, et al. Nondepleting anti-CD4 antibodies in transplantation. Evidence that modulation is far less effective than prolonged CD4 blockade. Transplantation 1994;57:1419–1426.

170. Shizuru JA, Seydel KB, Flavin TF, et al. Induction of donor-specific unresponsiveness to cardiac allografts in rats by pretransplant anti-CD4 monoclonal antibody therapy. Transplantation 1990;50:366–373.

171. Pearson TC, Madsen JC, Larsen CP, et al. Induction of transplantation tolerance in adults using donor antigen and anti-CD4 monoclonal antibody. Transplantation 1992;54:475–483.

172. Bushell A, Morris PJ, Wood KJ. Induction of operational tolerance by random blood transfusion combined with anti-CD4 antibody therapy. A protocol with significant clinical potential. Transplantation 1994;58:133–139.

173. Bretscher P. The two-signal model of lymphocyte activation twenty-one years later. Immunol Today 1993;13:74–76.

174. Alters SE, Song HK, Fathman CG. Evidence that clonal anergy is induced in thymic migrant cells after anti-CD4-mediated transplantation tolerance. Transplantation 1993;56:633–638.

175. Cosimi AB, Delmonico FL, Wright JK, et al. Prolonged survival of nonhuman primate renal allograft recipients treated only with anti-CD4 monoclonal antibody. Surgery 1990;108:406–413.

176. Riechmann L, Clark M, Waldmann H, et al. Reshaping human antibodies for therapy. Nature 1988;332:323–327.

177. Greenwood J, Clark M, Waldmann H. Structural motifs involved in human IgG antibody effector functions. Eur J Immunol 1993;23:1098–1104.

178. Powelson JA, Knowles RW, Delmonico FL, et al. CDR-grafted OKT4A monoclonal antibody in cynomolgus renal allograft recipients. Transplantation 1994;57:788–793.

179. Delmonico FL, Cosimi AB, Kawai T, et al. Non-human primate responses to murine and humanized OKT4A. Transplantation 1993;55:722–728.

180. Land W. Monoclonal antibodies in 1991: new potential options in clinical immunosuppressive therapy. Clin Transplant 1991;5:493–500.

181. Dantal J, Ninin E, Hourmant M, et al. Anti-CD4 MoAb therapy in kidney transplantation—a pilot study in early prophylaxis of rejection. Transplantation 1996;62:1502–1506.

182. Meiser BM, Reiter C, Reichenspurner H, et al. Chimeric monoclonal CD4 antibody—a novel immunosuppressant for clinical heart transplantation. Transplantation 1994;58:419–423.

183. Reinke P, Kern F, Fietze W, et al. Anti-CD4 monoclonal antibody therapy of late acute rejection in renal allograft recipients—CD4+ T cells play an essential role in the rejection process. Transplant Proc 1995;27:859–862.

184. Lazarovits AI, Rochon J, Banks L, et al. Human mouse chimeric CD7 monoclonal antibody for the prophylaxis of kidney transplant rejection. J Clin Invest 1993;150:5163.

185. Waldmann TA. The IL-2/IL-2 receptor system: a target for rational immune intervention. Immunol Today 1993;14:264–269.

186. Kupiec-Weglinski J, Diamantstein T, Tilney NL. Interleukin-2 receptor-targeted therapy—rationale and applications in organ transplantation. Transplantation 1988;46:785–792.

187. Kirkman RL, Shapiro ME, Carpenter CB, et al. A randomized prospective trial of anti-Tac monoclonal antibody in human renal transplantation. Transplantation 1991;51:107–113.

188. Soulillou JP, Cantarovish D, Le ML, et al. Randomized controlled trial of a monoclonal antibody against the interleukin-2 receptor (33B3.1) as compared with rabbit antithymocyte globulin for prophylaxis against rejection of renal allografts. N Engl J Med 1990;322:1175–1182.

189. Cantarovich D, Le Mauff B, Hourmant M, et al. Prevention of acute rejection episodes with an anti-interleukin-2 receptor monoclonal antibody. Results after combined pancreas and kidney transplantation. Transplantation 1994;57:198–203.

190. Reding R, Feyaerts A, Vraux H, et al. Prophylactic immunosuppression with anti-interleukin-2 receptor monoclonal antibody Lo-Tact-1 versus OKT3 in liver allografting. Transplantation 1996;61:1406–1413.

191. van Gelder T, Zietse R, Mulder AH, et al. A double-blind, placebo-controlled study of monoclonal anti-interleukin-2 receptor antibody (BT563) administration to prevent acute rejection after kidney transplantation. Transplantation 1995;60:248–252.

192. Nashan B, Schlitt HJ, Schwinzer R, et al. Immunoprophylaxis with a monoclonal anti-IL-2 receptor antibody in liver transplant patients. Transplantation 1996;61:546–554.

193. Langrehr JM, Nussler NC, Neumann U, et al. A prospective randomized trial comparing interleukin-2 receptor antibody versus antithymocyte globulin as part of a quadruple immunosuppressive induction therapy following orthotopic liver transplantation. Transplantation 1997;63:1772–1781.

194. van Gelder T, Balk AHMM, Jonkman FAM, et al. A randomized trial comparing safety and efficacy of OKT3 and a monoclonal anti-interleukin-2 receptor antibody (BT563) in the prevention of acute rejection after heart transplantation. Transplantation 1996;62:51–55.

195. Tinubu SA, Hakimi J, Kondas JA, et al. Humanized antibody directed to the IL-2 receptor β-chain prolongs primate cardiac allograft survival. J Immunology 1994;153:4330–4338.

196. Amlot PL, Rawlings E, Fernando ON, et al. Prolonged action of a chimeric interleukin-2 receptor (CD25) monoclonal antibody used in cadaveric renal transplantation. Transplantation 1995;60:748–756.

197. Nashan B, Moore R, Amlot P, et al. Randomized trial of basiliximab versus placebo for control of acute cellular rejection in renal allograft recipients. Lancet 1997;350:1193–1198.

198. Vincenti F, Kirkman R, Light SE, et al. Interleukin 2-receptor blockade with Daclizumab to prevent acute rejection in renal transplantation. N Engl J Med 1998;338:161–165.

199. Kahan BD, Rajagopalan PR, Hall M, et al. Reduction of the occurrence of acute cellular rejection among renal allograft recipients treated with basiliximab, a chimeric anti-interleukin-2-receptor monoclonal antibody. United States Simulect Renal Study Group. Transplantation 1999;67:276–284.

200. Nashan B, Light S, Hardie IR, et al. Reduction of acute renal allograft rejection by daclizumab. Daclizumab Double Therapy Study Group. Transplantation 1999;67:110–115.

201. Kovarik J, Breidenbach T, Gerbeau C, et al. Disposition and immunodynamics of basiliximab in liver allograft recipients. Clin Pharmacol Ther 1998;64:66–72.

202. Cantarovich D, Le Mauff B, Hourmant M, et al. Anti-interleukin 2 receptor monoclonal antibody in the treatment of ongoing acute rejection episodes of human kidney graft—a pilot study. Transplantation 1989;47:454–457.

203. Herbelin C, Stephan JL, Donadieu J, et al. Treatment of steroid-resistant acute graft-versus-host disease with an anti IL-2R monoclonal antibody (BT563) in children who received T-cell depleted, partially matched, related bone marrow transplants. Bone Marrow Transplant 1994;13:563–569.

204. Anasetti C, Hansen JA, Waldmann TA, et al. Treatment of acute graft-versus-host disease with humanized anti-Tac, an antibody that binds to the interleukin-2 receptor. Blood 1994;84:1320–1327.

205. Grisham MB, Hernandez LA, Granger DN. Xanthine oxidase and neutrophil infiltration in intestinal ischemia. Am J Physiol 1986;251:G567–G574.

206. Pober JS, Cotran RS. The role of endothelial cells in inflammation. Transplantation 1990;50:537–544.

207. Lasky LA. Selectins: interpreters of cell-specific carbohydrate information during inflammation. Science 1992;258:964–969.

208. Heemann UW, Tullius SG, Azuma H, et al. Adhesion molecules and transplantation. Ann Surg 1994;219:4–12.

209. Isobe M, Yagita H, Okumura K, et al. Specific acceptance of cardiac allograft after treatment with antibodies to ICAM-1 and LFA-1. Science 1992;255:1125–1127.

210. Qin L, Chavin KD, Lin J, et al. Anti-CD2 receptor and anti-CD2 ligand (CD48) antibodies synergize to prolong allograft survival. J Exp Med 1994;179:341–346.

211. Woodward JE, Qin L, Chavin KD, et al. Blockade of multiple costimulatory receptors induces hyporesponsiveness. Transplantation 1996;62:1011–1018.

212. Berlin PJ, Bacher JD, Sharrow SO, et al. Monoclonal antibodies against human T-cell adhesion molecules—modulation of immune function in nonhuman primates. Transplantation 1992;53:840–849.

213. Kaplon RJ, Hochman PS, Michler RE, et al. Short course single agent therapy with an LFA-3-IgG fusion protein prolongs primate cardiac allograft survival. Transplantation 1996;61:356–363.

214. Adams D. Therapeutic potential of inhibiting the ICAM-1/LFA-1 pathway of leukocyte adhesion. In: Salomon DR, Sollinger H, eds. Recent developments in transplantation medicine: adhesion molecules, fusion proteins, novel peptides and monoclonal antibodies. Glenview, IL: Physicians and Scientists, 1995:27–43.

215. Byrne JG, Smith WJ, Murphy MP, et al. Complete prevention of myocardial stunning, contracture, low-reflex and edema after heart transplantation by blocking neutrophil adhesion molecules during reperfusion. J Thorac Cardiovasc Surg 1992;104:1589–1596.

216. Kelly KJ, Williams WJ, Colvin RB, et al. Antibody to intercellular adhesion molecule 1 protects the kidney. Proc Natl Acad Sci USA 1994;91:812–816.

217. DeMeester SR, Molinari MA, Shiraishi T, et al. Attenuation of rat lung isograft reperfusion injury with a combination of anti-ICAM-1 and anti-β₂ integrin monoclonal antibodies. Transplantation 1996;62:1477–1485.

218. Davies MH, Tregunno GA, Scharschmidt L, Neuberger JM. Monoclonal anti-ICAM-1 antibodies in liver transplantation—preliminary results of a phase I trial. Hepatology 1993;18:75a.

219. Maraninchi D, Mawas C, Stoppa AM, et al. Anti LFA1 monoclonal antibody for the prevention of graft rejection after T cell-depleted HLA-matched bone marrow transplantation for leukemia in adults. Bone Marrow Transplant 1989;4:147–150.

220. Hourmant M, Bedrossian J, Durand D, et al. A randomized multicenter trial comparing leukocyte function-associated antigen-1 monoclonal antibody with rabbit antithymocyte globulin as induction treatment in first kidney transplantations. Transplantation 1996;62:1565–1570.

221. Le Mauff B, Hourmant M, Rougier JP, et al. Effect of anti-LFA-1 (CD11a) monoclonal antibodies in acute rejection in human kidney transplantation. Transplantation 1991;52:297–299.

222. Brown SA, Lucas BA, Waid TH, et al. T10B9 (MEDI-500) mediated immunosuppression: studies on the mechanism of action. Clin Transplantation 1996;10:607–613.

223. Ghetie MA, Vitetta ES. Recent developments in immunotoxin therapy. Curr Opinion Immunol 1994;6:707–714.

224. Thomas JM, Neville DM, Contreras JL, et al. Preclinical studies of allograft tolerance in rhesus monkeys. Transplantation 1997;64:124–135.

225. Lenschow DJ, Zeno Y, Hathcock KS, et al. Inhibition of transplant rejection following treatment with anti-B7-2 and anti-B7-1 antibodies. Transplantation 1995;60:1171–1178.

226. Eck SC, Chang D, Wells AD, Turka LA. Differential down-regulation of CD28 by B7-1 and B7-2 engagement. Transplantation 1997;64:1497–1499.

## COMMENTARY REFERENCES

1. Soulillou JP, Peyronnet B, Le Mauff B, et al. Prevention of rejection of kidney transplants by monoclonal antibody directed against interleukin 2 receptor. Lancet 1987;1:1339–1342.

2. Nashan B, Moore R, Amlot P, et al. Randomised trial of basiliximab versus placebo for control of acute cellular rejection in renal allograft recipients. Lancet 1997;350:1193–1198.

3. Dantal J, Hourmant M, Cantarovich D, et al. Effect of long-term immunosuppression in kidney-graft recipients on cancer incidence: randomised comparison of two cyclosporine regimens. Lancet 1998;351:623–628.

4. Kirk A, Harlan D, Armstrong N, et al. CTLA4Ig and anti-CD40 ligand prevent renal allograft rejection in primates. Proc Natl Acad Sci 1997;94:8789–8794.

5. Ossevoort M, Ringers J, Boon L, et al. Blocking of costimulatory pathways using monoclonal antibodies to prevent transplant rejection in a non-human primate model. 3rd International Conference on new trends in clinical and experimental immunosuppression. Geneva: Fevrier, 1998.

6. Qin L, Chavin KD, Lin J, et al. Anti-CD2 receptor and anti-CD2 ligand (CD48) antibodies synergized to prolong allograft survival. J Exp Med 1994;179:341–346.

7. Hourmant M, Bedrossian J, Durand D, et al. A randomized multicenter trial comparing leukocyte function-associated antigen-1 monoclonal antibody with rabbit antithymocyte globulin as induction treatment in first kidney transplantations. Transplantation 1996;62:1565–1570.

8. Rabb H, Martin JG. An emerging paradigm shift on the roll of leukocyte adhesion molecules. J Clin Inv 1997;100:2937–2938.

9. Larsen CP, Elwood ET, Alexander DZ, et al. Long-term acceptance of skin and cardiac allografts after blocking CD40 and CD28 pathways. Nature 1996;381:434–439.

10. Isobe M, Yagita H, Okumura K, Ihara A. Specific acceptance of cardiac allograft after treatment with antibodies to ICAM1 and anti LFA-1. Science 1992;255:1125–1127.

11. Thompson CB, Allison JP. The emerging role of CTLA4 as an immune attenuator. Immunity 1997;7:445–450.

12. Perez VL, Van Parijs L, Blucklans A, et al. Induction of peripheral T cell tolerance in vivo requires CTLA-4 engagement. Immunity 1997;6:411–417.

13. Chandraker M, Takada M, Nadeau K, et al. The role of the B7 costimulatory pathway in experimental cold ischemia/reperfusion injury. Kidney Int 1997;52:1678–1684.

14. François C, Dantal J, Sorel M, et al. Antibodies directed at mouse IL-2-R α and β chains act in synergy to abolish T cell proliferation in vitro and delayed type hypersensitivity reaction in vivo. Transplant Int 1996;9:46–50.

15. Audrain M, Boeffard F, Soulillou JP, Jacques Y. Synergistic action of monoclonal antibodies directed at p55 and p75 chain of the human IL-2-receptor. J Immunol 1991;77:780–786.

16. Hourmant M, Dantal J. Adhesion molecules in rejection and tolerance of allografts. Nephrol Dial Transplant 1996;11:1661–1666.

17. He XY, Xu Z, Melrose A, et al. Humanization and pharmacokinetics of a monoclonal antibody with specificity for both E- and P-selectin. J Immunol 1998;160:1029–1035.

18. Madsen JC, Superina RA, Wood KJ, Morris PJ. Immunological unresponsiveness induced by recipient cells transfected with donor MHC genes. Nature 1988;332:161–164.

19. Zavazova N, Kvonke M. Soluble HLA class I molecules induce apoptosis alloreactive cytotoxic T lymphocytes. Nat Med 1996;2:1005–1010.

20. Pichlmayer P, Cantarovich D, Soulillou JP, et al. European Mycophenolate Mofetil Cooperative Study Group. Placebo-controlled study of mycophenolate mofetil combined with cyclosporin and corticosteroids for prevention of acute rejection. Lancet 1995;345:1321–1325.

# Use of Irradiation and Photopheresis for Immunosuppression in Transplantation

Mark Waer

The basis of the immunosuppressive effects of ionizing radiation is complex and depends on various elements such as the irradiation dose, the dose per fraction, the emitting source used, and the status of the irradiated tissue. The timing of the irradiation is also important to the immunologic response; for example, a primary antibody response is more radiosensitive than a secondary one (1). It has been shown that lymphocytes are extremely sensitive to radiotherapy. In contrast to most other cells that die a mitotic death because of radiation-related damage of DNA structures, lymphocytes die a so-called interphase death. This occurs within one hour of an LD50 dose (2). In contrast to resting T lymphocytes, activated T lymphocytes are relatively radioresistant (3). B lymphocytes are more radiosensitive than T lymphocytes but, similar to T lymphocytes, can become extremely radioresistant when activated (1).

Photopheresis is based on the principle of activating inert 8-methoxypsoralen (8-MOP) by ultraviolet-A (UVA) irradiation. Subsequently, activated 8-MOP provokes a firm linkage of DNA strands in such a way that they cannot be separated, which is needed for cell division. The use of photopheresis after transplantation is based on the hypothesis that donor reactive lymphocytes will expand in the recipient peripheral blood. When peripheral blood is subjected to photopheresis, it is mainly this population of reactive lymphocytes that will be affected. Moreover, giving back inactivated donor reactive lymphocytes may "vaccinate" the recipient with these cells, which eventually may induce downregulatory (e.g., anti-idiotypic), immune circuits.

## TOTAL BODY IRRADIATION AND LOCAL GRAFT IRRADIATION

The immunosuppressive effects of ionizing radiation were noted early in the twentieth century (4,5), and total body irradiation has been used since the first days of human kidney transplantation (6). Unfortunately, it was soon learned that sublethal total body irradiation (TBI) was insufficient to provoke long-term survival of allografts and that higher doses would result in irreversible bone marrow aplasia and severe gastrointestinal toxicity (6). Other, more selective radiation techniques included irradiation of the graft implantation site (7), extracorporeal irradiation of the blood lymphocytes (7), and irradiation of thoracic duct lymphocytes (7,8). Still other approaches involved the injection of radioactive substances with high affinity for lymphoid tissues (9) or intravascular implantation of sources of high-energy beta emitters (7,10). However, due to technical difficulties, serious side effects, or lack of efficacy, none of these radiation procedures is routinely used in clinical organ transplantation.

Local graft irradiation has been used in many centers to treat acute rejection crises (11). As a favorable effect could never be substantiated in a controlled trial, this procedure has now been abandoned by most centers. The prophylactic effect of the postoperative administration of local graft irradiation, consisting of 600 Gy given in four fractions, was evaluated in a randomized trial (12). There was no apparent benefit in kidney function or time to first rejection episode in the group receiving local graft irradiation. Cadaver allograft survival was also not significantly different between the two treatment arms.

The most interesting form of irradiation for transplantation is total lymphoid irradiation (TLI). This procedure is still being extensively explored in experimental models and has been used for the past 15 years in transplant patients by several centers. TLI is therefore discussed in more detail in the sections that follow.

## TOTAL LYMPHOID IRRADIATION

### Discovery of TLI as an Immunosuppressant

TLI has been a standard form of therapy for treating patients with Hodgkin's disease (13). Irradiation is administered through two ports (Fig. 9.1): a thoracic "mantle" field, and an abdominal "inverted Y" encompassing the major lymph node areas, the thymus, and the spleen. In order to increase the hematologic tolerance of the procedure, the spleen is frequently removed before TLI. Usually a total dose of 40–50 Gy (1 Gy = 100 rad or cGy) is administered in daily fractions of 1.5–2.5 Gy. In a study of patients treated with TLI for Hodgkin's disease, it was found that cellular immunity was strikingly impaired for up to 10 years after TLI. The absolute number of T lymphocytes as well as their in

vitro reactivity to the mitogens phytohemagglutinin (PHA) and concanavalin A (ConA) or allogeneic stimulator cells in the mixed lymphocyte reaction (MLR) was significantly decreased (14). Interestingly, secondary hematologic tumors (15) or clinically important infections (16) were not increased after TLI. These clinical observations prompted researchers at Stanford to investigate the immunosuppressive potential of TLI in experimental models (17).

### TLI in Experimental Models

#### Induction of Specific Transplantation Tolerance in Rodents
A TLI irradiation technique similar to that used in Hodgkin's patients was developed for mice and rats. BALB/c mice were given 17 fractions of 2 Gy daily, delivered to the thoracic and abdominal fields concomitantly. Subsequently, their lymphocyte count as well as PHA, ConA, or MLR reactivity was decreased in a similar fashion as observed in Hodgkin's patients (17). Allogeneic C57BL skin grafts, transplanted one day after TLI, survived five times longer than in unirradiated mice. Interestingly, the infusion of $30 \times 10^6$ unmanipulated C57BL bone marrow (BM) cells resulted in stable bone marrow chimerism without graft-versus-host disease (GVHD). These chimeras became specifically tolerant to skin grafts originating from the bone marrow donor (17).

The rodent models clearly revealed that several variables determined the success rate of TLI. First, the width of the irradiation field seemed critical. In rats, shielding of even minor parts of the pelvic field prevented the induction of tolerance after TLI (17). Conversely, widening the TLI fields under the form of one or two total body irradiation fractions impressively increased the efficacy of TLI in mice (18). The effect of the total TLI dose was critical (17) and strain related (19). Another important finding with regard to clinical applications was that organ grafts had to be transplanted soon after TLI. Delaying skin graft transplantation to one week after TLI resulted in rapid rejection (17). Presensitization by blood transfusion, even to only minor transplantation antigens, abolished the capacity of TLI to induce stable chimerism (17). The absence of GVHD after TLI was not absolute and depended on the number of T cells present in the bone marrow inoculum (17) or on the level of gut decontamination of the recipient mice (19).

#### TLI in Large Animal Models
In dogs, although donor bone marrow infusion easily induced chimerism after TLI, it did not appear necessary to obtain long-term heart (20) or kidney allograft (21) survival. Therefore, TLI regimens without bone marrow infusion were further evaluated. A combination of TLI with azathioprine and antithymocyte globulin (ATG) led to an unacceptably high incidence of side effects (22). Addition of continuous high doses (17 mg/kg) of cyclosporine, although very effective, led to lethal lymphomas in 3 of 10 monkeys (22). A combination of 18 fractions of 1 Gy of TLI, followed

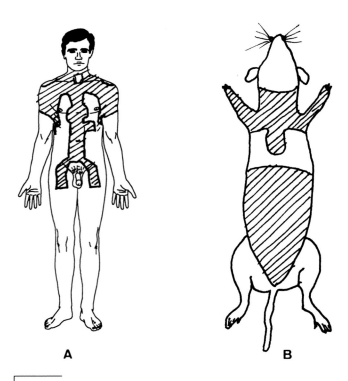

**A**                      **B**

**FIGURE 9.1.**    *TLI irradiation ports as used in patients (**A**) or in experimental studies in rodents (**B**). When no splenectomy is performed, the spleen is usually also included in the irradiation field in patients.*

by a 10-day course of postoperative ATG alone, induced specific transplantation tolerance in 40% of the transplanted dogs (23). A similar regimen was, however, much less effective in a kidney or a pancreas allograft model (24). Hence, from the overall experience in dogs it was not easy to determine which TLI-based regimen would be most suitable for patients.

In splenectomized rhesus monkeys, four to five TLI fractions of 125 cGy each were administered beginning on day 1 after kidney allografting. This was combined with five injections of ATG beginning on day 0. At the time of kidney grafting, recipients received DR– CD3– donor bone marrow cells. An actuarial one-year graft survival without chronic immunosuppression was obtained (25). Microchimerism was documented within skin only. Not depleting the CD3 cells from the donor bone marrow resulted in more generalized microchimerism but, unfortunately, also in subclinical GVHD and inferior one-year graft survival rates (25).

Eight fractions of 1 Gy of TLI delivered over four weeks, but administered through a very wide TLI field, was shown to be very effective in baboons (26). Such a TLI regimen was effective even without administering bone marrow or extra drugs. In two-thirds of the baboons, specific and permanent tolerance toward solid grafts was obtained (26). Altogether, the various experiments performed in monkeys seem to confirm the tolerogenic capacity of TLI as observed in small rodents.

### Mechanisms Involved in the Immunomodulatory Action of TLI

Many experiments were performed, mostly in the mouse model, to unravel the mechanisms facilitating tolerance induction after TLI. Suppressor cells were shown to be expanded in the spleen from mice soon after the end of TLI (27). These cells nonspecifically suppressed many immune reactions in vitro. These so-called natural suppressor cells were cloned and shown to express a surface phenotype similar to that of natural killer (NK) cells (i.e., Thy 1+, asialo GM+, Ig–, Lyt 1–, Lyt 2–, Ia–, MAC1–) (28). Nevertheless, these post-TLI suppressor cells did not display NK activity (28). Moreover, they expressed mRNA transcripts for the $\alpha$, $\beta$, and $\gamma$ T-cell receptor chains, indicating a T-cell–like origin (29). That these nonspecific suppressor cells played a role in the induction of stable BM chimerism after TLI was elaborated from various experiments. First, it was demonstrated that the level of induction of these cells after various TLI regimens correlated well with the relative capacity of these regimens to allow for induction of chimerism after TLI (18,19). Second, coinjection of cloned post-TLI natural suppressor cells was able to prevent the induction of GVHD in cotransfer experiments in mice (30). Third, injection of asialo GM1 antibodies after TLI resulted in the disappearance of post-TLI suppressor cells and concomitantly in the appearance of severe GVHD in a majority of BM transplanted mice (31,32). Whether these nonspecific suppressor

cells are also necessary to maintain tolerance after TLI is less clear. Moreover, their persistence or role in inducing specific suppressor cells has been difficult to demonstrate in long-term tolerant TLI-treated mice (33–35). Therefore, other tolerance mechanisms have been suggested to play a role as well.

The presence of clonal anergy in tolerant post-TLI T cells was demonstrated in various models (36,37). These anergized cells were incapable of proliferating, even in the presence of exogenous interleukin 2 (IL-2) (36). In some situations, clonal deletion was demonstrated as well. It was clearly shown that donor- and host-type thymocytes underwent clonal deletion for host and donor antigens, respectively, in the thymus of TLI-treated mice (37). It was also found that TLI-treated rats, developing tolerance for allogeneic antigens, had decreased precursor frequencies of antidonor cytotoxic T lymphocytes (CTLs) from three months post-TLI (38).

The most recent data suggest that "immunoredirection" may take place after TLI. It is suggested that the post-TLI environment facilitates the preferential development of $T_H2$-type lymphocytes (secreting IL-4, IL-5, IL-10) at the expense of $T_H1$ lymphocytes (secreting IL-2 or interferon gamma) (39–41). (See Chapter 7 for further discussion of $T_H1$ and $T_H2$ lymphocytes.) Apparently, alloantigen priming in the immediate post-TLI phase results in a shift of the allospecific cytokine pattern toward $T_H2$ cytokines by enhancing IL-4–producing CD4 cells and preventing maturation of interferon gamma (IFN-$\gamma$)-producing cells. In a study in baboons developing transplantation tolerance toward a kidney allograft, blocking low-affinity IgG antibodies directed at donor antigen presenting cells were demonstrated (42). As the formation of non-Fc binding, noncomplement-fixing IgG antibodies may be the expression of $T_H2$ activity, this observation may further indicate that TLI facilitates $T_H2$-type immune reactions.

## TLI in Xenotransplantation Experiments

One of the first major hurdles to overcome in xenotransplantation is the occurrence of early humoral rejection, which is mainly provoked by IgM xenoantibodies. These antibodies can be either preexisting, in the case of discordant, phylogenetically distant species combinations, or they can be rapidly induced in the case of closer, concordant combinations. Apparently, in most cases these IgM xenoantibodies are T-cell–independent. Although it had been previously shown that TLI was not very active in blocking T-cell–independent antibody formation, it seemed very active in suppressing the antihamster antibody formation in rats. When combined with cyclosporine (CsA) and splenectomy (43), with CsA and anti-CD4 monoclonal antibodies (44), or with deoxyspergualin (45), heart xenograft survival was significantly prolonged and xenoantibody formation was delayed and significantly suppressed. Also in the concordant cynomolgus monkey-to-baboon combination, TLI was exquisitely effective, especially when combined with CsA and methylprednisolone (46–48). Xenograft survival times of more than one year were obtained. Also in these primates, IgM xenoantibody formation was totally suppressed by TLI (46). Nevertheless, the total IgM or IgG blood levels were not altered. These data suggest that TLI may be specifically active on the B-lymphocyte subpopulations that are producing so-called natural xenoantibodies.

Several experiments were performed in order to determine whether TLI could also provoke a decrease of the titer of preexisting IgM xenoantibodies as seen in discordant combinations. In the guinea pig-to-rat combination, a three-week TLI treatment regimen together with azathioprine, cyclosporine, and methylprednisolone resulted in a significant decrease of the preexisting xenoantibody titer. This was unfortunately not accompanied with a prolongation of xenograft survival (49). In the pig islet-into-rat xenograft model, however, TLI was extremely effective when combined with deoxyspergualin (50). Also, in a discordant large animal model involving lamb heart transplantation into pigs, a one-week treatment regimen with TLI, CsA, and azathioprine resulted in a significant decrease of the xenoantibody titer and concomitantly a 30-fold increase of the mean xenograft survival time (51).

In view of the renewed interest in xenotransplantation, the capacity of TLI to influence natural xenoantibodies clearly deserves further exploration.

## TLI in Clinical Kidney Transplantation

### TLI and Low-Dose Prednisone in Diabetic Renal Allograft Recipients

Between the end of 1981 and the end of 1988, 54 insulin-dependent patients with end-stage renal disease due to diabetic nephropathy were transplanted at the University of Leuven. Twenty-seven of them were given pretransplant TLI followed by low-dose maintenance prednisone after transplantation. The 27 other patients were treated with CsA and a similar low-dose prednisone protocol. The details of the TLI and CsA protocols have been described elsewhere (52–54). TLI patients were given daily fractions of 1 Gy of TLI. In order to be able to irradiate the mantle and inverted Y fields concomitantly, a splenectomy was performed in 18 patients to lower the risk of leukopenia or thrombocytopenia. A minimal total dose of 20 Gy was given to all patients. When a crossmatch-negative donor was not available within two weeks of TLI, extra fractions were administered on a weekly basis, to a maximal cumulative dose of 30 Gy. In all patients, a donor kidney was found within one month after the last TLI fraction. As early transplantation after completion of TLI was considered a priority, only major blood group (ABO) and not histocompatibility matching was taken into account. After transplantation, only 20 to 30 mg of prednisone was given daily and tapered within two weeks to 10 mg per day, which was continued as maintenance therapy. Ten patients in each group

were included in a randomized controlled trial. Details and short-term results of this controlled trial have been published elsewhere (54). Here, the long-term results obtained in both groups, also including the patients of the controlled trial, are reported.

As can be seen from Figures 9.2A and 9.2B, patient and graft survival are significantly inferior in the TLI group (Wilcoxon $P < 0.05$ and $P < 0.006$, respectively). Clearly, the TLI regimen as used in this study was unable to provide acceptable graft and patient survival rates. This was also reflected by the fact that TLI-treated patients developed significantly more rejection crises than CsA-treated recipients. Only 4 of the 27 TLI patients did not develop a rejection crisis, and 9 of 27 underwent more than one rejection crisis. In contrast, 14 of 27 CsA patients were rejection free, and only 5 of 27 developed more than one rejection episode. This weak overall immunosuppressive effect of TLI explains why in TLI patients other maintenance immunosuppressants such as azathioprine (4) or CsA (5) had to be introduced. The primary aim of omitting maintenance immunosuppressants in TLI-treated patients was, therefore, not met in the majority of TLI-treated patients.

The major causes of death among the 15 deceased TLI patients were sepsis, which occurred in seven, and cardiovascular accidents, which occurred in five patients. One TLI patient, who was a heavy smoker, died because of lung cancer. In the CsA group, nine patients died of a cardiovascular accident, one of suicide, and three due to sepsis. In all the patients who died as a result of sepsis, high doses of steroids had been given to treat rejection. Hence, the excess mortality due to sepsis that was observed in the TLI patients was indirectly the consequence of the lower capacity of TLI to prevent the occurrence of rejection crises. The overall conclusion of this study is that TLI is insufficient by itself to guarantee good kidney graft survival rates in patients. Clearly, further manipulations such as the infusion of bone marrow cells or the addition of other immunosuppressants than steroids are needed. This experience actually confirms what was observed in most animal models: without the infusion of donor bone marrow or the administration of supplementary immunosuppressants, the induction of transplantation tolerance was rarely achieved with TLI.

### TLI with Low-Dose Prednisone and Postoperative ATG

The experience at the University of Leuven clearly showed that a combination of TLI with low-dose prednisone resulted in insufficient immunosuppression in most patients. Based on this preliminary experience and encouraged by the results obtained with TLI combined with ATG in dogs (23), a collaborative program involving preoperative TLI and postoperative ATG and low-dose prednisone (TAP) was initiated at Stanford University and Pacific Medical Center in San Francisco (55,56). Twenty fractions of 1 Gy were administered over a mean period of 12 weeks. A crossmatch-negative cadaver donor was found at a mean interval of nine days after the last TLI fraction. After transplantation, six

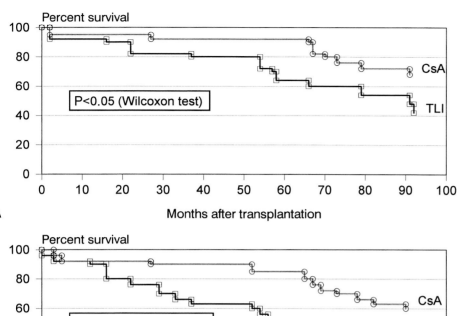

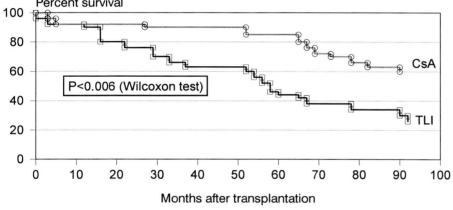

**FIGURE 9.2.** *Patient survival (**A**) and graft survival (**B**) in patients treated with TLI versus patients receiving CsA immunosuppression.*

courses of ATG were given and a low-dose prednisone maintenance therapy was initiated. Although the initial short-term results were very favorable (55), a long-term analysis in 52 patients receiving this TAP protocol showed that it was much less effective than a standard protocol of CsA and prednisone (three-year graft survival rates of 50% and 75%, respectively, were observed) (56). All immunosuppressive medication could be stopped in three patients who had remained rejection free for more than one year. Two of these showed specific nonreactivity to their donor cells in MLR (56,57). Unfortunately, two of the patients in whom all drugs were withdrawn developed a rejection six months later.

These results showed that the addition of prednisone and ATG is also not sufficient to increase the efficacy of TLI. Therefore, the same investigators added maintenance therapy with CsA to a similar TAP protocol in six patients. After more than two years, none of these patients underwent rejection crises (56). This protocol, therefore, may hold promise for the future.

### Wide-Field TLI with Cyclosporine
A wide-field TLI irradiation protocol was developed at the University of Johannesburg (58,59). The irradiation field involved the entire torso from the base of the skull down to and including the pelvis and proximal end of femora and

humeri. Ribs and lungs were shielded. In approximately one-half of baboons receiving this wide-field TLI regimen as eight fractions of 1 Gy over a four-week period, specific allotransplant tolerance without the need for extra drugs was achieved (26).

Fifty-six patients were treated using a similar TLI regimen before allogeneic cadaveric kidney transplantation. After transplantation, CsA and low-dose prednisone were given. The one- and five-year actuarial graft survival was 86% and 60%, respectively (59). In 12 patients, CsA elimination was attempted. However, in nine of them reinstitution of CsA or commencement of azathioprine was necessary.

This illustrates that with this TLI regimen, which was intensively investigated in a relevant baboon preclinical model, the aim of inducing specific tolerance was almost impossible to achieve. The authors suggested that presensitization, which was usually present in their patients, may be responsible for this inferior outcome. Indeed, among their patients, recipients with pretransplantation panel reactive antibodies (PRA) of more than 30% did significantly worse than the other patients (59).

### TLI Immunosuppression for Immunologic High-Risk Patients
Twenty patients who previously had rejected a first or second renal allograft were given TLI in a total dose ranging between 10 and 40 Gy at the University of Minnesota (60).

Historically, such patients had a two-year graft survival of less than 40% using an azathioprine-prednisone–based immunosuppression. After TLI, the patients were given post-operative azathioprine and prednisone. The graft survival was significantly increased to 70% at two years and did not change subsequently (61). Later, similarly improved second graft survival rates could be obtained using CsA as well. Because of the ease of the latter regimen, TLI was abandoned (61).

At the University of Rome, two TLI-based regimens were evaluated for treating highly sensitized recipients (62,63). When treated with azathioprine and prednisone, only 10% of similar patients had functioning grafts at one year after transplantation. In a first regimen, 14 patients were given 25–35 Gy of TLI, followed by antilymphocyte globulin (ALG), prednisone, and azathioprine. The one-year graft survival was 64%, and 7 of the 14 patients did not develop any rejection crises (62). A second group of 13 highly immunized patients (four due to blood transfusions and nine due to previous transplantation) was given 20 Gy of TLI, followed by low-dose steroids and CsA. The one-year graft survival in this group was 69%, and 6 patients remained rejection free (62). A follow-up report indicated that the eight-year actuarial graft survival remained at 69% (63).

## Post-transplantation TLI for the Treatment of Cardiac Allograft Rejection

Although it is generally accepted that TLI is most effective when administered before the alloantigen challenge, the use of post-transplantation TLI was investigated in a rat model and subsequently successfully explored in cardiac allograft recipients. In combination with anti-CD3 monoclonal antibodies, or with ATG together with donor-specific blood transfusions, post-transplantation TLI resulted in long-term specific transplantation tolerance in a strongly immunogenic heart transplant model in rats (64).

After some anecdotal reports of successful clinical use of post-transplantation TLI for the reversal of conventional therapy–resistant cardiac rejection (65,66), the efficacy of 10 fractions of 0.8 Gy of TLI was evaluated in 49 heart transplant patients suffering resistant rejection (n = 44) or early severe vascular rejection (n = 5) at the University of Alabama at Birmingham (67). A significant decrease of the rejection frequency ($P < 0.0001$) was observed in these patients. The reduced post-TLI rejection frequencies were maintained for at least two years. There was no increase in the frequency of infections after TLI, nor were there any deaths during or immediately following TLI (67). These results convinced the investigators that it would be unethical to deny high-risk patients the TLI treatment, despite the lack of appropriate control subjects. Along the same line, based on limited results in six patients, Valentine et al (68) suggested that TLI may be useful for the treatment of intractable acute allograft rejection following heart–lung and lung transplantation.

## Discussion

After demonstration of its safety and potential for inducing tolerance in animal models, TLI has been explored in clinical transplantation. The clinical experience reaffirms that TLI is indeed a safe procedure. In nearly all studies, the patient survival rates of the TLI groups were at least as good as in the control groups. Only in the Leuven study in diabetics did TLI-treated patients have significantly lower survival rates. However, as previously mentioned, this excessive mortality was probably related to steroid therapy for rejection crises, which were more common in the TLI group, rather than to intrinsic radiation-related risks.

The major concern when using irradiation in patients is the enhanced risk of tumor development. As could be expected from the experience in Hodgkin's patients, cancers were not more common during the early follow-up of TLI-treated renal transplant recipients. Among the more than 200 such recipients, only five neoplasia-related deaths were documented. Two patients of the Minnesota group developed a lethal lymphoma. As these patients had undergone retransplantation and had previously also received antithymocyte globulins, these deaths are more likely a consequence of overimmunosuppression in general than of TLI in particular. Two other deaths, one due to lung cancer in a heavy smoker in Leuven and one due to pelvic carcinoma in Johannesburg, are also unlikely to be related to irradiation. The only possible irradiation-related death may be the patient dying from myeloid leukemia in Johannesburg. However, in view of a recent report showing a high cumulative incidence of solid tumors in TLI-treated children with Hodgkin's disease starting from 15 years after TLI (69), a close follow-up of TLI-treated transplant patients seems indicated.

As far as the efficacy of TLI is concerned, a distinction must be made between its nonspecific action as an adjunct immunosuppressant and its capacity to induce transplantation tolerance. As an adjunct immunosuppressant added to standard regimens such as azathioprine-prednisone or CsA-prednisone, TLI seems to be extremely efficient. The best example of this comes from the heart transplantation experience. Here, TLI seemed exquisitely effective for the treatment of recurrent or severe vascular rejection. However, as several new immunosuppressive drugs seem able to decrease the incidence of rejection crises when added to CsA-based immunosuppressive schedules, it is unlikely that TLI will find widespread application as an adjunct immunosuppressant for clinical transplantation.

The primary aim of using TLI to achieve transplantation tolerance in a majority of patients has clearly not been achieved. In almost all centers, long-term maintenance immunosuppression was needed. Although the induction of specific transplantation tolerance without maintenance therapy was documented in a few patients, in the majority of other patients, interruption of maintenance immunosuppression was unsuccessful. This weak capacity to induce transplantation tolerance in patients as compared to animals was most striking in the Johannesburg experience. Although these investigators had carefully selected the most efficient TLI-based regimen in a very relevant preclinical model in baboons, a similar TLI schedule was not able to induce tolerance in their patients. Apparently, antigen disparity between donors and recipients is more pronounced in patients than in the less-outbred baboons. Moreover, pre-transplantation sensitization, which was shown in various models to hamper the tolerance-inducing capacity of TLI, is very likely more common in patients.

As multiple TLI regimens have now been explored in the clinic, it seems that a totally new approach is needed in order to achieve clinical tolerance with TLI. From that point of view, the East Carolina University experience in rhesus monkeys involving post-transplant TLI together with the infusion of DR– CD3– donor bone marrow is very appealing, but awaits confirmation in the clinic.

Xenotransplantation is now increasingly considered an achievable option to solve the lack of donor organs for clinical transplantation. Although it was known that the effects of TLI were strongest on T-cell immunity, it is fascinating to observe that TLI is very effective in suppressing or decreasing the formation of T-cell–independent IgM xenoantibodies as well. This suggests that TLI may specifically act on B-lymphocyte subpopulations responsible for the formation of these so-called natural antibodies. A confirmation that TLI suppresses xenoantibody formation will be important if and when xenotransplantation becomes a clinical reality.

## THE USE OF PHOTOPHERESIS FOR TRANSPLANTATION

Photopheresis, which includes a combination of leuko-pheresis and administration of the photosensitive drug 8-MOP followed by extracorporeal photoirradiation with long-wavelength UVA irradiation, was developed by Edelson et al (70) for the treatment of erythrodermic cutaneous T-cell lymphoma. As this treatment achieved remarkable remissions (70) and the proliferating malignant T lymphocytes were primarily of the T helper type, it was hypothesized that a similar treatment regimen may be of use for treating transplant recipients.

### Experimental Studies

The potential use of photopheresis was supported by positive experiments in mice (71,72). Spleen cells taken at the time of skin graft rejection were exposed to 8-MOP and UVA irradiation. When reinfused, these cells were able to provoke significant skin graft survival. Studies in a primate cardiac xenotransplantation model showed a synergistic action between CsA, steroids, and photopheresis resulting in extended xenograft survival (73,74).

### Clinical Studies

Photopheresis has been used successfully for the treatment of moderately severe heart transplant rejection. In this trial, eight of nine episodes could be reversed with one or two courses (75). However, interstitial T-cell infiltrates persisted longer as compared with steroid-treated control recipients.

Photopheresis was also successfully added to adjunct antibody therapy to prevent rejection of transplants in high-risk patients characterized by the presence of increased levels of lymphocytotoxic antibodies (76). In another study, photopheresis was used for adjunct immunosuppression without concomitant antibody therapy in 15 heart transplant recipients receiving standard triple drug immunosuppression (77). Ten or twenty photopheresis courses were given starting on the first day after heart transplantation. In this study, a new liquid form of 8-MOP was added directly to the buffy coat, resulting in reliable and sufficient drug levels in the cell suspension that is not always achievable after oral application of 8-MOP. Over the total observation time of about 10 months, both photopheresis regimens significantly reduced the number of acute rejection episodes by more than 50% as compared to the control group. Probably as a consequence of the lower need for rejection treatments, photopheresis patients developed significantly fewer infections than control patients. A subsequent multi-institution randomized trial has confirmed that addition of photopheresis to conventional immunosuppression significantly decreases the risk of cardiac rejection; however, survival was not improved in this study (78).

Overall, these first clinical experiences suggest that photopheresis is a safe and effective method of adjunct immunosuppression that should be further explored as an alternative for antibody-based adjunct immunosuppressive regimens.

---

## COMMENTARY

### J. A. Myburgh

Experience over some 30 years with experimental organ allotransplantation in the chacma baboon leaves the dominant impression of the uniquely potent tolerogenic effects of a modified regimen of total lymphoid irradiation (TLI), especially when compared with other methods of immune manipulation that are highly effective in rodent models but only modestly so in this primate. Nevertheless, the application of this method to the clinical situation has been rather disappointing, in both our experience and that of a few other centers. The reasons are not wholly clear, but several aspects are probably relevant.

The technique and regimen of TLI used in our baboons was developed from the pioneering work in rodents by Strober and his colleagues at Stanford. One aspect that we have repeatedly emphasized is the *necessity for a wide field of irradiation.* In essence, this includes irradiation of the entire torso from the base of the skull downward, including the pelvis and the upper ends of the humeri and femora (1). In the baboon, shielding to produce fields similar to the mantle and inverted-Y used in the treatment of Hodgkin's disease abolished tolerance production, as was observed in rodents. It is to be emphasized that in nearly all experimental reports from other laboratories and in all clinical series apart from ours, mantle and inverted-Y fields have been used. We believe that the use of the narrower fields is at least partially responsible for the failure of other laboratories to produce tolerance with TLI alone.

In terms of dosage of irradiation, the regimen used in the rodents, namely 17 fractions of 200 cGy each given five days per week, was found to be unacceptably toxic when given to the same wide field in the baboon. An exhaustive series of studies to determine a safe but effective regimen for the baboon resulted in a regimen of a total dose of 800 cGy given in fractions of 80 or 100 cGy twice a week. The dose response curve was parabolic, with lower or higher cumulative doses being less effective in terms of the proportion of recipients made tolerant (1).

The injection of donor bone marrow is certainly not necessary to achieve tolerance in the baboon, and in fact we found it consistently counterproductive whether whole bone marrow, several marrow fractions, or T cell–depleted bone marrow was used. This is in contradistinction to the original rodent experience and is of particular interest in the light of current work on the potential role of microchimerism in tolerance production.

The tolerance produced in baboons by TLI alone is highly specific and durable (2). Skin grafts from the kidney donor are permanently accepted while third-party skin or kidneys are rejected in an unmodified fashion. These baboons have maintained normal graft function for up to 10 years after transplantation, at which time they have been sacrificed for logistic reasons. However, tolerance is attained in only one-third to two-thirds of baboons in different groups and the likelihood of success has not been predictable in individual animals by in vitro tests. Accordingly, over the years we have studied a variety of additive measures in attempts to increase the predictability of tolerance induction and the fraction of tolerant animals obtained. These have included short post-transplant courses of immunosuppressive agents such as both anti-human and antibaboon antithymocyte globulin (ATG), prednisone, cyclosporine, mycophenolate mofetil, and deoxyspergualin; the injection of solubilized donor histocompatibility antigens; and the intrathymic injection of donor lymphoid cells (3). With none of these was there any evidence of a synergistic or even an additive effect to TLI. With all the immunosuppressive agents except ATG, and particularly with cyclosporine, the effect was, in fact, counterproductive in that tolerance was hardly ever

obtained. This suggests that these agents were opposing an active tolerogenic mechanism. This is further supported by our finding that the addition of two fractions of TLI after transplantation totally abrogated the tolerogenic effect of the pretransplant course. The addition of intrathymic donor glomeruli had no effect either positive or negative, but intrathymic donor lymphoid cells after pretransplant TLI sensitized the animals and produced accelerated acute rejection. The thymus of most mature adult baboons is atrophic and not encapsulated, and it is not possible to prevent extrathymic extravasation of the injectate. This may be the reason why the results were so different from those obtained in rodents.

It was the unpredictability of tolerance production in individual animals that led us, for obvious ethical reasons, to use conventional immunosuppressive agents following kidney transplantation for patients conditioned with pretransplant TLI. The recognized difference in actuarial survival between patients with panel reactive antibodies of more than 30% and those with less than 30%, and the fact that nearly one-third of our patients were so substantially presensitized (whereas none of our baboons were presensitized), may partially account for the less encouraging results obtained in our clinical trials. We also believe, however, that the results in the baboons showing the counterproductive effects of post-transplant immunosuppressive agents following pretransplant TLI may help to explain the lack of tolerance production in our patients. In addition, attention is drawn again to the fact that other clinical series did not use the wide-field irradiation found to be necessary for tolerance production in both rodents and baboons. While it is clear from the baboon studies that measures in addition to pretransplant TLI, or possibly a modification of the irradiation regimen, will be necessary for more consistent tolerance production, clinical studies without the initial use of additional immunosuppressive drugs after transplantation would appear to be justified and indicated. Attaining tolerance in even one-third of patients, thereby removing the need for post-transplant immunosuppressive drug therapy, would be a very important and most gratifying achievement.

A clearer understanding of the potential mechanisms of tolerance production by TLI should contribute to a more rational search for appropriate additional measures. Our studies in tolerant baboons have shown three patterns of mixed lymphocyte reactions (MLRs): 1) donor specific hypo- or unresponsiveness in 5 of 12 baboons studied up to 4.5 years after transplantation, 2) broad nonspecific hyporesponsiveness to both donor and third-party baboons in another 5 tolerant baboons, and 3) donor responsiveness with a nonspecific suppressor factor in the serum of the other 2 tolerant baboons (5). This suppressor factor was also demonstrated in the serum of three of the baboons with hyporesponsiveness. Nonspecific non-T suppressor cells expressing myeloid-associated antigens CD11b and CD38 were demonstrated by add-in experiments to be involved in most of the MLR suppression (6).

We have also studied this regimen of TLI in chacma baboon–to–vervet monkey kidney xenotransplantation (7,8). The results obtained have approximated those in baboon kidney allotransplantation. With pretransplant TLI alone, 2 of 6 monkeys survived for 364 and 550 days before the grafts were rejected. In a group that received an additional 10 mg/kg of ATG on days −1 and 0, 2 of 4 monkeys survived for 289 and 293 days. However, the additional administration of mycophenolate mofetil was counterproductive in terms of graft survival. As in the baboon allotransplantation studies, the intrathymic injection of donor spleen cells on day 7 abolished the graft-prolonging effect of pretransplant TLI.

Immunologic studies in the two long-surviving monkeys receiving TLI alone revealed the development of low levels of nonspecific cytotoxic antibodies against baboon but not monkey lymphocytes (15% to 29% cell lysis by $^{51}$Cr release assays) three weeks after transplantation. These persisted until three months after transplantation. Most of the cytotoxicity was due to IgM. Antibody-dependent cellular cytotoxicity with the use of normal monkey lymphocyte effectors paralleled complement-dependent cytotoxicity, and lymphocyte-mediated cytotoxicity was also present transiently during the antibody-positive period. TLI obliterated the proliferative response of monkey lymphocytes to IL-2, ConA, and PHA. MLR to baboon cells was markedly reduced after TLI, with slow recovery toward pre-TLI levels five months after transplantation. TLI inhibited mitogen-induced IL-2 synthesis to below measurable levels (10 fmol/mL) for two months. Synthesizing ability for IL-2 recovered fully by five months after transplantation without any immediate deterioration of graft function. Sera collected 32 days after transplantation blocked one-way donor-specific and nonspecific MLR using cryopreserved pre-TLI recipient lymphocytes as responders. Open-wedge biopsies of these two grafts three months after transplantation revealed only occasional periglomerular and interstitial foci of chronic inflammatory cells. Immunofluorescence staining revealed focal glomerular deposits of IgM and IgG but no complement.

These findings are of interest and potential relevance to the possibility of baboon-to-human transplantation, although direct extrapolation is clearly not yet possible. The possible impact of species differences is shown by our studies in which the same regimen of TLI was totally ineffective in the reciprocal interprimate combination of monkey-to-baboon kidney transplantation. We feel that TLI should also be studied in discordant combinations such as pig-to-baboon transplantation, in conjunction with measures directed toward the complement and natural antibody components of the immunologic reaction.

## CHAPTER REFERENCES

1. Anderson RE, Warner NL. Ionizing radiation and the immune response. Adv Immunol 1976;24:215–335.
2. Kaplan HS. Selective effects of total lymphoid irradiation (TLI) on the immune response. Transplant Proc 1981;13:425–428.
3. Sprent J, Anderson RE, Miller JFAP. Radiosensitivity of T and B lymphocytes. II. Effect of irradiation on response of T cells to alloantigens. Eur J Immunol 1974;4:204–210.
4. Heincke H. Uber die Einwirkung der Röntgenstrahlen auf Tiere. Muenc Med Wochenschr 1903;50:2090–2092.
5. Benjamin E, Sulka E. Antikörperbildung nach experimenteller Schadgung des haematopoietischen Systems durch Röntgenstrahlen. Wien Klin Wochenschr 1908;21:311–314.
6. Hamburger J, Vayse J, Crosnier J, et al. Renal homotransplantation in man after radiation of the recipient. Am J Med 1962;32:854–871.
7. Hume DM, Wolf JS. Abrogation of the immune response: irradiation therapy and lymphocyte depletion. Modification of renal homograft rejection by irradiation. Transplantation 1967;5:1174–1191.
8. Joel DD, Chanana AD, Cronkite EP, Schiffer LM. Modification of skin allograft immunity by extracorporeal irradiation of lymph. Transplantation 1967;5:1192–1197.
9. Hardy MA, Oluwole S, Fawwaz R, et al. Selective lymphoid irradiation. Transplantation 1982;33:237–242.
10. Wolf JS, Hume DM. Transplant immunity in animals with lymphocytopenia induced by indwelling beta irradiation. Surg Forum 1965;16:202–204.
11. Johnson HK, Malcolm A, Al-Abdulla S, et al. The effect of local graft irradiation upon the reversal of cadaveric renal allograft rejection. Transplant Proc 1985;17:2–31.
12. Torrisi JR, Dritschilo A, Harter KW, et al. A randomized study of the efficacy of adjuvant local graft irradiation following renal transplantation. Int J Radiat Oncol Biol Phys 1990;18:1027–1031.
13. Kaplan HS. Hodgkin's disease. 2nd ed. Cambridge, MA: Harvard University, 1980.
14. Fuks Z, Strober S, Bobrove AM, et al. Long term effects of radiation on T and B lymphocytes in peripheral blood of patients with Hodgkin's disease. J Clin Invest 1976;58:803–814.
15. Pedersen-Bjergaard J, Larsen SO. Incidence of acute nonlymphocytic leukemia, preleukemia, and acute myeloproliferative syndrome up to 10 years after treatment of Hodgkin's disease. N Engl J Med 1982;307:965–971.
16. Goffinet DR, Glatstein E, Merigan RD. Herpes zoster-varicella infections and lymphoma. Ann Inter Med 1970;76:235–239.
17. Strober S, Slavin S, Gottlieb M, et al. Allograft tolerance after total lymphoid irradiation (TLI). Immunol Rev 1979;46:87–112.
18. Waer M, Ang KK, van der Schueren E, Vandeputte M. Influence of radiation field and fractionation schedule of total lymphoid irradiation (TLI) on the induction of suppressor cells and stable chimerism after bone marrow transplantation in mice. J Immunol 1984;132:985–990.
19. Waer M, Ang KK, van der Schueren E, Vandeputte M. Allogeneic bone marrow transplantation in mice after total lymphoid irradiation: influence of breeding conditions and strain of recipient mice. J Immunol 1984;132:991–996.
20. Gottlieb M, Strober S, Hoppe RT, et al. Engraftment of allogeneic bone marrow without graft-versus-host disease in mongrel dogs using total lymphoid irradiation. Transplantation 1980;29:487–491.
21. Howard RJ, Sutherland DER, Lum CT, et al. Kidney allograft survival in dogs treated with total lymphoid irradiation. Ann Surg 1981;193:196–200.
22. Pennock JL, Reitz BA, Bieber CP, et al. Survival of primates following orthotopic cardiac transplantation treated with total lymphoid irradiation and chemical immune suppression. Transplantation 1981;32:467–473.
23. Koretz SH, Gottlieb MS, Strober S, et al. Organ transplantation in mongrel dogs using total lymphoid irradiation (TLI). Transplant Proc 1981;13:443–445.
24. Williamson P, Allen RD, Deane SA, et al. Canine pancreas and kidney transplantation following total-lymphoid irradiation. Transplantation 1990;50:576–579.
25. Thomas J, Alqaisi M, Cunningham P, et al. The development of a posttransplant TLI treatment strategy that promotes organ allograft acceptance without chronic immunosuppression. Transplantation 1992;53:247–258.
26. Myburgh JA, Smit JA, Browde S, Stark JH. Current status of total lymphoid irradiation. Transplant Proc 1983;11:659–667.
27. Strober S. Natural suppressor (NS) cells, neonatal tolerance, and total lymphoid irradiation: exploring obscure relationships. Ann Rev Immunol 1984;2:97–115.

28. Schwadron RB, Strober S. Cloned natural suppressor cells derived from the neonatal spleen: in vitro action and lineage. Transplant Proc 1987;19:533.

29. Hertel-Wulff B, Lindsten T, Schwadron R, et al. Rearrangement and expression of T cell receptor genes in cloned murine natural suppressor cell lines. J Exp Med 1987;166:1168.

30. Hertel-Wulff B, Palathumpat V, Schwadron RB, et al. Prevention of GVHD by natural suppressor cells. Transplant Proc 1987;19:536–538.

31. De Ruysscher D, Sobis H, Vandeputte M, Waer M. A subset of asialo GM1+ cells play a protective role in the occurrence of graft-versus-host disease in mice. J Immunol 1991;146:4065–4070.

32. Waer M, Salam A, Vandeputte M. Protective role of asialo GM1+, NK1.1⁻ cells in the occurrence of graft-versus-host disease after total lymphoid irradiation. Transplantation 1993;56:1049–1050.

33. Okada S, Palathumpat V, Strober S. Identification of donor-derived antigen-specific suppressor cells in murine bone marrow chimeras prepared with total-lymphoid irradiation. Transplantation 1983;36:417.

34. Slavin S, Morecki S, Weigensberg M, et al. Functional clonal depletion versus suppressor cell-induced transplantation tolerance in chimeras prepared with a short course of total-lymphoid irradiation. Transplantation 1986;41:680.

35. Morecki S, Leshem B, Weigensberg M, et al. Functional clonal deletion versus active suppression in transplantation tolerance induced by total-lymphoid irradiation. Transplantation 1985;40:201.

36. Field EH, Steinmuller D. Nondeletional mechanisms of tolerance in total-lymphoid irradiation-induced bone marrow chimeras. Transplantation 1993;56:250–253.

37. Salam A, Vandeputte M, Waer M. Clonal deletion and clonal anergy in allogeneic bone marrow chimeras prepared with TBI or TLI. Transplant Int 1994;7:S457–S461.

38. Florence LS, Jiang GL, Ang KK, et al. In vitro analysis of T cell-mediated cytotoxicity displayed by rat heart allograft recipients rendered unresponsive by total-lymphoid irradiation and extracted donor antigen. Transplantation 1990;49:436–444.

39. Bass H, Strober S. Deficits in T helper cells after total lymphoid irradiation (TLI): reduced IL-2 secretion and normal IL-2 receptor expression in the mixed leucocyte reaction MLR. Cell Immunol 1990;126:129.

40. Bass H, Mosmann T, Strober S. Evidence for mouse TH1 and TH2-like helper T cells in vivo. J Exp Med 1989;170:1495.

41. Field EH, Rouse TM. Alloantigen priming after total lymphoid irradiation alters alloimmune cytokine responses. Transplantation 1995;60:695–702.

42. Stark JH, Smit JA, Myburgh JA. Nonspecific mixed lymphocyte culture inhibitory antibodies in sera of tolerant transplanted baboons conditioned with total lymphoid irradiation. Transplantation 1994;57:1103–1110.

43. Yamaguchi Y, Halperin EC, Harland RC. Significant prolongation of hamster liver transplant survival in Lewis rats by total lymphoid irradiation, cyclosporine and splenectomy. Transplantation 1990;49:13.

44. Steinbrüchel DA, Madsen H, Nielsen B, et al. The effect of combined treatment with TLI, cyclosporine A and anti-CD4 monoclonal antibodies in a hamster-to-rat transplantation model. Transplant Proc 1991;23:579.

45. Marchman W, Araneda D, DeMasi R, et al. Prolongation of xenograft survival after combination therapy with 15-deoxyspergualin and total-lymphoid irradiation in the hamster-to-rat cardiac xenograft model. Transplantation 1993;53:30–34.

46. Roslin MS, Tranbaugh RE, Panza A, et al. One-year monkey heart xenograft survival in cyclosporine-treated baboons. Suppression of the xenoantibody response with total-lymphoid irradiation. Transplantation 1992;54:949–955.

47. Sadeghi AM, Laks H, Drinkwater DC, et al. Heart-lung xenotransplantation in primates. J Heart Lung Transplant 1991;10:442–447.

48. Panza A, Roslin M, Coons M, et al. Successful cardiac xenogeneic transplantation in primates using total lymphoid irradiation. Eur J Cardiothorac Surg 1991;5:161–163.

49. Kaplan E, Dresdale AR, Diehl JT, et al. Total lymphoid irradiation and discordant cardiac xenografts. J Heart Transplant 1990;9:11–13.

50. Thomas F, Pittman K, Ljung T, Cekada E. Deoxyspergualin is a unique immunosuppressive agent with selective utility inducing tolerance to pancreas islet xenografts. Transplant Proc 1995;27:417–419.

51. Tixier D, Levy C, Le Bourgeois JP, et al. Discordant heart xenografts. Experimental study in pigs conditioned by total lymphoid irradiation and cyclosporine A. Presse Med 1992;21:1941–1944.

52. Waer M, Vanrenterghem Y, Ang KK, et al. Comparison of the immunosuppressive effect of fractionated total lymphoid irradiation (TLI) vs conventional immunosuppression (CI) in renal cadaveric allotransplantation. J Immunol 1984;132:1041–1048.

53. Waer M, Vanrenterghem Y, Roels L, et al. Immunological and clinical observations in diabetic kidney graft recipients pretreated with total-lymphoid irradiation. Transplantation 1987;43:371–379.

54. Waer M, Vanrenterghem Y, Roels L, et al. Renal cadaveric transplantation in diabetics using total lymphoid irradiation or cyclosporin A. A controlled randomized study. Transplant Int 1988;1:64–68.

55. Levin B, Collins G, Waer M, et al. Treatment of cadaveric renal transplant recipients with total lymphoid irradiation, antithymocyte globulin, and low-dose prednisone. Lancet 1985;2:1321.

56. Levin B, Bohannon L, Warvariv V, et al. Total lymphoid irradiation (TLI) in the cyclosporine era—use of TLI in resistant cardiac allograft rejection. Transplant Proc 1989;21:1793–1795.

57. Strober S, Dhillon M, Schubert M, et al. Acquired immune tolerance to cadaveric renal allografts: a study of three patients treated with total lymphoid irradiation. N Engl J Med 1989;321:28.

58. Myburgh JA, Meyers AM, Botha JR, et al. Wide field low-dose total lymphoid irradiation in clinical kidney transplantation. Transplant Proc 1987;19: 1974–1977.

59. Myburgh JA, Meyers AM, Margolius L, et al. Total lymphoid irradiation in clinical renal transplantation—results in 73 patients. Transplant Proc 1991;23:2033–2034.

60. Najarian JS, Ferguson RM, Sutherland DER, et al. Fractionated total lymphoid irradiation as preparative immunosuppression in high risk renal transplantation. Ann Surg 1982;196:442–452.

61. Kaufman DB, Kim TH, Slavin S, et al. Long term clinical studies of high-risk renal retransplant recipients given total lymphoid irradiation. Transplant Proc 1989;21:1798.

62. Cortesini R, Molajoni ER, Monari C, et al. Total lymphoid irradiation in clinical transplantation: experience in 30 high-risk patients. Transplant Proc 1985;92:1291–1293.

63. Molajoni ER, Bachetoni A, Cinti P, et al. Eight-year actuarial graft and patient survival of kidney transplants in highly immunized recipients pretreated with total lymphoid irradiation: a single-center experience. Transplant Proc 1993;25:776–777.

64. Woodley SL, Gurley KE, Hoffmann SL, et al. Induction of tolerance to heart allografts in rats using posttransplant total lymphoid irradiation and anti-T cell antibodies. Transplantation 1993;56:1443–1447.

65. Evans MA, Schomberg PJ, Rodeheffer RJ, et al. Total lymphoid irradiation: a novel and successful therapy for resistant cardiac allograft rejection. Mayo Clin Proc 1992;67:785–790.

66. Hunt SA, Strober S, Hoppe RT, Stinson EB. Total lymphoid irradiation for treatment of intractable cardiac allograft rejection. J Heart Lung Transplant 1991;10:211–216.

67. Salter SP, Slater MM, Kirklin JK, et al. Total lymphoid irradiation in the treatment of early or recurrent heart transplant rejection. Int J Radiation Oncol Biol Phys 1995;33:83–88.

68. Valentine VG, Robbins RC, Wehner JH, et al. Total lymphoid irradiation for refractory acute rejection in heart-lung and lung allografts. Chest 1996;109:1184–1189.

69. Bhatia S, Robison L, Oberlin O, et al. Breast cancer and other second neoplasms after childhood Hodgkin's disease. N Engl J Med 1996;334:745–751.

70. Edelson R, Berger C, Gasparro F, et al. Treatment of cutaneous T cell lymphoma by extracorporeal photochemotherapy: preliminary results. N Engl J Med 1987;316:297.

71. Perez M, Edelson R, Lori J, et al. Inhibition of antiskin allograft immunity by infusions with syngeneic photoinactivated effector lymphocytes. J Invest Dermatol 1989;92:669.

72. Perez M, Edelson R, Laroche L. Inhibition of antiskin allograft immunity by infusions with photoinactivated effector T-lymphocytes (PET cells). Yale J Biol Med 1989;62:595.

73. Pepino P, Berger CL, Fuzesi L, et al. Primate cardiac allo- and xenotransplantation: modulation of the immune response with photochemotherapy. Eur Surg Res 1989;21:105.

74. Berger C. Experimental murine and primate models for dissection of the immunosuppressive potential of photochemotherapy in autoimmune disease and transplantation. Yale J Biol Med 1989;62:611.

75. Kraemer KH, Haywood LW, Cohen LF, et al. Effects of 8-methoxypsoralen and ultraviolet radiation on human lymphoid cells in vitro. J Invest Dermatol 1981;76:80.

76. Edelson RL. Light-activated drugs. Sci Am 1988;259:68.

77. Meiser BM, Kur F, Reichenspurner H, et al. Reduction of the incidence of rejection by adjunct immunosuppression with photochemotherapy after heart transplantation. Transplantation 1994;57:563.

78. Barr ML, Meiser BM, Eisen HJ, et al. Photopheresis for the prevention of rejection in cardiac transplantation. Photopheresis Transplantation Study Group. N Engl J Med 1998;339:1744–1751.

## COMMENTARY REFERENCES

1. Myburgh JA, Smit JA, Meyers AM, et al. Total lymphoid irradiation in renal transplantation. World J Surg 1986;10:369–380.
2. Myburgh JA, Smit JA. Delineation, durability, predictability and specificity of operational tolerance with total lymphoid irradiation in baboon kidney transplantation. Transplant Proc 1985;17:1442–1445.
3. Smit JA, Stark JH, Myburgh JA. Intrathymic donor antigen in baboon kidney allotransplantation. Afr J Health Sci 1995;2:344–348.
4. Myburgh JA, Meyers AM, Margolius L, et al. Total lymphoid irradiation in clinical renal transplantation—Results in 73 patients. Transplant Proc 1991;23:2033–2034.
5. Stark JH, Smit JA, Myburgh JA. Nonspecific mixed lymphocyte culture inhibitory antibodies in sera of tolerant transplanted baboons conditioned with total lymphoid irradiation. Transplantation 1994;57:1103–1110.
6. Gray CM, Smit JA, Myburgh JA. Identification of non-T suppressor cells with possible contra-interleukin-2 properties in non-human primates tolerant to their renal allografts. Afr J Health Sci 1995;2:354–358.
7. Myburgh JA, Smit JA, Stark JH. Transplantation tolerance following total lymphoid irradiation in baboon-to-monkey kidney xenotransplantation. Transplant Proc 1994;26:1080–1081.
8. Myburgh JA, Smit JA, Stark JH. Experimental concordant kidney xenotransplantation in primates. In Cooper DKC, ed. Xenotransplantation. 2nd ed. Heidelberg, Germany, Pro Edit GmbH 1997:316–322.

Note: Page numbers followed by *f* indicate figures; those followed by *t* indicate tables.